European Monitoring Centre
for Drugs and Drug Addiction

EMC

MO

Hepatitis
impact, c

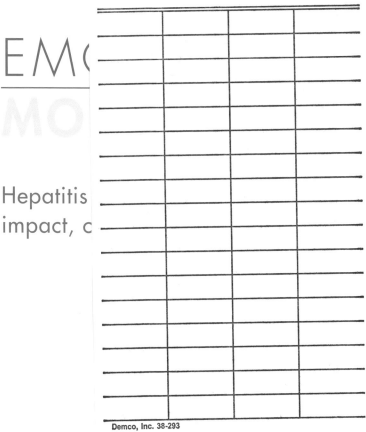

Editors

Johannes Jager, Wien Limburg, Mirjam Kretzschmar,
Maarten Postma, Lucas Wiessing

7

Legal notice

This publication of the European Monitoring Centre for Drugs and Drug Addiction
(EMCDDA) is protected by copyright. The EMCDDA accepts no responsibility or liability for
any consequences arising from the use of the data contained in this document. The contents
of this publication do not necessarily reflect the official opinions of the EMCDDA's partners,
any EU Member State or any agency or institution of the European Union or European
Communities.

A great deal of additional information on the European Union is available on the Internet.
It can be accessed through the Europa server **(http://europa.eu.int)**.

Europe Direct is a service to help you find answers
to your questions about the European Union

Freephone number:
00 800 6 7 8 9 10 11

Cataloguing data can be found at the end of this publication.

Luxembourg: Office for Official Publications of the European Communities, 2004

ISBN 92-9168-168-7

© European Monitoring Centre for Drugs and Drug Addiction, 2004
Reproduction is authorised provided the source is acknowledged.

Printed in Belgium

PRINTED ON WHITE CHLORINE-FREE PAPER

European Monitoring Centre
for Drugs and Drug Addiction

Rua da Cruz de Santa Apólonia 23–25, P-1149-045 Lisbon
Tel. (351) 21 811 30 00 • Fax (351) 21 813 17 11
info@emcdda.eu.int • http://www.emcdda.eu.int

Contents

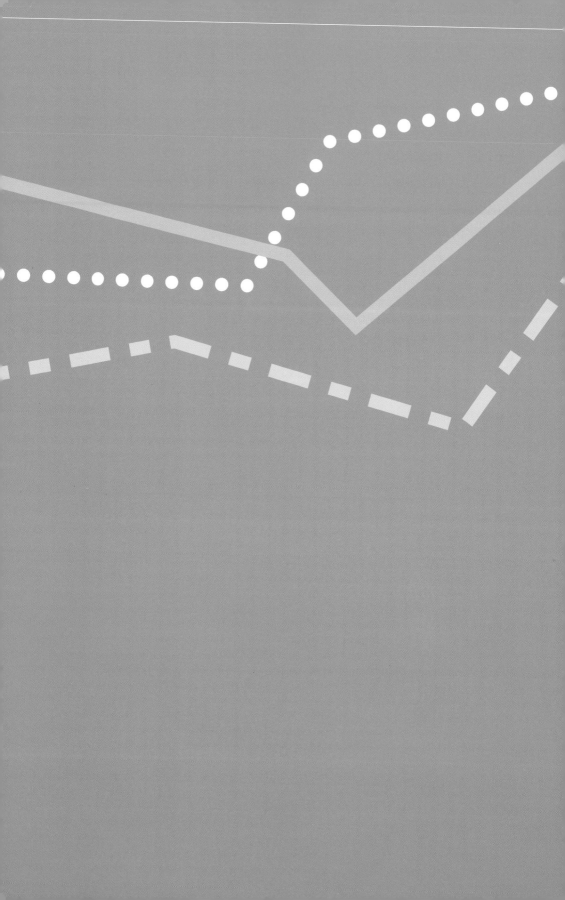

Foreword

It is a great pleasure to present the scientific monograph 'Hepatitis C and injecting drug use: impact, costs and policy options'. Earlier monographs of the European Monitoring Centre for Drugs and Drug Addiction (EMCDDA) have focused on issues such as prevalence estimation, qualitative research methods and dynamic modelling in the field of drugs, thereby exploring tools for the analysis of the often scarcely available drugs data. This publication aims to provide evidence for potential action on a major health problem in the EU: hepatitis C infection. Hepatitis C is not only a vast problem within the field of drugs, even if drug users are currently the largest population at risk, it may also be a high priority in the wider domain of public health, considering that it will lead to very substantial and increasing costs for European healthcare systems.

This monograph pulls together state-of-the-art knowledge in treatment, natural history and prevention. It provides the first European data on epidemiological trends in injecting drug users, presents modelling results that give early indications to which interventions could be the most effective at the population level, as well as estimates of the future costs of healthcare, what part of these costs are avoidable, and the cost-effectiveness of existing interventions such as needle and syringe exchange and methadone treatment.

The monograph reflects the close collaboration of the EMCDDA and the National Institute of Public Health and the Environment in the Netherlands, as part of a European research project funded by the European Commission (European drugs modelling network, funded by the Directorate-General for Research, 'Targeted socioeconomic research' programme, Project No ERB 4141 PL 980030, see http://www.emcdda.eu.int/?nnodeid=1376).

I wish to thank the following people for their contribution: Fernando Antoñanzas, Nicolas Blanchard, Jasper Bos, Ardine de Wit, Nicolino Esposito, Graham Foster, David Goldberg, Gordon Hay, Richard Hartnoll, Robert Heimer, Johannes Jager, Claude Jeanrenaud, Hans-Helmut König, Pierre Kopp, Mirjam Kretzschmar, Reiner Leidl, Wien Limburg, Harold Pollack, Maarten Postma, Thierry Poynard, Roberto Rodríguez, Carla Rossi, Kirsty Roy, David Sapinho, Uwe Siebert, Diana Sylvestre, Avril Taylor, Gernot Tragler, María Velasco, Robert Welte, Lucas Wiessing, and John Wong; and Rosemary de Sousa, Peter Fay and Deborah Burrows, who were responsible for coordination of the publication and the final text editing.

Georges Estievenart
Executive Director, EMCDDA

General introduction

General introduction

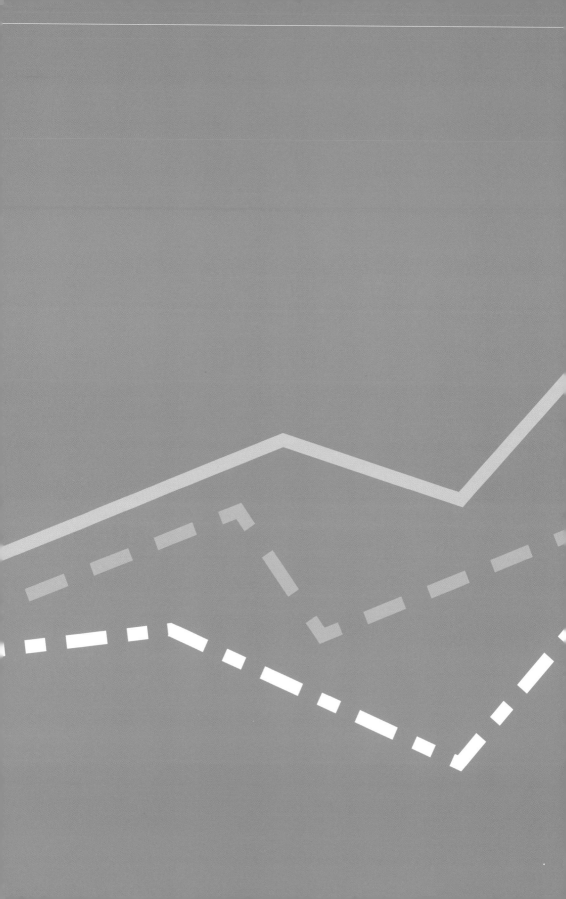

General introduction

One of the major aims of the EMCDDA is the collection of information on drugs and drug addiction and their consequences, as a basis for policy-making and prevention. For policies to be effective and rational, they need up-to-date, evidence-based information. This monograph is an attempt to bridge the gap between research and policy-making by integrating research findings and current knowledge and presenting the results in an accessible way.

Infectious diseases, such as hepatitis A, B and C and HIV, are an important health consequence of drug addiction, especially in IDUs. Hepatitis C, in IDUs the most common infectious disease, is the central focus of the monograph. A broad approach is attempted, by also describing the dynamics, consequences and costs of the underlying drug use epidemic. The monograph thus aims to present an overview of current knowledge on the impact and costs of hepatitis C in IDUs, within a broad context, as a basis for future policy formulation. Injecting drug use, through sharing injection equipment, is currently the major risk factor for hepatitis C. The great majority of new hepatitis C cases are related to injecting drug use and the prevalence and incidence of hepatitis C in IDUs are extremely high.

An adequate assessment of hepatitis-C-related costs of illness in IDUs requires information on the prevalence and incidence of injectors, unhealthy behaviours and transmission routes and dynamics, the course of the disease and related healthcare needs, and treatment-effectiveness and costs. More specific information is needed concerning the effectiveness and costs of interventions to prevent transmission, including needle and syringe programmes (NSPs) and methadone maintenance programmes, their indirect costs and effects, and private and social costs. Eventually, this information will be an important input for the formulation of recommendations and policy options regarding the prevention and management of hepatitis C in IDUs. The methods and approaches explored in this monograph may in the future, however, be equally applied to other aspects of the problem of injecting drug use.

Structure of the monograph

Part I: Natural history, treatment, quality of life, epidemiology and prevention

Much of the general information on hepatitis C and hepatitis C in IDUs is provided in the first part of the monograph. As such, it serves as an introductory section to the rest of the book.

Chapter 1, a literature overview, focuses on the natural history, treatment and prevention of hepatitis C. Recently, questions have arisen as to the percentage of patients that spontaneously clear the virus, and the severity of the natural history of hepatitis C in different patient groups. Major advances have been made in the treatment of hepatitis C. However, accessibility of treatment to IDUs, currently the major risk group for hepatitis C virus (HCV) infection, is less evident. Important prevention and harm reduction interventions of hepatitis C in IDUs include screening, counselling and education, methadone maintenance treatment (MMT), and needle and syringe programmes. Questions relate to the effectiveness of the interventions and how to optimise this.

Chapter 2 explores in detail the diagnostics, treatment, and treatment indications and contraindications of hepatitis C. It shows how, over the last decade, approved treatment has evolved through several stages with dramatically increasing rates of success. In addition, the treatment options for relapsers, non-responders and patients coinfected with the human immunodeficiency virus (HIV) are discussed.

Hepatitis C is known as an 'asymptomatic' disease. Whether this also applies to the quality of life of hepatitis C patients is discussed in Chapter 3. It also addresses the effect of treatment on quality of life and the factors that may contribute to the impairment of quality of life.

Reliable and up-to-date epidemiological data are a prerequisite for modelling activities and cost-of-illness studies. Chapter 4 provides data on the prevalence and incidence of HCV infection among IDUs in the European Union (EU) as collected by the EMCDDA. Data were obtained from 63 sources in 111 sites in 14 EU countries. Although the available data are not comprehensive, it is clear that the size of the problem is considerable. Still, reported prevalences may vary considerably between and within countries. Time trends suggest that changes in HCV prevalence may have occurred in several countries and regions.

Part II: Models of hepatitis C, injecting drug use and policy options

To equal the success of modelling as a tool to support AIDS policy, modelling hepatitis C in relation to injecting drug use still requires much work. Three models are introduced here, one for the transmission of hepatitis C in IDUs, one for injecting drug use and one for determining the optimal mix of prevention strategies.

The first model, presented in Chapter 5, is a 'simple' mathematical model, which includes the numbers of susceptibles and persons in the various stages of the disease, the recruitment and mortality rates, transmission in relation to infectivity and risk behaviour, and duration of injecting as main parameters. This model allows a preliminary evaluation of the effects of prevention measures and treatment in terms of avoided new and secondary infections.

In Chapter 6, a model for injecting drug use is developed. It mathematically describes the dynamics of injecting drug use by relevant parameters and the (inter)relationships between these parameters. It is extended to include an infectious disease epidemic like hepatitis C. It is used to carry out a tentative evaluation as to the effectiveness of various prevention programmes.

A fundamental question in drug policy relates to the allocation of scarce resources between control strategies like prevention, treatment and law enforcement. In Chapter 7, an attempt is made to answer this question by developing an optimal model that enables the determination of the optimal mix of such control strategies. The model draws tentative conclusions as to which strategies to apply at which stages of a drug use epidemic and what strategies should be allocated maximum resources. The model is flexible enough to incorporate the spread of blood-borne diseases such as hepatitis C in IDUs. It is pointed out that the lack of appropriate data seriously limits the applicability of the model.

Part III: Healthcare costs of drug-related hepatitis C infection

Cost-effectiveness ratios are an increasingly important consideration in the selection of treatment and prevention strategies for infectious diseases. An estimation of patient-related, direct healthcare costs that can be avoided by prevention is therefore required. Part III consists of two studies on the medical costs of hepatitis C treatment in IDUs based on the cost-of-illness design.

In Chapter 8, a cost-of-illness study, lifetime treatment costs of an IDU diagnosed with HCV at the age of 25 are assessed, using a Markov model for disease progression. Treatment costs are assessed with both full and no access to combination treatment for IDUs for 10 EU countries.

In Chapter 9, the cost-of-illness design is used in a cost-effectiveness and cost–utility analysis of the treatment of treatment-naive (ex-)IDUs with moderate hepatitis or cirrhosis with a combination of interferon and ribavirin. The incremental cost-effectiveness ratio is compared to other medical interventions, also when, for example, allowing for an accelerated disease progression due to comorbid alcoholism, or a decreased sustained response rate due to non-adherence.

Part IV: Wider costs of drug use

In this part, drug-use-related costs are extended to include social costs other than patient-related direct healthcare costs. It reflects the current discussion on cost studies concerning the cost categories that make up social costs, which categories are relevant from which perspective ('who pays what'), which is the most appropriate method to use with a specific perspective, and what are the merits of the various methods. Most authors stress the need for methodological standardisation and explicit formulation of relevant cost categories, although they may disagree on what these should entail.

In Chapter 10, the indirect costs of injecting drug use are explored from the perspective of the IDU, his/her family, employer, social insurance and society for both the paid and unpaid work sectors, in relation to various methods used to evaluate these costs. Until standardisation is in place, reporting of the results obtained by all the various approaches seems best.

On the basis of a literature review, the lack of consensus on relevant cost categories and best method is demonstrated in Chapter 11. It is stressed how important it is to distinguish between social and private costs, and the lack of adequate epidemiological data is pointed out.

In Chapter 12, the cost-of-illness method is used to estimate the tangible social costs of illicit drug use in France in 1997. Estimates of healthcare costs, costs of a wide range of public organisations involved in the fight against problem drug use, income and production losses, tax losses and lost added values are presented. Eventually, the costs borne by the community due to illegal drug use are compared with the costs of the legal drugs, alcohol and tobacco.

After careful consideration of the pros and cons of the various methods to assess the tangible and intangible costs of illicit drug use, a method that combines the human capital approach and the willingness-to-pay approach is proposed in Chapter 13. This proposed method allows the estimation of both tangible costs due to production losses and intangible costs related to the decrease in the quality of life of drug users. It is shown that methodological choices and the definition of social costs lead to an underestimation of the benefits of a Swiss programme for the medical prescription of heroin.

Part V: Cost-effectiveness of needle and syringe programmes and methadone maintenance

In Part V of the monograph, two prevention measures, that is NSPs and MMT, are evaluated from an economic point of view.

On the basis of a literature review, the cost-effectiveness of NSPs is assessed in Chapter 14. Originally designed as a tool to prevent the spread of HIV in IDUs, NSPs appear to be cost-effective. The average costs per averted HIV infection are still far below lifetime treatment costs. However, as to containing the spread of hepatitis C, NSPs' effectiveness is compromised by the high infectivity and consequently high incidence and prevalence in IDUs. It is suggested that the most cost-effective prevention strategy combines several prevention interventions simultaneously.

In Chapter 15, the question as to whether MMT is effective and cost-effective in reducing HCV transmission is explored by means of a relatively simple mathematical model. MMT may result in less risk behaviour, that is less injecting and less sharing, and may also link IDUs to other treatment services. MMT proves to be highly cost-effective as a means of HIV prevention in IDUs. The outcome of the model shows that the cost-effectiveness of MMT as an HCV prevention measure is less favourable. MMT effectiveness increases with better treatment quality, with high accessibility, and when offered in conjunction with other services.

The monograph ends with general conclusions and a policy-centred evaluation of the results that have been presented in, or can be inferred from, the preceding chapters. To do justice to the complexity of this relatively new research and policy field, a multidisciplinary approach has been chosen. In addition, various authors have adopted their particular perspectives within the framework of the aims of the monograph as formulated above. The consequent heterogeneity is reflected in the varying emphasis with which the various subjects have been presented and elaborated.

Wien Limburg, Lucas Wiessing and Johannes Jager
EMCDDA

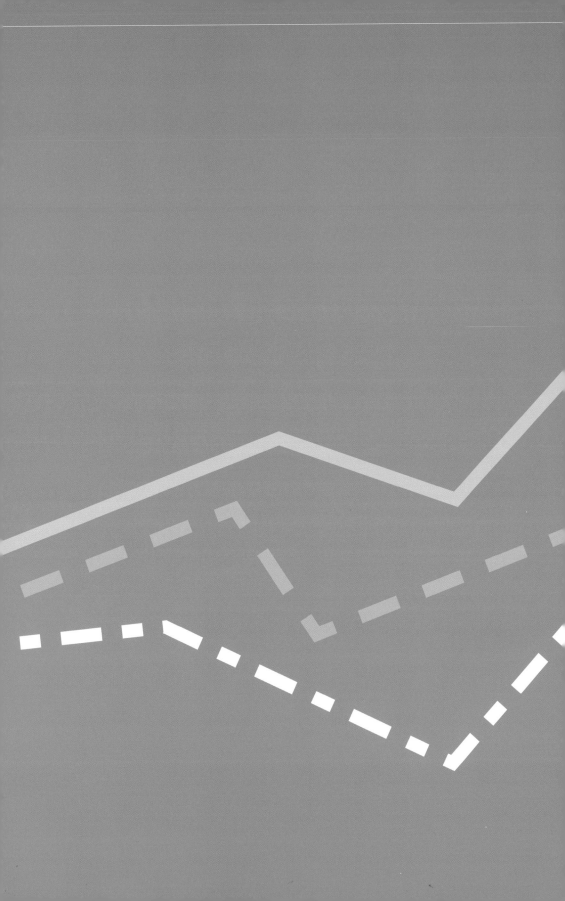

Natural history, treatment, quality of life, epidemiology and prevention

PART I

Introduction

Part I serves as an introductory section to this monograph on hepatitis C in injecting drug users (IDUs).

Chapter 1 presents a concise overview of the natural history of the disease and the treatment modalities, and touches upon prevention and harm reduction interventions for hepatitis C in IDUs. The natural history of hepatitis C may be less serious than has recently been assumed. There are indications that a higher percentage of acute patients clear the virus and that for young, chronic patients it takes longer to develop severe liver disease.

At present, IDUs are the major risk group for hepatitis C virus (HCV) infection. Unfortunately, they seem to profit little from the advances that have been made in the management of chronic hepatitis. Although some official guidelines have recently become less strict, most guidelines still express reluctance to treating active IDUs. It seems that, in practice, few European Union (EU) countries offer treatment to active IDUs; other countries offer treatment under very strict conditions only, such as a one-year period of abstinence prior to treatment.

Controlling HCV in IDUs proves to be extremely difficult. Offering various prevention and harm reduction interventions simultaneously instead of one at a time seems to increase the likelihood of success. In addition, young and new injectors should be specifically targeted, as a larger proportion of them may not yet be infected.

Chapter 2 focuses on the latest diagnostic and treatment modalities for chronic hepatitis C patients, including relapsers and non-responders. It presents a detailed account of their efficacy in terms of both viral and histologic endpoints, in relation to the various stages of the disease and different genotypes of the virus. Major advances have been made in the last decade in the management of chronic hepatitis C patients. Treatment modalities evolved from standard interferon monotherapy through a combination therapy with standard interferon with ribavirin to a combination therapy of pegylated (PEG) interferon with ribavirin, with dramatically increased rates of success.

Chapter 3 deals with the quality of life of hepatitis C patients. It convincingly shows that for many so-called 'asymptomatic' hepatitis C patients, and maybe even more so for IDUs, the label 'asymptomatic' is misleading. Although they may not yet have developed serious liver disease, they may experience a variety of other severe symptoms and show a marked reduction in quality of life.

Chapter 4 provides recent data on prevalence of HCV infection among IDUs in the EU. Data were obtained from 63 sources in 111 sites in 14 countries. Although the available data are not comprehensive, it is clear that prevalence in IDUs, including young and new injectors, continues to be high, strongly suggesting continued transmission. Reported prevalence, however, varied considerably between and within countries. Time trends suggest that changes in HCV prevalence may have occurred in several countries and regions. It is too early yet to fully understand these changes or even to relate them to prevention and harm reduction measures, but improved and expanded data collection should in the future enable improved evaluation of such measures.

Wien Limburg

Chapter 1
Natural history, treatment and prevention of hepatitis C in injecting drug users: an overview

Wien Limburg

This chapter presents a concise overview of the natural history, treatment and prevention of hepatitis C in IDUs. It focuses primarily on the various disease stages and disease progression, diagnostics, and treatment modalities. Prevention measures taken to control the spread of the disease among IDUs, in particular so-called 'harm reduction measures', are also addressed. The epidemiology, risk factors and modes of transmission of HCV in IDUs are only discussed briefly in so far as they are relevant for prevention.

Introduction

Hepatitis C is a blood-borne viral infection that affects the liver. It is a relatively recently discovered disease, of which the causative agents were identified only in 1989. They proved to be responsible for 90 % of cases of what was then referred to as non-A-non-B hepatitis. In the late 1980s, the incidence of non-A-non-B hepatitis was at its peak. The development and subsequent improvement of diagnostic assays in the early 1990s, enabling the screening of donated blood, reduced the transfusion-associated incidence of hepatitis C to virtually zero (CDC, 1998; Alter, 1999). Since then, by far the largest proportion of notified cases are IDUs (European Monitoring Centre for Drugs and Drug Addiction (EMCDDA), unpublished data). The World Health Organisation (WHO) estimated that about 170 million people worldwide, and about 8.9 million people in Europe, are infected with hepatitis C (WHO, 2000).

Chronic HCV infection may cause substantial health problems. In the long run, it is a major cause of liver cirrhosis and end-stage liver diseases, second only to alcohol (Wong et al., 1998), and the main reason for liver transplantation. The healthcare demand and concomitant costs are considerable. For one year of drug-related HCV, hepatitis B virus (HBV) and HIV infections for 10 EU countries, the future healthcare costs were assessed at EUR 1.89 billion (Postma et al., see Chapter 8), with HCV accounting for almost 40 %.

In many EU countries, hepatitis C is a notifiable disease. By 1996, 12 of the 15 EU countries had made HCV infection notifiable (Nalpas et al., 1998). However, since the notification requirements are by no means uniform and many cases of HCV infection go unnoticed for a long time, notification data do not lend themselves to international comparison, nor is notification very adequate as a form of surveillance.

Transmission and risk factors

HCV is predominantly parenterally transmitted. It is far more infectious than HIV in terms of blood-borne transmission and shows much higher seroprevalences. Major routes of transmission are blood transfusion (before 1991), injecting drug use, and, to a much lesser degree, healthcare-related procedures, needle-stick accidents in healthcare, tattooing, and vertical transmission from mother to child. Transmission through especially high-risk sex practices that involve blood-to-blood contact occurs, although it is not a very efficient mode of transmission (Wasley and Alter, 2000). It is, however, a potential route of transmission from IDUs to non-IDUs (Vidal-Trécan et al., 2000). A recent study (Tortu et al., 2001) suggests that HCV may also be transmitted through non-injecting drug use by the shared use of crackpipes and cocaine straws, although existing evidence is not conclusive.

At present, the HCV prevalence rates in IDUs are high; in western Europe they range from 40 to 90 % among different subgroups. The limited data on new injectors (injecting for less than two years) in general indicate prevalence rates of 40 % or even higher in this group, although some local and regional studies report much lower rates (EMCDDA, 2002; see also Chapter 4). A positive HCV status in IDUs seems to be associated with syringe sharing and the sharing of injecting paraphernalia like cookers and cotton, number of injecting years, frequency of injecting, older age, level of drug consumption, HBV coinfection, excessive alcohol consumption, imprisonment, and male gender (Stark et al., 1997; Crofts et al., 1999a; Keppler and Stover, 1999). Because of its high prevalence in IDUs and high infectivity, even short-term recreational injecting drug use may lead to HCV infection (Novick, 2000).

Natural history

Genotypes

HCV is a ribonucleic acid (RNA) virus and belongs to the family of flaviviruses. Within an infected person, replication of the virus is extremely high and not totally faithful, resulting in the rapid evolution of diverse but related quasispecies. This makes HCV a difficult target for the immune system as well as treatment and slows down the development of a vaccine.

There are at least six genotypes (1 to 6) and many subtypes of HCV (Lauer and Walker, 2001). In western Europe and the United States (US), the subtypes 1a, 1b, 2a, 2b and 3a are the most common. Subtype 1b is strongly associated with transfusion-related HCV and therefore the most common in patients older than 50. HCV in IDUs is mainly associated with genotypes 1a and 3a, with genotype 3a being far more frequent in IDUs than in other populations (Stark et al., 1995; Beld et al., 1998; Pol et al., 1998; Webster et al., 2000). In the south-east of France, genotypes 1a and 3a in IDUs increased between 1970 and 1990, with genotype 1a being predominant (Bourlière et al., 2002). Infection with different genotypes is possible.

It is not yet clear what influence HCV genotypes have on the course of the disease or on the occurrence of extrahepatic diseases. They show, however, a different response to antiviral therapy; genotypes 2 and 3 are associated with a much better response than the other genotypes (Mondelli and Silini, 1999; Hoofnagle, 2000).

Acute hepatitis C

The symptoms in the acute stage, if any, are fatigue, malaise, abdominal pain, loss of appetite and jaundice, and may last for two to twelve weeks. Within one to two weeks after exposure, HCV RNA may become detectable in the serum, and in about six weeks, serum alanine aminotransferase (ALT) levels begin to increase. However, in the acute stage, HCV infection often (66 to > 80 %) goes unnoticed (Seeff, 1997; Lam, 1999).

Spontaneous recovery does occur, with reported rates ranging from 15 to 20 % (Ryder and Beckingham, 2001a) to 15 to 30 % (Hoofnagle, 2001). Higher recovery rates have been reported in children, in young adults — particularly in young women — and in persons with jaundice. Clearance of the virus may in time lead to the disappearance of HCV antibodies.

Acute HCV is hardly ever fulminant, but, when it is, it is often lethal. Fulminant HCV is seen with concurrent HBV.

Chronic hepatitis C

Hepatitis C is marked as chronic when HCV RNA persists for at least six months after infection. Recent estimates of the percentage of acute HCV infection becoming chronic are 55 to 85 %. The chronic stage is often indolent and symptoms may show only in an advanced stage of liver cirrhosis decades after the initial infection (Gross, 1998; Lam, 1999). Because of its asymptomatic manifestation and because not all HCV carriers develop chronic hepatitis, there is an unidentified group of HCV carriers that may for years constitute a potential source of transmission.

In the chronic stage, the ALT levels tend to be elevated, but they may fluctuate and be intermittently normal.

The disease stages of chronic HCV are no, mild, moderate and severe liver fibrosis, liver cirrhosis, end-stage liver disease and hepatocellular carcinoma (HCC). Factors that promote liver fibrosis are duration of infection, age, male gender, alcohol abuse, HIV coinfection and low CD4 count. The progression to cirrhosis is strongly influenced by gender and age (Poynard et al., 2000). Conservative estimates of the percentage of people with chronic HCV developing liver cirrhosis range from 20 to 30 % in approximately 30 years (Ryder and Beckingham, 2001b). At present, there is discussion that these estimates are too high. It is, as yet, unclear whether the lower estimates are true, in particular, for certain subgroups, like young women or children, or for all people with HCV (Seeff et al., 2000). On the basis of a review of studies on the natural history of hepatitis C, Freeman et al. (2001) conclude that there is a strong indication that the younger the age at infection, the longer it takes for the disease to progress and the lower the risk of developing end-stage liver disease. As IDUs often get infected at a young age, this may indicate that they are in the low range of those who progress to severe disease (if their condition is not exacerbated by heavy alcohol use).

Factors that may promote HCC are cirrhosis, alcohol abuse, and coinfection with HBV (Booth et al., 2001). Patients with cirrhosis have a heightened risk of developing HCC of 1 to 4 % per year (Hoofnagle, 1997; Flamm et al., 1998; Gross, 1998; Lam, 1999). Complications of cirrhosis mark end-stage liver disease. Approximately 15 to 20 % of patients with HCV-related cirrhosis progress to this stage (Seeff, 2000). It is as yet unclear if, and if so, what influence viraemia, genotype and quasispecies have on disease progression.

Disease activity of chronic HCV is graded into minimal, mild, moderate and severe, usually by means of the Knodell score, which indicates the degree of necroinflammatory change. It is a tool that provides information on the likelihood of progression to cirrhosis, and on the response to and the effect of treatment (Dienes et al., 1999). Although there is a correlation between disease activity and disease stage, there is no known one-to-one relationship.

Hepatitis C is a non-specific disease, which means that there are no symptoms that lead exclusively to the diagnosis of the disease. Many patients show extrahepatic symptoms and may complain of fatigue, muscle ache, anorexia, right upper quadrant pain and nausea (Booth et al., 2001). Chronic HCV may also manifest itself in non-hepatic symptoms like arthritis and essential mixed cryoglobulinaemia.

Crofts et al. (1999b) note that a major gap in our knowledge of HCV concerns the natural history of infection, and that our understanding of the rate at which people can and do progress through the stages of HCV disease is poor. This poor understanding may be partly explained by the relatively recent discovery of HCV and the lack of well-designed, comprehensive natural history studies of hepatitis C. Such studies are quite difficult to design as the onset of HCV infection goes unnoticed in more than 80 % of patients and must be inferred, HCV is often asymptomatic with normal ALT levels, and the time between onset and overt chronic liver disease can span 20 to 40 years (Seeff, 1999). Hence, it may not come as a surprise that even less is certain about the course of the disease in IDUs, a population that is hard to follow up. Thus, it is not known whether the disease progression and time of progression differ essentially between IDUs and non-IDUs (Crofts, 2001).

Diagnosis and treatment

Diagnosis

As the symptoms of HCV are not disease specific, HCV infection is diagnosed by testing for either the presence of the virus RNA or the presence of antibodies to the virus. If acute hepatitis C is suspected, testing for the presence of virus RNA is indicated, as antibodies to the HCV may become detectable only up to three months after infection (window period) (Ryder and Beckingham, 2001a). For screening purposes, testing for antibodies precedes testing for HCV RNA.

The antibody test involves a third-generation enzyme immunosorbant assay (ELISA-3) which can detect antibodies within 4 to 10 weeks after infection. If positive, it is followed by a confirmation test with a recombinant immunoblot assay (e.g. RIBA-3) especially in low-risk settings (Lauer and Walker, 2001). Despite improved sensitivity, the results of a RIBA-3 test may be indeterminate, necessitating evaluation of the patient for evidence of viral replication and liver disease (Booth et al., 2001).

To test whether a person is an HCV carrier, two types of tests are used — qualitative and quantitative. As a qualitative test, a polymerase chain reaction (PCR) assay is the most sensitive for detecting HCV in the blood, but, because it is not standardised, it may be unreliable. These tests are indicated when transaminases are normal, within the window period of suspected acute HCV, to confirm viraemia, and to assess treatment response (Lauer and Walker, 2001). Quantitative RNA tests measure the level of viral RNA in the blood. They are less sensitive than qualitative PCR assays and should therefore not be used for screening (Gross, 1998). People can be carriers without having antibodies (Touzet et al., 2000).

To monitor HCV infection and the efficacy of treatment in between the abovementioned tests, the measurement of the ALT level is relatively cheap and easy. It is, however, not conclusive evidence, as ALT levels may be normal or fluctuate even with liver cirrhosis.

A liver biopsy is used to confirm the HCV diagnosis and to determine the severity of the disease (Knodell score), the stage of the disease and the response to treatment. As biopsy is not without risk, it is not recommended when treatment is indicated, for example when acute HCV is diagnosed (Poynard et al., 2000).

Treatment

Because acute HCV infection often goes unnoticed, treatment is rare and little is known about its efficacy. The European Association for the Study of the Liver (EASL, 1999), however, recommends treatment in this stage, in particular, because of the high risk of developing chronic HCV with limited treatment efficacy in later stages. In the acute stage, treatment with interferon alpha, a protein with immuno-modulating and -regulating characteristics, may reduce the rate of chronicity from about 80 % to less than 50 % (Ryder and Beckingham, 2001a) or even by 98 % (Jaeckel et al., 2001). In a comment to this latter study, Hoofnagle (2001) is highly critical of this outcome and he is by no means convinced that all patients with acute HCV should receive treatment.

Treatment-effectiveness is expressed in 'sustained virological response', that is treatment is considered to have been effective if, six months after ending treatment, HCV RNA is still undetectable in the blood or serum. Until a few years ago, treatment modalities were recombinant interferon alpha 2b for 6 to up to 24 months, recombinant interferon alpha 2a for 12 months and 'consensus' interferon for 6 months. Treatment was recommended for patients who did not yet have, but who were likely to develop, liver cirrhosis. Discontinuation of treatment was often followed by relapse. Only 15 to 20 % of patients showed a sustained response in the serum ALT level, and a mere 10 to 15 % HCV RNA clearance (Lam, 1999). Combination therapy with interferon and ribavirin proved to be far more effective than with just interferon, as it showed a sustained response in 30 to 50 % of the patients treated and reduced the risk of relapse. At present, a 24- or 48-week course of the combination therapy of ribavirin and PEG interferon is the most effective treatment option for genotypes 2 and 3, and other genotypes, respectively. It shows a sustained response of 55 % for genotypes other than 2 and 3, and up to 85 % for genotypes 2 and 3. For the latest developments in combination therapy and their efficacy, see Chapter 2 of this monograph by Poynard. Treatment with interferon alone is indicated when ribavirin is contraindicated.

Combination therapy is likely to have side effects, which may include the cumulative side effects of both drugs. The side effects to interferon include influenza-like symptoms, fatigue, myalgia (muscle pain), headache, emotional lability and forgetfulness, and to ribavirin haemolysis (anaemia), nausea, sore throat, dyspnoea (laboured breathing), and pruritus (itching). Rare but serious side effects include bacterial infections, severe depression, relapse into alcohol or substance abuse, seizures, and foetal abnormalities. The side effects may be considerable, even to the extent that dose reduction or even cessation of treatment is required (20 % of cases) (Hoofnagle, 2000). HCV treatment of both men and women is absolutely contraindicated around (desired) pregnancy, as it is teratogenic and may harm the foetus.

Liver transplantation

Liver transplantation is about the only treatment option in end-stage liver disease due to chronic hepatitis C. Contraindications include HCC with multiple tumours or a tumour greater than 5 cm, extrahepatic malignancy, systemic sepsis, and suspected non-compliance with drug treatment (Prasad and Lodge, 2001). Reinfection with HCV after liver transplantation, thought to be due to circulating virus, is almost universal. The clinical course of the disease after transplantation is not uniform. Short- to medium-term survival (< 10 years) is similar to that of patients who have had transplants for other forms of chronic liver disease (EASL, 1999). Long-term survival, though, is more problematic, which may be due to comorbidity or faster disease progression, with the presence of HCC prior to transplantation as a main risk factor (Crosbie and Alexander, 2000; Bahr et al., 2001).

Treatment and IDUs

Since the implementation of testing of donated blood in 1991–92, the number of people newly infected with HCV through blood transfusions or blood products has declined dramatically. At present, IDUs show by far the highest HCV incidence.

However, if clinical guidelines are anything to go by, IDUs are not the most likely or the most important treatment candidates.

Clinical guidelines on the management of HCV, including recommendations on who to treat and who not to treat, have been developed by various organisations in most European countries and at the European level (EASL, 1999). The recommendations made as to the treatment of IDUs come down to more or less the same thing, i.e. active IDUs should not be treated and ex-IDUs or IDUs on substitution, like methadone, may be treated only under strict conditions. If given at all, the main reasons for these recommendations are possible poor compliance, fear of relapse, possible exacerbation of psychiatric disorders, drug interaction, and reinfection. However, things may be changing.

Recommendations may differ in the leeway they allow as to the treatment of IDUs and this leeway seems to be increasing. In 2002, there were two consensus meetings, in the US and in France. The National Institute of Health (2002) recommends 'that treatment of active injection drug use be considered on a case-by-case basis, and that active injection drug use in and of itself is not to be used to exclude such patients from antiviral therapy'. The French guidelines (ANAES, 2002) state that 'given the higher frequency of factors favouring a satisfactory virological response, the therapeutic indications should be broader in active intravenous drug users. These patients should be taken charge of by a multidisciplinary team ... Occasional intraveneous drug use by an otherwise stabilised patient does not contraindicate treatment'. However, it is by no means clear whether and to what extent guidelines are adhered to in practice.

The treatment, or seeming lack of treatment, of IDUs is quite a controversial issue. Davis and Rodrigue (2001) more or less agree to the recommendation of abstinence as they subscribe to the reasons given above. Conversely, Edlin et al. (2001) argue that guidelines recommending withholding treatment to IDUs are not based on empirical evidence, and may be discriminatory and unfair; poorer compliance by IDUs has never conclusively been proven, and poor compliance can best be improved by an individualised approach rather than used as an excuse not to treat. Empirical studies on the HCV treatment of active drug users (Backmund et al., 2001; Gölz et al., 2001; Jowett et al., 2001; Dalgard et al., 2002) show that treatment success is feasible and comparable to that of non-IDUs. In a comment on Edlin et al. and Davis and Rodrigue, Wiessing (2001) reports that, in practice, the treatment of IDUs in EU countries seems limited. Only Luxembourg, Greece and, possibly, Germany seem to offer treatment to IDUs; other countries may provide treatment only after years of abstinence, or as part of clinical trials, or in addition to methadone treatment. He also argues that improved availability of prevention measures like needle and syringe programmes (NSPs), and combining HCV treatment and addiction services are likely to enhance the access to HCV treatment for IDUs.

Liver transplantation and IDUs

Next to the general contraindications to liver transplantation, as mentioned above, circumstances that are considered to have an adverse effect on survival may be regarded as contraindications in individual patients (Crosbie and Alexander, 2000). Such circumstances include AIDS, alcohol abuse and illicit drug abuse. Despite reports of successful transplantations in IDUs on methadone, the shortage of donor organs and the supposedly poor compliance of IDUs to drug regimens are not likely to enhance their chance of becoming donor recipients.

Prevention and harm reduction

General strategies to curtail the spread of an infectious disease such as hepatitis C are vaccination and screening. Other, primarily drug-use-centred strategies include healthcare interventions like substitution treatment and counselling, healthcare protection interventions like NSPs, and health promotion interventions like education on hygienic injecting practices. Many of these interventions can be labelled both 'prevention of HCV infection' and 'harm reduction among IDUs'. The term 'harm reduction' is often used in an imprecise manner indicating health services for drug users which do not have the primary aim of abstinence, and including the prevention of infectious diseases such as HCV, HBV and HIV.

Vaccine

The best way to prevent an infectious disease from spreading in any population, including IDUs, is to immunise against the source of infection by means of a vaccine. Unfortunately, there is as yet no vaccine against HCV, nor is it expected to become available in the near future. Serious attempts have been made to develop a vaccine and, although the future is looking brighter, its development is hampered by the high mutation rate of the virus, the failure to grow the virus in laboratory conditions, and the ill-understood response of the immune system to the virus (Crabb, 2001).

Screening

Screening for HCV serves multiple purposes: to prevent the transmission of HCV and to identify HCV-positive patients and thus to get an insight into the prevalence and incidence of the disease; to identify target groups for prevention and harm reduction measures; and to evaluate the effectiveness of prevention interventions. As a prevention measure, screening has proven particularly successful in the case of donated blood. Since the early 1990s, the screening of donated blood by means of diagnostic assays has been mandatory in the EU countries and has become common practice. Consequently, transfusion-associated incidence of hepatitis C has been reduced to virtually zero. The screening of donor organs and tissue is also mandatory in most EU countries (Nalpas et al., 1998).

Most European (as well as the National Institutes of Health and Center for Disease Control) guidelines agree that, to identify HCV-positive persons, the screening of risk groups especially is indicated. These risk groups include recipients of blood and blood products before 1991, haemophilia and haemodialysed patients, (ex-)IDUs, and children of HCV-positive mothers. Other 'lower-risk' groups that may be screened include sex partners of HCV-positive people, non-injecting illicit drug users, and people with a tattoo or body-piercings. Testing for HCV is often routinely offered to IDUs when needing medical treatment or when entering a drug treatment programme or NSP. Other attempts to identify HCV-positive IDUs are to approach IDUs through outreach programmes or special studies with street recruitment (Roy et al., 2002) and offer them testing. Repeated testing of IDUs and monitoring seroconversion rates are a means of assessing the effectiveness of such programmes.

Counselling and education

Testing should always be accompanied by counselling and education: if a person proves to be HCV negative, to prevent him or her from getting infected, or if a person proves to be HCV positive, to teach him or her how to cope with the disease, to inform him or her of medical treatment options, and to prevent transmission to others. Irrespective of the outcome of an HCV test, IDUs should be made aware of the risks of certain injecting behaviours for the transmission of the disease. Ideally, they should be convinced to stop (injecting) drug use and enter a substance abuse treatment, but this often proves difficult. A more realistic option might be to offer substitution treatment by, for example, methadone. If people continue to inject drugs, they should be urged to adhere to hygienic injecting practices and avoid sharing injecting paraphernalia, for example by enrolling in an NSP. IDUs who test positive for HCV should be strongly advised to refrain from taking alcohol and, if indicated, to get vaccinated against hepatitis A virus (HAV) and HBV, as these may promote disease progression and exacerbate liver damage. Abstaining from alcohol may prove quite a problem as many IDUs also abuse alcohol. To reduce the risk of transmission by blood-to-blood contact, it is also advisable not to share personal care utensils like razors and toothbrushes, not to dress the cuts and wounds of others, and to avoid risky sexual practices (Moyer et al., 1999; Zarski and Leroy, 1999). Peer group education and counselling may be especially helpful considering the social nature of much risk behaviour (Crofts, 2001).

HCV-positive IDUs should be informed about the disease, possible disease progression, diagnostic and treatment procedures, and treatment outcomes. As was discussed earlier, treatment of HCV is never simple and this is also true for IDUs. Counsellors may then guide the HCV-positive IDUs through the overwhelming amount of information, support them in coming to terms with the diagnosis and in their decision-making concerning treatment and lifestyle changes, and in putting these decisions into practice. As such, counselling may enhance the effect of other prevention activities and treatment.

Methadone maintenance treatment

Substitution treatment is an important harm-reducing healthcare intervention in dealing with substance abuse, in particular of opioids, and its effects. In all EU countries, some form of substitution treatment has become available, with MMT being the most frequent (EMCDDA, 2001). Methadone is a synthetic opioid agonist and can be taken as a liquid, a tablet or intravenously. Its main effects are relief of craving for heroin, blocking of the narcotic effect of heroin, and relief of withdrawal symptoms for 24 to 36 hours (Joseph et al., 2000). A major drawback of methadone as an opiate substitute is that, as soon as the administration of methadone is stopped, the craving and withdrawal symptoms manifest themselves again. As a consequence, people may be on methadone for a very long time, if not a lifetime, and the relapse rate after stopping methadone is extremely high.

For methadone to have the required effects, a minimum dose is needed, which may differ considerably for different individuals. The required dose may be so high as to meet with reluctance from those who prescribe it. However, too low a dose increases the risk of people continuing to take illicit drugs along with methadone (Strain et al., 1999). MMT reduces injection-related risk behaviour, that is both the frequency of injecting and of needle sharing (Leavitt et al., 2000), and the longer people remain in treatment the more so (Drucker et al., 1998). Still, MMT seems little effective in reducing HCV incidence and prevalence in IDUs as many have already been infected when entering MMT, occasionally shoot drugs while on methadone, or show gaps in their methadone treatment (Crofts et al., 1997).

Being in MMT seems in itself to be beneficial to IDUs as it tends to keep them in contact with specialised addiction services and other medical and social services (Serfaty et al., 1997), and reduces involvement in commercial sex work and criminal behaviour and thereby rates of imprisonment (Drucker et al., 1998).

Needle and syringe programmes

The major route of transmission of HCV in IDUs is through needle and syringe sharing. Although injecting drug use has strongly declined in some EU countries (EMCDDA unpublished data), it is high in others and is unlikely to disappear. In most EU countries, there are NSPs, initially set up with the aim to curtail the spread of HIV, but the scale of them differs considerably between countries. The provision of syringes is not always without controversy (EMCDDA, 2001); in the US it is still officially banned, and pharmacies may be unwilling to dispense or distribute syringes. To be effective, a sufficient coverage of distributed syringes per IDU per year is required. Preliminary estimates indicate that England and Wales have a relatively high coverage with 180 to 540 syringes per IDU per year, but many other west European countries score much lower (Wiessing et al., 2001). In general, NSPs have a beneficial effect on injecting drug use and injecting risk behaviours (Heimer et al., 1998; Vlahov et al., 1997). Their effect on a blood-borne infection like HIV has been pronounced and highly beneficial, but their effect on HCV is less clear. Outcomes of studies on HCV transmission and NSPs vary considerably. Drucker et al. (1998) report a beneficial effect, although more so with HIV than with HCV. Hagan et al. (1995) found the risk of hepatitis C among IDUs participating in the Tacoma NSP to be reduced. This finding was not confirmed in a later study by Hagan et al. (1999) on HCV infection in an NSP in Seattle. Studies by Goldberg et al. (1998) and Taylor et al. (2000) in Glasgow suggest a positive, although small, effect on HCV prevalence in IDUs since the introduction of NSPs, but the prevalence and thereby the incidence remain high. In their Australian study among IDUs, MacDonald et al. (2000) come to a similar conclusion. An Australian, worldwide study (Commonwealth Department of Health and Ageing, 2002) reports extensively on the incidence and prevalence of HIV and HCV in IDUs with and without NSPs. It is estimated that by the year 2000, approximately 21 000 HCV infections would have been prevented among IDUs since the introduction of NSPs in 1988. A major difficulty is the usually high prevalence rate among IDUs including recently started injectors at the introduction or joining of an NSP. Therefore, a special effort should be made to target comprehensive prevention interventions at young and new injectors.

Final remarks

Worldwide, hepatitis C poses a serious threat to public health. A considerable part of the HCV-positive population is asymptomatic, remains hidden and constitutes a potential source of infection with high infectivity. Only a small proportion of those infected with HCV are diagnosed — the proverbial tip of the iceberg.

Because the majority of those infected with HCV are diagnosed years after the time of infection, disease progression is still unclear, and is even more so in IDUs, who are a difficult population to monitor.

At present, IDUs are a major risk group for hepatitis C infection and the prevalence of infection in this population is extremely high. However, they are still not the most likely treatment candidates. Many guidelines exclude active IDUs from treatment, and physicians may be reluctant to treat this population because of supposedly poor compliance, drug interactions and reinfection after treatment.

Harm reduction measures like MMT and NSPs are successful in that they reduce injecting risk behaviour. In containing the spread of HCV, the success of these measures is less pronounced and does not equal their success with HIV. Because of its high infectivity, many IDUs have already been infected with HCV when they enter these programmes. Therefore, a special effort should be made to target harm reduction interventions at the newest injectors. However, being in MMT or an NSP is in itself beneficial to IDUs, as it tends to keep them in contact with specialised addiction services and other medical and social services.

References

Agence nationale d'accréditation et d'evaluation en santé (ANAES) (2002), 'Consensus conference: "Treatment of hepatitis C" ', Paris, France, 27 and 28 February 2002, *Gastroenterologie Clinique et Biologique* 26 (Special Issue No 2): B302–3.

Alter, H. (1999), 'Discovery of non-A, non-B hepatitis and identification of its etiology', *American Journal of Medicine* 107(6B):16S–20S.

Backmund, M., Meyer, K., von Zielonka, M., Eichenlaub, D. (2001), 'Treatment of hepatitis C infection in injection drug users', *Hepatology* 34: 188–93.

Bahr, M. J., Böker, K. H. W., Manns, M. P. (2001), 'Hepatitis C und Lebertransplantation', *Bundesgesundheitsblat, Gesundheitsforschung und Gesundheitsschutz* 44(6): 527–77.

Beld, M., Penning, M., van Putten, M. et al. (1998), 'Hepatitis C virus serotype-specific core and NS4 antibodies in injecting drug users participating in the Amsterdam cohort studies', *Journal of Clinical Microbiology* 36: 3002–6.

Booth, J. C. L., O'Grady, J., Neuberger, J., on behalf of the Royal College of Physicians of London and the British Society of Gastroenterology (2001), 'Clinical gu.   ..s on the management of hepatitis C', *Gut* 49 (Suppl. I): i1–i21.

Bourlière, M., Barberin, J. M., Rotily, M. et al. (2002), 'Epidemiological changes in hepatitis C virus genotypes in France: evidence in intravenous drug users', *Journal of Viral Hepatitis* 9: 62–70.

Center for Disease Control (CDC) (1998), 'Recommendation for prevention and control of hepatitis C virus (HCV) infection and HCV-related chronic disease', *MMWR Morbidity and Mortality Weekly Report Recommendations and Reports* 47 (RR-19): 1–40.

Commonwealth Department of Health and Ageing (2002), *Return of investment in needle and syringe programs in Australia — Report*, Health Outcome International Pty Ltd in association with the National Centre for HIV Epidemiology and Clinical Research, and M. Drummond, Centre of Health Economics, York University, Commonwealth Department of Health and Ageing, Canberra.

Crabb, C. (2001), 'Hard-won advances spark excitement about hepatitis C', *Science* 294: 506–7.

Crofts, N. (2001), 'Going where the epidemic is. Epidemiology and control of hepatitis C among injecting drug users', *Australian Family Physician* 30: 420–5.

Crofts, N., Nigro, L., Oman, K., Stevenson, E., Sherman, J. (1997), 'Methadone maintenance and hepatitis C virus infection among injecting drug users', *Addiction* 92: 999–1005.

Crofts, N., Thompson, N., Kaldor, J. M. (1999a), *Epidemiology of the hepatitis C virus*, Communicable Diseases Network Australia and New Zealand, Communicable Disease Intelligence, Technical Report Series No 3, Commonwealth Department of Health and Aged Care, Canberra.

Crofts, N., Aitken, C. K., Kaldor, J. M. (1999b), 'The force of numbers: why hepatitis C is spreading among Australian injecting drug users while HIV is not', *Medical Journal of Australia* 170: 220–1.

Crosbie, O. M., Alexander, G. J. M. (2000), 'Liver transplantation for hepatitis C virus related cirrhosis', *Baillière's Clinical Gastroenterology* 14 (2): 307–25.

Dalgard, O., Bjoro, K., Hellum, K., Myrvang, B., Skaug, K., Gutigard, B., Bell, H., the Construct Group (2002), 'Treatment of chronic hepatitis C in injecting drug users: 5 years' follow-up', *European Addiction Research* 8: 45–9.

Davis, G. L., Rodrigue, J. (2001), 'Treatment of chronic hepatitis C in active drug users', *New England Journal of Medicine* 345: 215–7.

Dienes, H. P., Drebber, U., von Both, I. (1999), 'Liver biopsy in hepatitis C', *Journal of Hepatology* 31 (Suppl. 1): 43–6.

Drucker, E., Lurie, P., Wodak, A., Alcabes, P. (1998), 'Measuring harm reduction: the effects of needle and syringe exchange programs and methadone maintenance on the ecology of HIV', *AIDS* 12 (Suppl. A): S217–30.

EASL International Consensus Conference on Hepatitis C (1999), 'Consensus statement', Paris, 26 to 28 February 1999, *Journal of Hepatology* 30: 956–61.

Edlin, B. R., Seal, K. H., Lorvick, J., Kral, A. H., Ciccarone, D. H., Moore, L. D., Lo, B. (2001), 'Is it justifiable to withhold treatment for hepatitis C from illicit-drug users?', *New England Journal of Medicine* 345: 211–5.

European Monitoring Centre for Drugs and Drug Addiction (EMCDDA) (2001), *Annual report on the state of the drugs problem in the European Union 2001*, Office for Official Publications of the European Communities, Luxembourg (available at http://ar2001.emcdda.eu.int).

European Monitoring Centre for Drugs and Drug Addiction (EMCDDA) (2002), *Annual report on the state of the drugs problem in the European Union and Norway 2002*, Office for Official Publications of the European Communities, Luxembourg (available at http://www.emcdda.eu.int/?nnodeid=419).

Flamm, S., Parker, R. A., Chopra, S. (1998), 'Risk factors associated with chronic hepatitis C virus infection: limited frequency of an unidentified source of transmission', *American Journal of Gastroenterology* 93: 597–600.

Freeman, A. J., Dore, G. J., Law, M. G., Thorpe, M., von Overbeck, J., Lloyd, A. R., Marinos, G., Kaldor, J. M. (2001), 'Estimating progression to cirrhosis in chronic hepatitis C virus infection', *Hepatology* 34: 809–16.

Gölz, J., Moll, A., Klausen, G., Schleehauf, D., Prziwara, D. (2001), 'Therapie der chronischen HCV-Infektion bei drogenabhängigen Patienten', *Bundesgesundheitsblatt, Gesundheitsforschung, Gesundheitsschutz* 44: 478–85.

Goldberg, D., Cameron, S., McMenamin, J. (1998), 'Hepatitis C virus antibody prevalence among injecting drug users in Glasgow has fallen but remains high', *Communicable Disease and Public Health* 1: 95–7.

Gross, J. B. (1998), 'Clinician's guide to hepatitis C', *Mayo Clinic Proceedings* 73: 355–61.

Hagan, H., Des Jarlais, D. C., Friedman, S. R., Purchase, D., Alter, M. J. (1995), 'Reduced risk of hepatitis B and hepatitis C among injecting drug users participating in the Tacoma syringe exchange program', *American Journal of Public Health* 85: 1531–7.

Hagan, H., McGough, J. P., Thiede, H., Weiss, N. S., Hopkins, S., Alexander, E. R. (1999), 'Syringe exchange and risk of infection with hepatitis B and C viruses', *American Journal of Epidemiology* 149: 201–13.

Heimer, R., Khoshnood, K., Bigg, D., Guydish, J., Junge, B. (1998), 'Syringe use and reuse: effects of syringe exchange programs in four cities', *Journal of Acquired Immune Deficiency Syndromes and Human Retrovirology* 18 (Suppl. 1): S37–S44.

Hoofnagle, J. H. (1997), 'Hepatitis C: the clinical spectrum of the disease', *Hepatology* 26 (3 Suppl. 1): 15S–20S.

Hoofnagle, J. H. (2000), 'Therapy for hepatitis C', in Liang, T. J. (moderator), 'Pathogenesis, natural history, treatment and prevention of hepatitis C', *Annals of Internal Medicine* 132: 300–3.

Hoofnagle, J. H. (2001), 'Therapy for acute hepatitis C', *New England Journal of Medicine* 345: 1495–7.

Jaeckel, E., Cornberg, M., Wedemeyer, H., Santantonio, T., Mayer, J., Zankel, M., Pastore, G., Dietrich, M., Trautwein, C., Manns, M. P., German Acute Hepatitis C Therapy Group (2001), 'Treatment of acute hepatitis C with interferon Alfa-2b', *New England Journal of Medicine* 345: 1452–7.

Joseph, H., Stancliff, S., Langrod, J. (2000), 'Methadone maintenance treatment (MMT): a review of historical and clinical issues', *The Mount Sinai Journal of Medicine* 67: 347–64.

Jowett, S. L., Agarwal, K., Smith, B. C., Craig, W., Hewett, M., Bassendine, D. R., Gilvarry, E., Burt, A. D., Bassendine, M. F. (2001), 'Managing chronic hepatitis C acquired through intravenous drug use', *Quarterly Journal of Medicine* 94: 153–8.

Keppler, K., Stover, H. (1999), 'Ubertragungen von Infektionskrankheiten im Justizvollzug: Ergebnisse einer Untersuchung und Vorstellung eines Modellprojektes zur Infektionsprophylaxe in Niedersachsen', *Gesundheitswesen* 61: 207–13.

Lam, N. P. (1999), 'Hepatitis C: natural history, diagnosis and management', *American Journal Health-Systems Pharmacy* 56: 961–73.

Lauer, G. M., Walker, B. D. (2001), 'Hepatitis C virus infection', Review article, Medical progress, *New England Journal of Medicine* 345: 41–52.

Leavitt, S. B., Shinderman, M., Maxwell, S., Eap, C. B., Paris, P. (2000), 'When "enough" is not enough. New perspectives on optimal methadone maintenance dose', *The Mount Sinai Journal of Medicine* 67: 404–11.

MacDonald, M. A., Wodak, A. D., Dolan, K. A., van Beek, I., Cunningham, P. H., Kaldor, J. M. (2000), 'Hepatitis C virus antibody prevalence among injecting drug users at selected needle and syringe programs in Australia, 1995–1997', *Medical Journal of Australia* 172: 57–61.

Mondelli, M. U., Silini, E. (1999), 'Clinical significance of hepatitis C virus genotypes', *Journal of Hepatology* 31 (Suppl. 1): 65–70.

Moyer, L. A., Mast, E. E., Alter, M. J. (1999), 'Hepatitis C: Part II: Prevention counselling and medical education', *American Family Physician* 59: 349–54.

Nalpas, B., Desenclos, J. C., Delarocque-Astagneau, E., Drucker, J. (1998), 'State of epidemiological knowledge and national management of hepatitis C virus infection in the European Community, 1996', *European Journal of Public Health* 8: 305–12.

National Institutes of Health (2002), 'Consensus development conference statement. Management of hepatitis C', 10 to 12 June 2002, *Gastroenterology* 123: 2082–99.

Novick, D. M. (2000), 'The impact of hepatitis C infection on methadone maintenance treatment', *The Mount Sinai Journal of Medicine* 67: 437–43.

Pol, S., Lamorthe, B., Thi, N. T. et al. (1998), 'Retrospective analysis of the impact of HIV infection and alcohol use on chronic hepatitis C in a large cohort of drug users', *Journal of Hepatology* 28: 945–50.

Poynard, T., Ratziu, V., Benhamou, Y., Di Martino, V. D., Bedossa, P., Opolon, P. (2000), 'Fibrosis in patients with chronic hepatitis C: detection and significance', *Seminars in Liver Disease* 20: 47–55.

Prasad, K. R., Lodge, J. P. A. (2001), 'ABC of diseases of liver, pancreas, and biliary system. Transplantation of the liver and pancreas. Clinical review', *British Medical Journal* 322: 845–7.

Roy, K., Hay, G., Andragetti, R., Taylor, A., Goldberg, D., Wiessing, L. (2002), 'Monitoring hepatitis C virus infection among injecting drug users in the European Union: a review of the literature', *Epidemiology and Infection* 129: 577–85.

Ryder, S. D., Beckingham, I. J. (2001a), 'ABC of diseases of liver, pancreas, and biliary system. Acute hepatitis. Clinical review', *British Medical Journal* 322: 151–3.

Ryder, S. D, Beckingham, I. J. (2001b), 'ABC of diseases of liver, pancreas, and biliary system. Chronic viral hepatitis. Clinical review', *British Medical Journal* 322: 219–21.

Seeff, L. B. (1997), 'Natural history of hepatitis C', *Hepatology* 26 (3 Suppl. 1): 21S–8S.

Seeff, L. B. (1999), 'Natural history of hepatitis C', *American Journal of Medicine* 107: 10S–5S.

Seeff, L. B. (2000), 'Natural history of hepatitis C', in Liang, T. J. (moderator), 'Pathogenesis, natural history, treatment and prevention of hepatitis C', *Annals of Internal Medicine* 132: 299–300.

Seeff, L. B., Miller, R. N., Rabkin, C. S., Buskell-Bales, Z., Straley-Eason, K. et al. (2000), '45 year follow-up of hepatitis C virus infection in healthy young adults', *Annals of Internal Medicine* 132: 105–11.

Stark, K., Schreier, E., Muller, R., Wirth, D., Driesel, G., Bienzle, U. (1995), 'Prevalence and determinants of anti-HCV seropositivity and of HCV genotype among intravenous drug users in Berlin', *Scandinavian Journal of Infectious Diseases* 27: 331–7.

Stark, K., Bienzle, U., Vonk, R., Guggenmoos Holzmann, I. (1997), 'History of syringe sharing in prison and risk of hepatitis B virus, hepatitis C virus, and human immunodeficiency virus infection among injecting drug users in Berlin', *International Journal of Epidemiology* 26: 1359–66.

Strain, E. C., Bigelow, G. E., Liebson, I. A., Stitzer, M. L. (1999), 'Moderate- vs high-dose methadone in the treatment of opioid dependence: a randomised trial', *Journal of the American Medical Association* 281: 1000–5.

Taylor, A., Goldberg, D., Hutchinson, S., Cameron, S., Gore, S. M., McMenamin, J., Green, S., Pithie, A., Fox, R. (2000), 'Prevalence of hepatitis C virus infection among injecting drug users in Glasgow 1990–1996: are current harm reduction strategies working?', *Journal of Infectious Diseases* 40: 176–83.

Thorpe, L. E., Ouellet, L. J., Levy, J. R., Williams, I. T., Monterosso, E. R. (2000), 'Hepatitis C virus infection: prevalence, risk factors, and prevention. Opportunities among young injection drug users in Chicago, 1997–1999', *Journal of Infectious Diseases* 182: 1588–94.

Tortu, S., Neaigus, A., McMahon, D., Hagan, D. (2001), 'Hepatitis C among non-injecting drug users: a report', *Substance Use and Misuse* 36: 523–34.

Touzet, S., Kraemer, L., Colin, C. et al. (2000), 'Epidemiology of hepatitis C virus infection in European Union countries: a critical analysis of the literature', *European Journal of Gastroenterology and Hepatology* 12: 667–78.

Vidal-Trécan, G., Cost, J., Varescon-Pousson, I., Christoforov, B., Boissonnas, A. (2000), 'HCV status knowledge and risk behaviours amongst intravenous drug users', *European Journal of Epidemiology* 16: 439–45.

Vlahov, D., Junge, B., Brookmeyer, R. et al. (1997), 'Reductions in high-risk drug use behaviours among participants in the Baltimore needle exchange program', *Journal of Acquired Immune Deficiency Syndromes and Human Retrovirology* 16: 400–6.

Wasley, A., Alter, M. J. (2000), 'Epidemiology of hepatitis C: geographic differences and temporal trends', *Seminars in Liver Disease* 20: 1–16.

Webster, G., Barnes, E., Brown, D., Dusheiko, G. (2000), 'HCV genotypes — role in pathogenesis of disease and response to therapy', *Ballière's Clinical Gastroenterology* 14: 229–40.

WHO (2000), 'Hepatitis C', Fact Sheet No 164, World Health Organisation (available at http://www.who.int/inf-fs/en/fact164.html).

Wiessing, L. (2001), 'The access of injecting drug users to hepatitis C treatment is low and should be improved', *Eurosurveillance Weekly* 5: 010802 (available at http://www.eurosurv.org/2001/010802.html).

Wiessing, L. G., Denis, B., Guttormsson, U. et al. (2001), 'Estimating coverage of harm reduction measures for injection drug users in the European Union', *Proceedings of 2000 global research network meeting on HIV prevention in drug using populations*, Third annual meeting, Durban, South Africa, 5 to 7 July 2000, National Institute on Drug Abuse, National Institutes of Health, US Department of Health and Human Services (available at http://www.emcdda.eu.int/?nnodeid=1375).

Wong, J. B., Bennett, W. G., Koff, R. S., Pauker, S. G. (1998), 'Pretreatment evaluation of chronic hepatitis C: risks, benefits and costs', *Journal of the American Medical Association* 280: 2088–93.

Zarski, J.-P., Leroy, V. (1999), 'Counselling patients with hepatitis C', *Journal of Hepatology* 31 (Suppl. 1): 136–40.

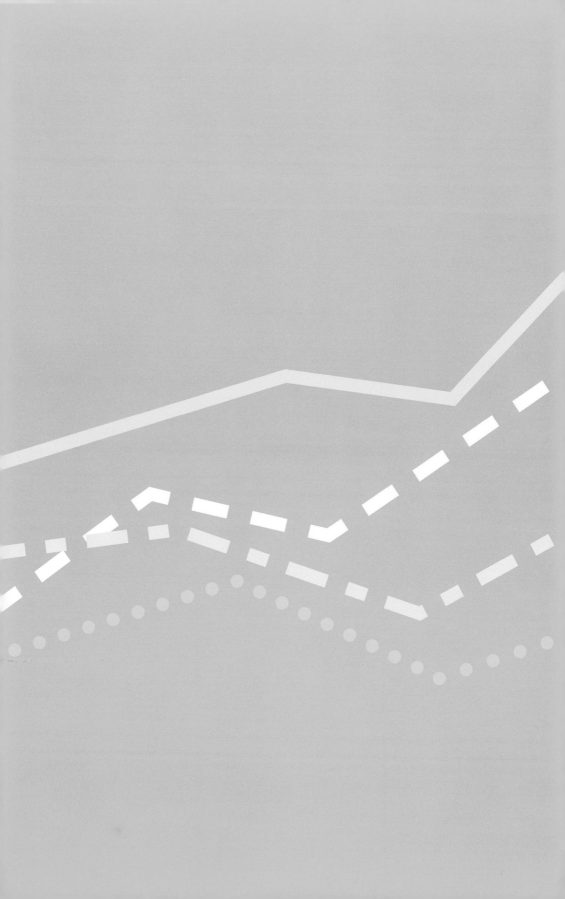

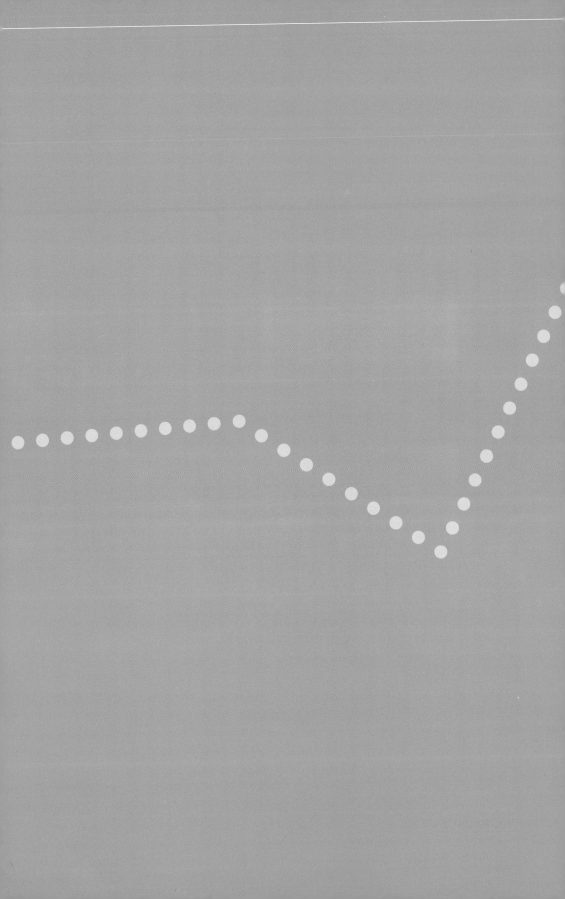

Chapter 2
Recent developments in hepatitis C diagnostics and treatment

Thierry Poynard

Introduction

Chronic HCV infection is a major cause of chronic liver disease with increasing mortality throughout the world (Alter et al., 1999; Deuffic et al., 1999a; El-Serag and Mason, 1999; Lauer and Walker, 2001). There are now very potent treatments which enable eradication of the virus in 60 % of cases and which reduce progression to cirrhosis in the remainder. Therefore, this infection should be detected and treated when necessary.

This chapter presents a contemporary approach to recent developments in the diagnostics (clinical and biological manifestations, and diagnostic tests) and management of chronic HCV infection.

Diagnostics of hepatitis C

There are no specific clinical or biological manifestations of HCV infection. Diagnostics are based on large-scale screening using serum anti-HCV antibody detection. Patients usually complain most of extrahepatic manifestations which impair their quality of life.

Clinical manifestations

Extrahepatic clinical manifestations are particularly frequent (Gumber and Chopra, 1995; Cacoub et al., 1999); 74 % of patients present with at least one of these, with a preponderance of rheumatic (i.e. arthralgia, myalgia, paraesthesia) and cutaneous-mucous (pruritus, sicca syndrome, Raynaud's phenomenon) symptoms (Cacoub et al., 1999) (Table 1). Six manifestations had a prevalence of above 10 % including, in decreasing order, fatigue, arthralgia, paraesthesia, myalgia, pruritus and sicca syndrome. This may include non-specific prevalence of these symptoms, as there is no control population matched for age and sex. Systemic lupus erythematosus, Sjögren's syndrome, rheumatoid arthritis or dermatomyositis are uncommon in HCV-positive patients, suggesting a fortuitous association.

Table 1: Prevalence of clinical and biological extrahepatic manifestations in HCV-positive patients (decreasing order). Adapted with permission (Cacoub et al., 1999)		
Extrahepatic manifestation	%	95 % CI
Clinical manifestation (tested in 1 614 patients)		
Fatigue	53	51–56
Arthralgia	23	21–26
Paraesthesia	17	15–19
Myalgia	15	14–17
Pruritus	15	13–17
Sicca syndrome	11	10–13
Arterial hypertension	10	8–11
Diabetes	7	5–8
Raynaud's phenomenon	3.5	2.6–4.5
Abnormal thyroid function	3.4	2.0–4.0
Psoriasis	3	2–4
At least one clinical manifestation	74	72–77
Biological manifestation (total tested)		
Cryoglobulin (1 083)	40	37–43
Antinuclear antibodies (874)	10	8–12
Low thyroxin (661)	10	8–13
Anti-smooth-muscle antibodies (873)	7	5–9
Antimicrosomal thyroid antibodies (451)	5	3–8
Elevated creatininemia (1 614)	3	2–4

Note: CI = confidence interval.

Systemic vasculitis, which is the severe symptomatic manifestation of cryoglobulinaemia, although rare (1 %), is the most frequent systemic inflammatory disease observed.

Biological manifestations

Four biological abnormalities have prevalences above 5 %: cryoglobulin, antinuclear antibodies, low thyroxin level and anti-smooth-muscle antibodies. At least one biological abnormality is present in 50 % of patients (Gumber and Chopra, 1995; Cacoub et al., 1999).

Mixed cryoglobulins are the predominant extrahepatic biological manifestation, identified in 40 % of the 1 083 patients tested (Cacoub et al., 1999). All cryoglobulin-positive patients have mixed type II cryoglobulins (65 %) or type III (35 %). Five independent factors are significantly associated with the presence of a cryoglobulin: female sex, alcohol consumption above 50 g/day, HCV genotype 2 or 3, and extensive liver fibrosis. Cryoglobulin-positive patients present with more arthralgia, arterial hypertension, purpura, and systemic vasculitis. However, considering the high frequency of positive cryoglobulin in HCV patients, severely symptomatic mixed cryoglobulinaemia with vasculitis is rare, noted in 2 to 3 % of cryoglobulin-positive patients.

Most systematic searches for biological extrahepatic manifestation in HCV-infected patients revealed high prevalences of antinuclear (20 to 40 %), anti-smooth-muscle cell (20 %), anti-thyroid (8 to 12 %) and anti-cardiolipin (20 %) antibodies. No association was observed between biological and clinical symptoms and autoantibody positivity (Gumber and Chopra, 1995; Cacoub et al., 1999).

Numerous thyroid abnormalities have been observed among patients chronically infected by HCV. In our experience, clinically relevant thyroid abnormalities at the first visit — that is before any interferon or other anti-HCV treatment — are rare. Low thyroxin levels are found in 10 % of patients but elevated thyroid-stimulating hormone levels are noted in only 1 %. Prevalences of anti-thyroid antibodies are in accordance with the age and sex ratio of the population studied (Gumber and Chopra, 1995; Cacoub et al., 1999).

The following extrahepatic manifestations were present in less than 2 % of patients: purpura 1.5 %, vasculitis 1 %, lichen planus 1 %, porphyria cutanea tarda 0.2 %, anti-thyroglobulin antibody 2 %, anti-liver-kidney microsomal antibody 2 %, anti-mitochondrial antibody 1 %, elevated thyroid-stimulating hormone 1 %, low thyroid-stimulating hormone 1 %, elevated thyroxin 1 %.

Diagnostics

Diagnostic tests for HCV infection are divided into serologic assays for antibodies and molecular tests for viral particles. Screening assays based on antibody detection have markedly reduced the risk of transfusion-related infection, and once a person seroconverts, they usually remain positive for antibodies. However, recent data indicate that the level of HCV antibodies decreases gradually over time in the few patients in whom infection spontaneously resolves (Takaki et al., 2000). Therefore, it is possible that the spontaneous rate can be underestimated.

Diagnostic tests: ELISA

Anti-HCV antibody is detected by ELISA. The third-generation test is usually very sensitive and very specific. The currently used third-generation ELISAs contain core protein as well as non-structural proteins 3, 4 and 5 and can detect antibodies 4 to 10 weeks after infection. If false positive or false negative results are suspected, the best test for confirmation of HCV infection is HCV RNA PCR. In low-risk populations, the test misses only 0.5 to 1 % of cases. False negative tests can occur in persons with compromised immunity, such as HIV-1 infection, patients with renal failure, and those with HCV-associated essential mixed cryoglobulinaemia. Anti-HCV antibody is still detectable during and after treatment, whatever the response, and should not be retested.

Diagnostic tests: PCR amplification

In the past few years, assays based on the molecular detection of HCV RNA have been introduced. These tests can be categorised as qualitative and quantitative. Samples to be tested should be separated and frozen within three hours of phlebotomy. Qualitative HCV RNA tests are based on the PCR technique and have a lower limit of detection of less than 100 copies of HCV RNA per ml of serum. These are the tests of choice for the confirmation of viraemia and the assessment of treatment response. Testing for HCV RNA is a reliable way of demonstrating HCV infection and is the most specific test of infection.

A qualitative PCR assay is particularly useful when: transaminases are normal; several causes of liver disease are possible (i.e. alcohol consumption); in immunosuppressed patients (i.e. after transplantation, in HIV coinfected patients); and in acute hepatitis C before occurrence of antibodies.

Diagnostic tests: genotype and serotype

There are six genotypes of hepatitis C and more than 50 subtypes. Knowing the genotype or serotype (genotype-specific antibodies) is helpful when choosing the interferon–ribavirin treatment duration. Response rates to treatment are around 88 % for genotypes 2 and 3, and around 48 % for genotypes 1, 4, 5 and 6. Genotypes do not change during the course of infection and must not be tested again. Serotyping (1, 2, etc.) is cheaper than genotyping but does not allow assessment of the subtype, which is only determined by genotype (1a,1b, 2a, 2b, etc.). Knowing the subtypes (i.e. 1a versus 1b) is currently not clinically helpful and therefore serotyping could be more cost-effective. There is no relationship between the severity of the disease (fibrosis stage) and genotypes.

Diagnostic tests: quantification of HCV RNA in serum

Methods for measuring the level of virus in serum used quantitative PCR and a branched DNA (bDNA) test (Pawlotsky et al., 2000). In the more recent studies, the median of viral load ranged from 2 to 4 million copies/ml ('Superquant' assay, National Genetics Institute, Los Angeles, California). Knowing the viral load is helpful for the choice of interferon–ribavirin treatment duration. Patients with a high initial viral load have higher relapse rates and benefit more from a 48-week treatment regimen than patients with a lower viral load. In contrast to HIV infection, viral load does not correlate with the severity of hepatitis (fibrosis progression).

Recently, an effort was made to define clinically relevant HCV RNA loads in standardised international units (IU) for use in routine clinical and research applications based on standardised quantitative assays validated with appropriate calibrated panels (Pawlotsky et al., 2000). Two HCV RNA quantitative assays have already been assessed: the 'Superquant' assay, for which possibly relevant thresholds were established; and the semi-automated 'Cobas Amplicor HCV Monitor' assay version 2.0 (Cobas v2.0, Roche Molecular Systems, Pleasanton, California), which measures HCV RNA loads in IU/ml. A value of 2 000 000 copies/ml (6.3 $\log^{10}$ copies/ml) with 'Superquant' was converted to nearly 800 000 IU/ml (5.9 $\log^{10}$ IU/ml), and 3 500 000 copies/ml (6.5 $\log^{10}$ copies/ml) to nearly 1 300 000 IU/ml (6.1 $\log^{10}$ IU/ml). To simplify diagnosis, we recommend a decision threshold of 1 000 000 IU/ml (6.0 $\log^{10}$ IU/ml) to tailor the interferon-alpha/ribavirin treatment duration.

Diagnostic tests: liver biopsy

PCR HCV RNA testing can diagnose hepatitis C infection. Biopsy is generally recommended for the initial assessment of persons with chronic HCV infection (Consensus statement, 1999). Biopsy is necessary for staging the severity of disease (fibrosis stage) and grading the amount of necrosis and inflammation (Metavir Cooperative Study Group, 1994; Bedossa and Poynard, 1996). Biopsy is also helpful in ruling out other causes of liver disease such as alcoholic features, non-alcoholic steatohepatitis, autoimmune hepatitis, medication-induced, coinfection with HBV, HIV or iron overload.

Liver biopsy is helpful before treating a patient, as an aid to the choice and duration of therapy. Biopsy is usually not helpful when cirrhosis is clinically or biologically obvious. Liver biopsy is usually performed by the intercostal route. In the case of clotting disorders, the transjugular route is used.

Complications of liver biopsy

From nine large-scale observations, gathering 98 445 cases of liver biopsy, the incidence of severe adverse events was 3.1 per 1 000 (95 % confidence interval: 2.8–3.5) with a 0.3 per 1 000 mortality (95 % confidence interval: 0.2–0.5) (Poynard et al., 2000a). Factors associated with severe adverse events and mortality were cirrhosis, age of the patient, and the presence of liver cancer.

Biochemical markers of liver fibrosis and activity

In the next decades, liver biopsy indications should decrease because of the validation of serum markers (Poynard et al., 2000b, 2002a; Imbert-Bismut et al., 2001). We recently made a prospective assessment of the predictive value of a combination of six simple serum biochemical markers for the diagnosis of significant fibrosis (ranging from few septa to cirrhosis) and necroinflammatory activity (Imbert-Bismut et al., 2001). From these results, we suggested that biochemical markers could lead to a significant reduction in the number of liver biopsies performed in patients with chronic

Figure 1: Longitudinal assessment of biochemical markers of liver fibrosis (fibrosis index) according to virological response. Adapted with permission (Poynard et al., 2002a)

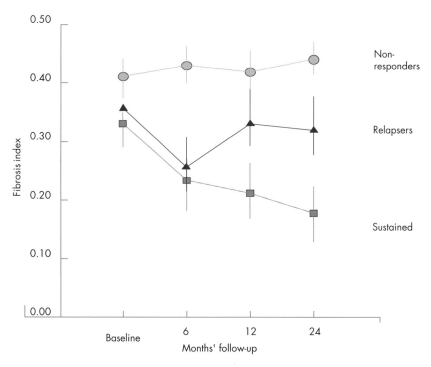

hepatitis C. Several studies confirmed the diagnostic value of these fibrosis and activity indices in different multicentre populations including longitudinal assessment with two liver biopsies (Poynard et al., 2002a, 2003) (Figure 1) and in patients coinfected with HIV (Myers, 2003).

Management protocols

In the last 10 years, considerable progress has been achieved in the management of chronic hepatitis C, both in terms of viral endpoints and histologic endpoints.

Several main treatment regimens have been assessed in large trials, the first being approved in 1990 (standard interferon regimen monotherapy with three injections three times a week (tiw)) and the last in 2002 (combination of ribavirin and PEG interferon). The specifics of these treatments are: (i) standard interferon alpha (alpha 2a or 2b, 3 million units (MU) tiw) for 24 weeks and then 48 weeks (Thevenot et al., 2001); (ii) a combination of standard interferon (3 MU tiw) and ribavirin (1 000–1 200 mg/day) for 24 weeks or 48 weeks (Poynard et al., 1998a, 2000c; McHutchison et al., 1998); (iii) PEG interferon for 48 weeks (alpha 2a 180 µg, or alpha 2b at three doses: 0.5, 1.0 or 1.5 µg/kg) (Heathcote et al., 2000; Zeuzem et al., 2000; Lindsay et al., 2001); and (iv) 48 weeks of combination PEG interferon and ribavirin (different doses of PEG and ribavirin) (Manns et al., 2001; Fried et al., 2002; Hadziyannis et al., 2002). Combination therapy has always been more effective than interferon monotherapy, even PEG interferon monotherapy.

Two PEG interferons are currently licensed. The first is a 12 kD PEG interferon alpha 2b that is dosed according to bodyweight (1.5 µg/kg, once a week) and combined with ribavirin adjusted also by weight (11 mg/kg) (Manns et al., 2001), which is a dose ranging from 800 to 1 400 mg/day. The second is a 40 kD PEG interferon alpha 2a which is used at a fixed dose of 180 µg/week and is combined with ribavirin at a dose of 1 000 or 1 200 mg/day (Fried et al., 2002; Hadziyannis et al., 2002). There has been no direct comparison of efficacy, but results from the published trials suggest that the two compounds have similar response rates and similar adverse events.

A summary of treatment progress is shown in Figure 2. Results are presented according to HCV genotype, the main factor associated with viral response. The histological impacts of these 10 different regimens on fibrosis stage and necroinflammatory grade have been demonstrated (Poynard et al., 2002c). All regimens significantly reduced fibrosis progression rates in comparison with rates

before treatment. The reversal of cirrhosis was observed in 75 of 153 patients
(49 %) with baseline cirrhosis (Poynard et al., 2002a).

The choice of 24 or 48 weeks for combination therapy has been clarified for the
former combination therapy of interferon and ribavirin but is as yet unknown for
the current one including PEG interferon and ribavirin. In one study using PEG
interferon alpha 2a in combination with ribavirin for 24 or 48 weeks, patients
with HCV genotype 1 significantly improved their sustained virological response
with longer treatment, independent of pretreatment viral load. No such difference
was seen for patients with HCV genotype 2 or 3, independent of pretreatment
HCV-RNA levels. Furthermore, patients with HCV genotype 1 responded better to
higher dosages (1 000–1 200 mg/daily) of ribavirin (Hadziyannis et al., 2002).

Based on previous results, it would not be prudent to recommend a strategy based
only on virological characteristics. Besides viral load or viral kinetics, several
independent response factors have been identified. Taking into account only the
viral factors is an oversimplification that could lead to errors in different populations
(Poynard et al., 2000c). Therefore, both the other independent factors of response

Figure 2: Progress in the treatment of chronic hepatitis C. Percentage of patients with
undetectable HCV RNA at the end of follow-up, according to genotype
(G1-4-5-6, G2-3)

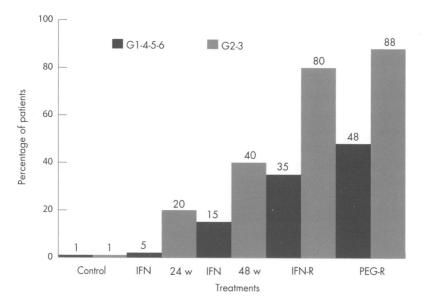

and the tolerance to treatment should be taken into account when deciding the length of therapy. Because of the antifibrotic effect of interferon, it is possible that a longer duration of treatment could benefit patients with extensive fibrosis or rapid fibrosis progression (Shiffman et al., 1999; Sobesky et al., 1999; Poynard et al., 2002d). Because of the economic burden of cirrhosis complications, treatments are cost-effective (Siebert et al., 2003).

The new standard treatment is the combination of PEG interferon with ribavirin, but there is so far just one comparison between 48 and 24 weeks' treatment duration (Hadziyannis et al., 2002). Therefore, a detailed analysis of the combination of interferon and ribavirin is still useful for the clinician.

Efficacy of the ribavirin and standard interferon combination regimen: lessons from the past

Efficacy of combination regimens on viral endpoints

When the results of two pivotal trials of a ribavirin and interferon combination were combined (McHutchison et al., 1998; Poynard et al., 1998a), the database included 1 744 treatment-naive patients. At the end of treatment, the percentage of patients with undetectable HCV RNA was significantly higher in the combination groups: 51 % in the IFN-R 48 week, 55 % in the IFN-R 24 week, 29 % in the IFN 48 week, and 29 % in the IFN 24 week group (Figure 3a). At the end of the follow-up, the percentage of patients with sustained undetectable HCV RNA was

Figure 3: Efficacy of combination ribavirin (Riba)-interferon (IFN) (a) at the end of the treatment and (b) at the end of 24 weeks' (w) follow-up. Adapted with permission (Poynard et al., 1998a, 2000c; McHutchison et al., 1998)

   (a) End-of-treatment response   (b) 24 weeks' follow-up

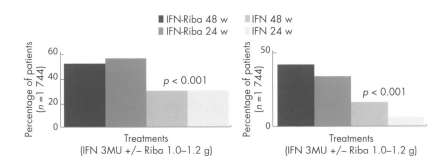

Figure 4: (a) ALT and (b) virological response to combination ribavirin–interferon in 536 patients treated for 48 weeks. Adapted with permission (Poynard et al., 1998a, 2000c; McHutchison et al., 1998)

(a) ALT response   (b) Virological response

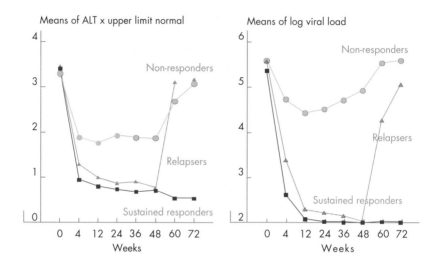

also higher in the combination groups 41, 33, 16 and 6 % respectively, with significant differences between all these groups (Figure 3b).

These results demonstrated that there was a combination effect without duration effect on the end-of-treatment response and that there was both a combination effect and a duration effect on the sustained response.

Efficacy of combination regimens on transaminases

There was a strong correlation between the impact of treatment on viral load and transaminases (Figure 4). However, transaminases' activity had a lower specificity for sustained response than viral load. In all, 12 % of patients with normal ALT levels at the end of follow-up were PCR positive.

Efficacy of combination regimens on histologic endpoints

There was a significant improvement in activity grades (Figure 5a) and fibrosis progression rates (Figure 5b) when biopsies performed 24 weeks after the end of treatment were compared to baseline biopsies. Improvement was greater in sustained responders.

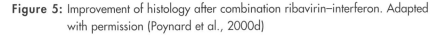

Figure 5: Improvement of histology after combination ribavirin–interferon. Adapted
with permission (Poynard et al., 2000d)

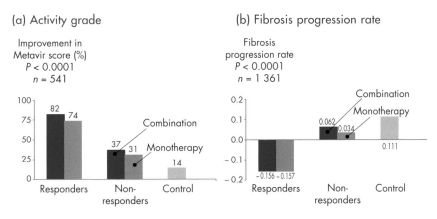

(a) Activity grade

(b) Fibrosis progression rate

Factors associated with treatment response and 'a la carte' regimen

Careful analysis of pivotal trials has confirmed the independent prognostic values
of five baseline characteristics (Poynard et al., 2000c). HCV genotypes 2 and 3
were associated with better response to the combination than other genotypes. For
viral load, the receiver operating characteristics curves showed that there was no
threshold that had either a positive or negative predictive value. Therefore, the
simplest way to classify viral load into 'high' or 'low' values was to take the
median value, which was 3.5 million copies. For age, the threshold of 40 years
seemed to have the best accuracy. Because the multivariate analysis showed that
these five factors could only explain 20 % of the variability of the sustained
response, we need to identify the other independent factors. These analyses have
excluded the possibility that the kinetics of viral load at 4 or 12 weeks allow very
early therapeutic decisions to be made.

Is a treatment with interferon alone sufficient among patients with many favourable factors?

It has been demonstrated that there is no place for interferon monotherapy (PEG
or non-PEG) for either 24 or 48 weeks, even in patients with the most favourable
risk profile. Among patients with genotype 2 or 3 and low viral load, the sustained
response rate was much greater with 24 weeks' combination regimen (71 %) than
with 48 weeks of interferon monotherapy (40 %, $p < 0.001$). Even for PEG
interferon, the results were lower than for the combination (Heathcote et al., 2000;
Zeuzem et al., 2000; Lindsay et al., 2001).

Duration of the combination regimen: 12, 24 or 48 weeks?

The first question is whether treatment can be stopped at 12 weeks in some subgroups of patients because of a high probability of non-response (Consensus statement, 1999). There is now much evidence in patients treated with PEG interferon and ribavirin to stop treatment at 12 weeks in non-responders without extensive fibrosis (Pawlotsky, 2002).

From data concerning non-PEG interferon with ribavirin, this approach could not be recommended because in the 48-week regimen, among the patients who had a positive PCR at 12 weeks, we observed a sustained response in 10 % of patients. Even the 24-week regimen induces a sustained response in 4 % of these patients (Poynard et al., 2000c). Furthermore, the antifibrotic effect of 24 to 48 weeks' treatment in non-responders is a benefit for patients with extensive fibrosis (Shiffman et al., 1999; Poynard et al., 2000d, 2002b). The choice of 24 or 48 weeks for combination therapy using non-PEG interferon has been clarified (Table 2). In patients who are PCR negative at 24 weeks (59 % of the patients in these studies), the goal is to reduce the relapse rate. There was an overall highly significant improvement with 48 weeks of treatment (74 % sustained responders) versus 24 weeks (59 % sustained responders). Since patients with many favourable response factors benefit less from 48 weeks of treatment, consideration can be given to stopping at 24 weeks for these patients. A simple strategy could be to consider only the HCV genotype, and stop treatment at week 24 in genotype 2 and 3 responders, since the sustained response was 82 % in patients treated for 24 weeks versus 84 % in patients treated for 48 weeks. However, from our results, it seems hazardous to recommend a strategy based only on virological characteristics. There were, in fact, five independent response factors, and to take into account only one factor among these five is an oversimplification that could lead to errors in different populations or subgroups (Poynard et al., 2000c). For example, we have identified that patients with genotype 2 or 3 who are PCR negative at 24 weeks and who have extensive fibrosis will have a better sustained response with 48 weeks of treatment: 80 %, compared with 65 % in patients whose treatment is stopped at 24 weeks. For a population of older men with extensive fibrosis, the choice of 48 weeks' duration in responders should not be based only on genotype and viral load. The decision should be based on both the number of independent factors and the tolerance to the combination.

Table 2: Sustained virological response to different durations of interferon (IFN) and ribavirin combination according to baseline characteristics (%)

Baseline characteristic	IFN–ribavirin 48 weeks	IFN–ribavirin 24 weeks
Genotype	65	67
2 or 3	30	18
1, 4, 5 or 6		
Mean HCV RNA		
≤ 3.5 x 10^6 copies/ml	44	40
> 3.5 x 10^6 copies/ml	38	26
Age		
≤ 40 years	48	40
> 40 years	34	26
Fibrosis stage		
No or portal fibrosis	43	36
Septal fibrosis or more	36	23
Gender		
Female	46	39
Male	38	30
Combination of virological factors		
Genotypes 2, 3 ≤ 3.5 x 10^6	65	71
Genotypes 2, 3 > 3.5 x 10^6	65	62
Genotypes 1, 4, 5, 6 ≤ 3.5 x 10^6	33	26
Genotypes 1, 4, 5, 6 > 3.5 x 10^6	27	10
Combination of non-virological factors		
Women ≤ 40 years, no or portal fibrosis	57	56
Men > 40 years, septal fibrosis or more	34	25
Extreme favourable population		
Women ≤ 40 years, no or portal fibrosis, genotypes 2, 3 ≤ 3.5 x 10^6 copies	79	69
Extreme unfavourable population		
Men > 40 years, septal fibrosis or more, genotypes 1, 4, 5, 6 > 3.5 x 10^6 copies	9	8

Efficacy of PEG interferon

Rationale

Pegylation of proteins decreases clearance and thereby increases half-life and may extend biological activity. The PEG interferons, either alpha 2b or alpha 2a, have pharmacokinetic profiles that allow one injection per week (Figure 6) (Algranati et al., 1999; Glue et al., 2000).

Efficacy of PEG interferon in comparison with standard interferon

PEG interferon alpha 2b (0.5, 1.0 and 1.5 µg/kg) has shown a greater efficacy than the standard interferon regimen (3 MU tiw) on virological endpoints, particularly at the end of treatment (Figure 7) (Lindsay et al., 2001). When genotype and viral load were taken into account, the efficacy was low in patients with genotype 1 and high viral load (Figure 8).

Figure 6: Pharmacokinetic single-dose profiles of PEG interferon alpha 2b (PEG-IFN) versus standard interferon alpha 2b (IFN 3 MU). Adapted with permission (Glue et al., 2000)

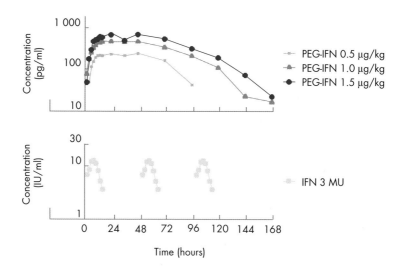

Figure 7: Efficacy of PEG interferon alpha 2b: loss of HCV RNA over time. Adapted with permission (Lindsay et al., 2001)

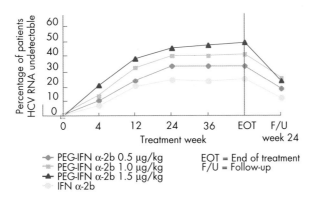

Figure 8: Efficacy of PEG interferon alpha 2b according to genotype and viral load. Adapted with permission (Lindsay et al., 2001)

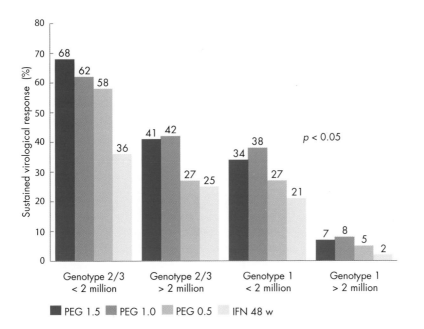

Figure 9: Efficacy of PEG interferon alpha 2a in patients with bridging fibrosis or
cirrhosis

(a) Comparison of PEG-IFN 180
with standard interferon (IFN).
Adapted with permission
(Zeuzem et al., 2000)

(b) Comparison of PEG-IFN 180
with PEG-IFN 90 and standard IFN.
Adapted with permission
(Heathcote et al., 2000)

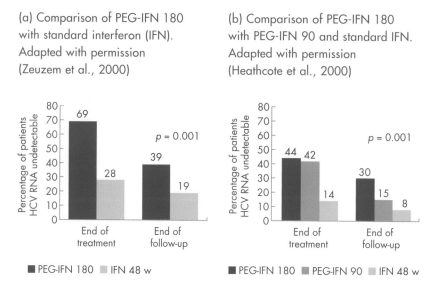

PEG interferon alpha 2a (180 µg or 90 µg once a week) for 48 weeks has shown
a greater efficacy than the standard interferon regimen (6 MU tiw alpha 2a for 12
weeks and then 3 MU tiw for the remaining 36 weeks of treatment) (Heathcote et
al., 2000; Zeuzem et al., 2000) (Figure 9).

Efficacy on histologic endpoints

Figure 10 shows that there was an improvement compared with baseline values
but that there was no significant difference between PEG interferons and standard
interferons (Heathcote et al., 2000; Zeuzem et al., 2000; Lindsay et al., 2001).

Efficacy on extrahepatic manifestations and on quality of life

Figure 11 shows that there were less adverse events in patients receiving lower
doses of PEG interferon alpha 2b in comparison with standard interferon (Lindsay
et al., 2001).

There was significantly less anorexia, insomnia and irritability in patients receiving
PEG 0.5 in comparison with standard interferon.

Figure 10: Efficacy of PEG interferons on histologic features. Adapted with permission (Lindsay et al., 2001; Zeuzem et al., 2000)

(a) PEG interferon alpha 2b. Inflammation grade expressed by the Knodell histological index without a fibrosis score

(b) PEG interferon alpha 2a. Knodell histological index including fibrosis score

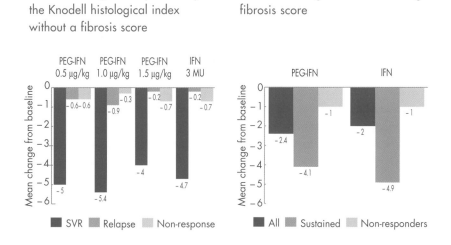

Figure 11: Adverse events in patients treated with PEG interferon alpha 2b. Adapted with permission (Lindsay et al., 2001)

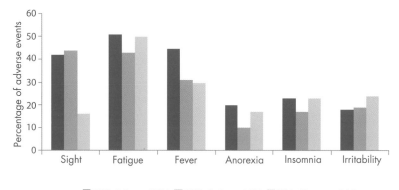

Efficacy of combination of PEG alpha 2 interferon and ribavirin

A randomised trial including 1 530 patients has compared three regimens, two combinations of PEG interferon alpha 2b and ribavirin, and the standard interferon–ribavirin combination (Manns et al., 2001). There was a significant difference in favour of the PEG interferon 1.5 µg/kg combination with ribavirin (Figure 12). In contrast to the other groups, this group had a fixed dose of ribavirin (800 mg) which was found retrospectively not to be optimised for patients with a weight of 65 kg or more (Figure 13). When the patients receiving the optimised dose (greater than 10.6 mg/kg, that is more than 800 mg/day for a 75-kg person) were compared, there was a very significant difference in favour of PEG interferon 1.5 µg versus the standard combination. Among patients infected with genotype 1 HCV with an increase of sustained response from 33 to 48 % (Figure 14), there was a significant impact on histological activity (Figure 15).

Factors associated with response

The same factors were associated with non-response and relapse (Manns et al., 2001) as for the standard combination (Poynard et al., 2000c). Therefore, post-approval studies must now establish one 'a la carte' regimen for an optimised combination treatment.

Figure 12: Efficacy of the PEG interferon and ribavirin combination. Analysis without adjusting for patient weight. Adapted with permission (Manns et al., 2001)

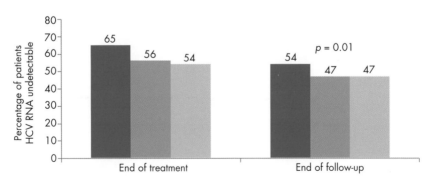

Figure 13: Effect of patient weight on sustained virological response when treated with PEG interferon alpha 2b and ribavirin. Adapted with permission (Manns et al., 2001)

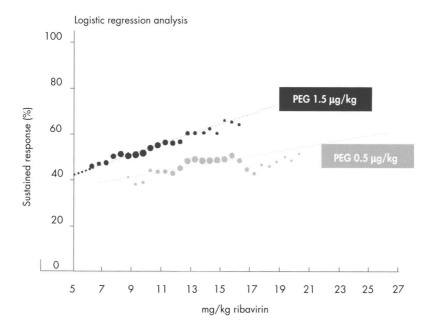

Figure 14: Efficacy of the PEG interferon and ribavirin optimised combination. Analysis adjusted for patient weight. Adapted with permission (Manns et al., 2001)

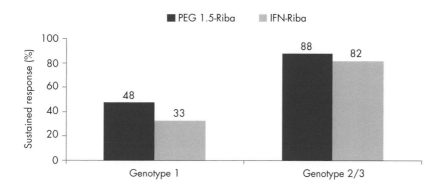

Figure 15: Efficacy of combination PEG interferon alpha 2b and ribavirin on histologic features. Inflammation grade expressed by the Knodell histological index without fibrosis score. Adapted with permission (Manns et al., 2001)

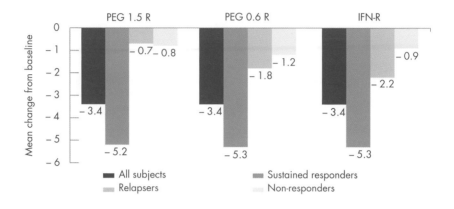

Management of relapsers and non-responders

Relapsers

A relapser is defined as a patient with undetectable HCV RNA in the serum at the end of the treatment but in whom HCV RNA is detectable afterwards. When this treatment was interferon, randomised trials have demonstrated that a ribavirin–interferon, 24-week combination achieved a 55 % sustained response rate versus 5 % of patients retreated by interferon alone (Davis et al., 1998).

If relapse occurs after a ribavirin–interferon combination, the best strategy is to treat with the optimised combination of PEG interferon 1.5 µg/kg and ribavirin, adjusted by bodyweight. If relapse occurs after the optimised ribavirin–interferon combination, the best strategy is unknown: a longer treatment duration or tri-therapy with amantadine could be discussed.

Non-responders

A non-responder is defined as a patient with still detectable HCV RNA in the serum at the end of the treatment.

A non-responder after interferon alone (administered for 24 or 48 weeks) or after the combination of ribavirin and standard interferon should be treated by the optimised combination of PEG interferon 1.5 µg/kg and ribavirin adjusted for bodyweight.

The best strategy is unknown for non-responders treated with the optimised combination of ribavirin–interferon for at least 24 weeks. These patients should be included in randomised trials. If this is not possible, one option is to treat the patients with extensive fibrosis by PEG interferon alone in order to decrease the progression rate to cirrhosis, while waiting for the development of a new generation of drugs. A small dose of PEG interferon, i.e. 0.5 µg, is an interesting treatment in this indication because of its good tolerance and once-weekly injection regimen. This concept of maintenance (suppressive therapy) has been developed with standard interferon monotherapy (Sobesky et al., 1999; Shiratori et al., 2000) showing a decrease in fibrosis progression rates (Figure 16) and an improvement in necrosis and inflammation in non-responders (Figure 17). Maintenance therapy with interferon should probably be repeated as after cessation of interferon fibrosis progression restarted (Figure 18).

Figure 16 shows that interferon reduced the fibrosis progression among viral non-responders in comparison with spontaneous progression without treatment. Interferon was given for 24 to 48 weeks in total, without stopping treatment if ALT was still elevated after three months of treatment.

Figure 16: Suppressive (or maintenance) concept. Adapted with permission (Sobesky et al., 1999)

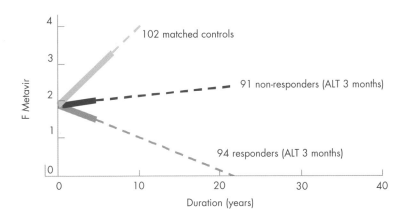

Figure 17 shows that virological non-responders to six months of interferon were randomised to 24 more months (maintenance therapy *n* = 27) versus no more treatment (*n* = 26). There was a significant histological improvement in patients receiving maintenance therapy.

Figure 18 shows that interferon improved the fibrosis stages both in viral responders and in viral non-responders in comparison with untreated patients.

Figure 17: Histological benefit of maintenance therapy with interferon (IFN). Adapted with permission (Shiffman et al., 1999)

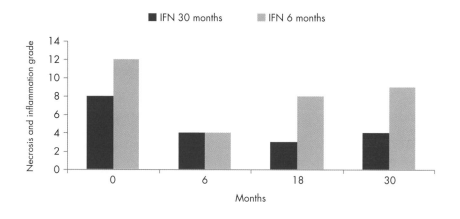

Figure 18: Suppressive (or maintenance) concept. Adapted with permission (Shiratori et al., 2000)

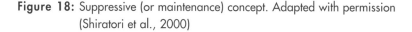
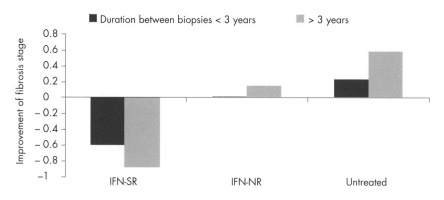

Abbreviations: SR = sustained response; NR = non-response.

When the duration between biopsies was longer than three years, the improvement was greater in sustained responders. In viral non-responders, fibrosis progression restarted after three years. In untreated patients, fibrosis progression was time dependent.

Management of patients with cirrhosis

Interferon alone

Overviews of randomised trials clearly demonstrate that compensated cirrhosis belongs to the full indication of interferon treatment (Thevenot et al., 2001). Although lower than in non-cirrhotic patients, there was a significant improvement with interferon compared with control in randomised trials. The histologic response could reach 80 % with 18 months' treatment. The effect on HCV RNA seems even better than that observed for ALT. From these results, and taking into account the severity of the disease, we think that it is mandatory to treat these patients, as the tolerance is roughly similar to that in non-cirrhotic patients. Interferon seems to be able to reduce the four-year mortality by 16 % and the incidence of HCC by 13 %. The number of randomised studies is small, but meta-analyses of controlled retrospective studies with many more patients are impressive, showing a similar reduction in HCC and mortality (Nishiguchi et al., 1995; Poynard et al., 1998b; Yoshida et al., 1999) (Table 3).

The results of PEG interferon in patients with extensive fibrosis or cirrhosis are also very encouraging (Heathcote et al., 2000).

Table 3: **Risk factors for hepatocellular carcinoma in 2 400 patients treated by interferon. Adapted with permission (Yoshida et al., 1999)**

Type of response to interferon	Risk ratio	p value
Virological		
Sustained	0.20	$p < 0.001$
Non-sustained	0.63	$p < 0.001$
Biochemical ALT		
Sustained	0.20	$p < 0.001$
Mildly elevated	0.36	$p < 0.001$
Highly elevated	0.91	NS

Abbreviation: NS = not significant.

Figure 19: Efficacy of ribavirin (Riba)-interferon (IFN) therapy in patients with cirrhosis in (a) pivotal randomised trials or (b) a pooled European database. Patients were given 1–1.2 g ribavirin plus 3 MU alpha 2 interferon tiw, or 3 MU tiw alone. Adapted with permission (Poynard et al., 1998b; Schalm et al., 1999)

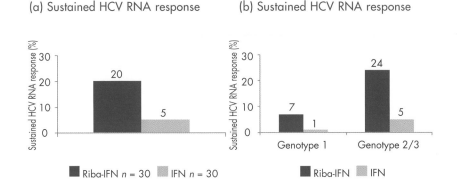

(a) Sustained HCV RNA response   (b) Sustained HCV RNA response

Combination regimen

In patients with cirrhosis, a ribavirin–interferon combination achieved a sustained virological response (below 100 copies/ml six months after the end of the treatment) in 20 % versus 5 % by interferon alone ($p = 0.01$) (Figure 19) (Schalm et al., 1999). An optimised combination of PEG interferon 1.5 µg/kg and ribavirin in patients with compensated cirrhosis is logically the new first-line treatment with 55 % of sustained response rate (24 of 44) (Manns et al., 2001) (Figure 20). Interferon toxicity on platelets and neutrophils must be carefully monitored.

Management of patients coinfected by HCV and HIV

Among patients infected by HIV, HCV coinfection must be systematically screened (anti-HCV antibodies) and treatment of HCV must be discussed when fibrosis is observed at liver biopsy (Benhamou et al., 1999). When transaminase activity is increased in a patient infected by HIV, a serum HCV PCR must be performed as false negatives for antibodies are possible in immunodepressed patients.

The mean prevalence of HCV antibodies fluctuates between 10 and 30 % in a large cohort of patients infected by HIV, is 8 % among sexually infected patients, and 80 % among IDUs.

An increase in the survival of HIV-infected persons related to active antiretroviral therapies highlights the problem of chronic hepatitis C. The prevalence of cirrhosis

Figure 20: Efficacy of optimised combination of PEG interferon and ribavirin in patients with extensive fibrosis or cirrhosis. Adapted with permission (Manns et al., 2001)

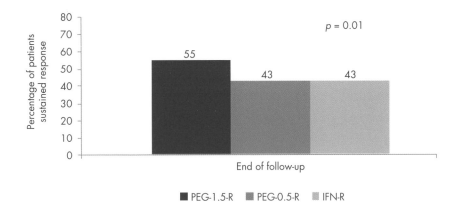

is three times higher in HIV–HCV coinfected patients than in HIV-negative HCV-infected patients and one third of coinfected patients are at risk of dying of liver disease. The progression of fibrosis is more rapid in coinfected patients in comparison with matched controls infected by HCV alone. In coinfected patients, a low CD4 count ($\leq$ 200 cells/μl), alcohol consumption (> 50 g/day) and age at HCV infection are associated with a higher liver fibrosis progression rate (Benhamou et al., 1999).

Anti-HIV treatments (i.e. D4T, DDI, abacavir, nevirapine, and protease inhibitor) are often associated with transaminase increases. When the increase is clinically significant, another liver biopsy must be discussed and compared with the biopsy before treatment. The following factors can be involved: alcohol consumption, illicit IV drug injection, substitution drug toxicity, anti-HIV drug toxicity, coinfection with HBV or Delta virus, liver opportunistic infection, immune restoration, and sclerosing cholangitis. The impact of immune reconstitution on liver fibrosis progression is unknown. However, we have observed a slower fibrosis progression rate in patients receiving anti-protease than in patients not receiving anti-protease. This difference persisted after adjustment for confounding factors (Benhamou et al., 2001).

Because of the severe aetiology, the most effective treatment of hepatitis C should be given to coinfected patients. The results and tolerance are similar to those of patients infected by HCV only, but the benefit–risk ratio is probably higher (Zylberberg et al., 2000).

Safety of the PEG interferon and ribavirin combination

Patients should be fully informed of the potential adverse events before starting therapy. The adverse event profiles of PEG interferon alpha 2b plus ribavirin and standard interferon plus ribavirin were si.. ... There were no new or unique adverse events.

Severe adverse events

For interferon, the main severe adverse events are depression, suicidal ideation, suicide and sustained hypothyroidism. For ribavirin, the main severe adverse events are anaemia and teratogenic effects. There is a 3 g/dl mean drop in haemoglobin concentration occurring in the first four weeks of treatment (Figure 21). Blood cell count must be checked at least two and four weeks after starting therapy and every four weeks thereafter. In the case of haemoglobin levels being lower than 10 g/dl, the ribavirin dose should be reduced by 50 %. If haemoglobin is lower than 8 g/dl, ribavirin should be stopped altogether.

Frequent adverse events (Table 4)

For interferon, the most frequent adverse events are flu-like symptoms and alopecia. For ribavirin, the most frequent adverse events are anaemia, and less frequently pharyngitis, insomnia, dyspnoea, pruritus, rash, nausea and anorexia.

Figure 21: Impact of optimised PEG interferon and ribavirin combination on neutrophils, platelets and haemoglobin. Adapted with permission (Manns et al., 2001)

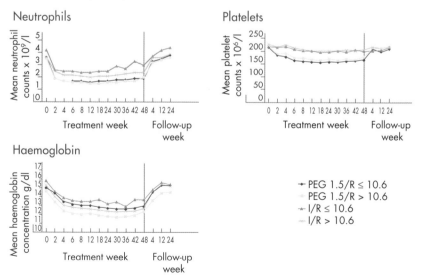

Uncommon and rare adverse events

Side effects occurring in less than 2 % of patients treated by combination therapy include autoimmune disease (especially thyroid disease), severe bacterial

Table 4: Adverse events observed in randomised PEG-ribavirin trials at 48 weeks (%)		
	Interferon/ ribavirin	Optimised PEG interferon plus ribavirin
Discontinuation for adverse events	13	14
Dose reduction for any adverse events	34	42
Dose reduction for anaemia	13	9
Dose reduction for neutropenia	8	18
Flu-like symptoms		
Fatigue	60	64
Headache	58	62
Myalgia	50	56
Fever	33	46
Arthralgia	28	34
Weight decrease	20	29
Musculoskeletal pain	19	21
Psychiatric symptoms		
Insomnia	41	40
Depression	34	31
Irritability	34	35
Impaired concentration	21	17
Gastrointestinal symptoms		
Nausea	33	43
Anorexia	27	32
Diarrhoea	17	22
Vomiting	12	14
Dermatological symptoms		
Alopecia	32	36
Pruritus	28	29
Rash	23	24
Dry skin	23	24
Inflammation at injection site	18	25
Respiratory tract symptoms		
Dyspnoea	24	26
Cough	13	17

infections, marked neutropenia, seizures, retinopathy with microhaemorrhages, hearing loss and tinnitus.

Contraindications to treatment

Contraindications to alpha interferon therapy include psychosis, severe depression, active injecting drug or alcohol abuse (when a reduction in drug or alcohol abuse has been achieved, a treatment can be discussed on a case-by-case basis including the benefit of preventing contamination), severe heart disease, severe neutropenia or thrombocytopenia, organ transplantation (except liver), decompensated cirrhosis, uncontrolled seizures, pregnancy, and non-reliable method of contraception. In fact, with the advice of a psychiatrist, it is sometimes possible to treat patients with psychosis or depression. Patients with bone marrow compromise or cytopenias, such as neutrophils < 1 000 and < 75 000 platelet count/mm^3, should be treated cautiously with frequent monitoring of cell counts. Relative contraindications are uncontrolled diabetes, uncontrolled autoimmune disorders (such as rheumatoid arthritis, lupus erythematosus, psoriasis and thyroiditis).

Absolute contraindications to ribavirin are pregnancy, non-reliable method of contraception, haemodialysis, end-stage renal failure, severe anaemia, and haemoglobinopathies. Relative contraindications are medical conditions in which anaemia can be dangerous especially coronary heart disease and cerebrovascular disease. Fatal myocardial infarctions and strokes have been reported during combination therapy. Patients with a pre-existing haemolysis or anaemia (haemoglobin < 11 g/dl) should not receive ribavirin.

There was an increased incidence (greater than 5 %) in flu-like symptoms in the PEG interferon 1.5 µg/kg group compared with standard interferon (Manns et al., 2001). As previously reported with PEG interferon monotherapy, there was a significant increase in injection site reaction. This reaction was generally mild, with a localised erythema, and was not treatment limiting.

The impact of ribavirin dose optimisation was minor, with few, more frequent adverse events (> 5 % difference) in the optimised group for asthenia, cough and alopecia. A decrease in haemoglobin to less than 10 g/dl occurred in 14 % of the optimised combination. A dose reduction for neutropenia (< 750 x 10^9/l) occurred in 21 % of the optimised combination, with less than 1 % of discontinuation (< 500 x 10^9/l).

The profiles of neutrophils, haemoglobin and platelet counts are shown in Figure 21.

Algorithms and decisions

Algorithms for treatment decision (Figure 22)

Considering the natural development of hepatitis C, there are three different goals for treatment: (i) to prevent the occurrence of cirrhosis and its complications; (ii) to reduce the extrahepatic manifestations; and (iii) to prevent the contamination of other people (e.g. the surgeon or drug user).

Suggested algorithms for treatment duration decision (Figure 23)

Finally, present recommendations take into account the lessons learnt from the combination of interferon and ribavirin and the results of the combination of PEG interferon and ribavirin. From these data, treatment-naive patients must be treated with PEG interferon and ribavirin combination for 12 weeks and the HCV PCR must be tested at this point.

If HCV RNA is undetectable at 12 weeks, the decision to continue the combination for a total of 48 weeks should be taken at 24 weeks according to the number of favourable factors. The official recommendation from the European approval is to continue treatment in patients with genotype 1 (Figure 23). The European approval also recommends taking into account the response factors. Therefore, it seems reasonable to stop treatment in the case of the presence of almost all the favourable factors, i.e. four or five factors. For patients with less than four factors, who represented almost 50 % of the trial's population, it seems useful to continue the treatment for a total of 48 weeks.

For patients who remain PCR positive at 12 weeks, the choice of whether to treat them for 24 or 48 weeks has not been fully resolved. From the perspective of HCV eradication, the combination can be stopped at 12 weeks as the probability of obtaining a sustained virological response is lower than 2 %. The remaining question concerns the usefulness of continuing the treatment in order to reduce histologic damage, since interferon and ribavirin have not only antiviral, but also antifibrotic and immuno-modulatory effects (Shiffman et al., 1999; Sobesky et al., 1999; Poynard et al., 2000d, 2002b). Studies are needed to assess whether patients who fail to respond to combination therapy will benefit from either long-term PEG interferon monotherapy or combination therapy. In patients with detectable HCV RNA after 24 weeks of interferon monotherapy, a randomised trial demonstrated that maintenance therapy for 48 weeks improved necrosis and inflammation in comparison with controls (Shiffman et al., 1999). Follow-up recommendations are summarised in Figure 24.

Figure 22: Algorithms for treatment decision

(a) Usual recommendation

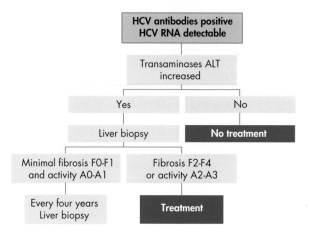

(b) Pragmatic algorithm to be tested

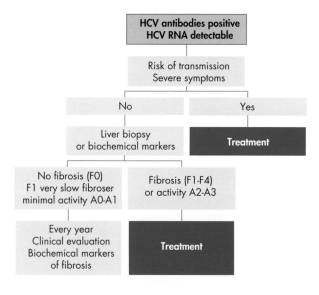

Figure 23: Algorithms for treatment duration decision

(a) Usual recommendation

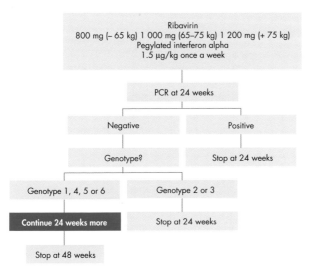

(b) Pragmatic algorithm to be tested

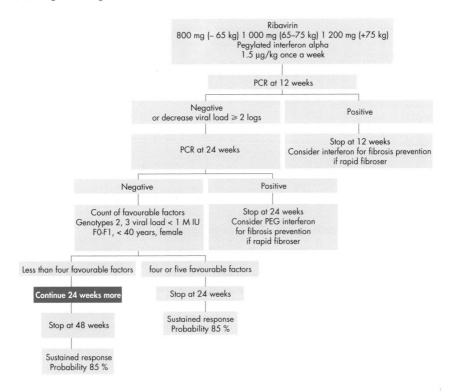

Figure 24: Proposed follow-up of treated patients

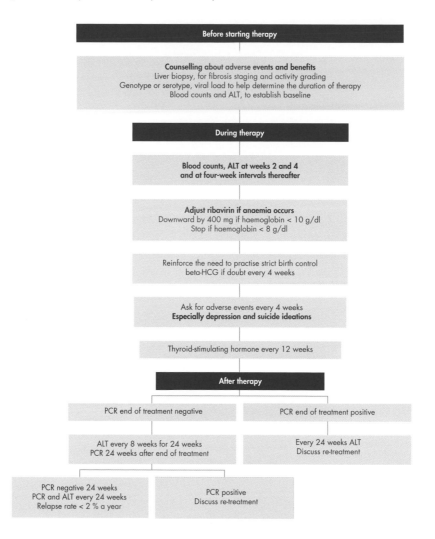

Is there a group of patients for whom the treatment is useless?

If the patient is not at risk of progress to cirrhosis, has no symptoms, and is not at risk of transmitting the virus, there is no need to treat him or her (for example a 60-year-old asymptomatic subject contaminated 30 years ago and without fibrosis at biopsy). Patients without any fibrosis (Metavir F0) represented only 7 % of a study of 4 552 patients.

If the patient has decompensated cirrhosis, the benefit of treatment is unknown. Because of the adverse event profile and particularly because of leucopenia, interferon and ribavirin are not recommended. Prospective trials are needed in these patients, especially before transplantation.

References

Algranati, N. E., Sy, S., Modi, M. (1999), 'A branched methoxy 40 kDa polyethylene glycol (PEG) moiety optimises the pharmacokinetics (PK) of peginterferon (alpha)-2a (PEG-IFN) and may explain its enhanced efficacy in chronic hepatitis C (CHC)', Journal of Hepatology 30 (Suppl. 109A), Abstract.

Alter, M. J., Kruszon-Moran, D., Nainan, O. V. et al. (1999), 'The prevalence of hepatitis virus infection in the United States, 1988 through 1994', New England Journal of Medicine 341: 556–62.

Bedossa, P., Poynard, T. (1996), 'An algorithm for the grading of activity in chronic hepatitis C. The Metavir Cooperative Study Group, Hepatology 24: 289–93.

Benhamou, Y., Bochet, M., Di Martino, V. D., Charlotte, F., Azria, F., Coutellier, A. et al. (1999), 'Liver fibrosis progression in human immunodeficiency virus and hepatitis C virus-coinfected patients', The Multivirc Group, Hepatology 30: 1054–8.

Benhamou, Y., Di Martino, V. D., Bochet, M. et al. (2001), 'Factors affecting liver fibrosis in human immunodeficiency virus- and hepatitis C virus-coinfected patients: impact of protease inhibitor therapy', Hepatology 34: 283–7.

Cacoub, P., Poynard, T., Ghillani, P., Charlotte, F., Olivi, M., Piette, J. C., Opolon, P. (1999), 'For the Multivirc Group. Extrahepatic manifestations in patients with chronic hepatitis C', Arthritis and Rheumatism 42: 2204–12.

Consensus statement (1999), EASL International Consensus Conference on Hepatitis C, Journal of Hepatology 30: 956–61.

Davis, G. L., Esteban-Mur, R., Rustgi, V. et al. (1998), 'Interferon alfa 2b alone or in combination with ribavirin for the treatment of relapse of chronic hepatitis C', New England Journal of Medicine 339: 1493–99.

Deuffic, S., Buffat, L., Poynard, T., Valleron, A. J. (1999a), 'Modelling the hepatitis C virus epidemic in France', Hepatology 29: 1596–601.

Deuffic, S., Poynard, T., Valleron, A. J. (1999b), 'Correlation between HCV prevalence and hepatocellular carcinoma mortality in Europe', Journal of Viral Hepatitis 6: 411–3.

El-Serag, H. B., Mason, A. (1999), 'Rising incidence of hepatocellular carcinoma in the United States', New England Journal of Medicine 341: 745–50.

Fried, M., Shiffman, M. L., Reddy, K. R., Smith, C., Marinos, G., Gonzales, F. L., Haussinger, D. T., Diago, M., Carosi, G., Dhumeaux, D., Craxi, A., Lin, A., Hoffman, J., Yu, J. (2002), 'Peginterferon alfa-2a plus ribavirin for chronic hepatitis C virus infection', New England Journal of Medicine 347: 975–82.

Glue, P., Fang, J. W., Rouzier-Panis, R. et al. (2000), 'PEG interferon-alpha 2b: pharmacokinetics, pharmacodynamics, safety, and preliminary efficacy data. Hepatitis C Intervention Therapy Group', Clinical Pharmacology and Therapeutics 68: 556–67.

Gumber, S. C., Chopra, S. C. (1995), 'Hepatitis C: a multifaceted disease. Review of extrahepatic manifestations', *Annals of Internal Medicine* 123: 615–20.

Hadziyannis, S. J., Cheinquer, H., Morgan, T., Diago, M., Jensen, D. M., Sette, H. et al. (2002), 'Peginterferon alfa-2a (40kD) in combination with ribavirin (RBV): efficacy and safety results from a phase III, randomised, double-blind multicentre study examining effect of duration of treatment and RBV dose', *Journal of Hepatology* 36 (Suppl. 1): 3.

Heathcote, E. J., Shiffman, M. L., Cooksley, W. G. E. et al. (2000), 'Peginterferon alfa-2a in patients with chronic hepatitis C and cirrhosis', *New England Journal of Medicine* 343: 1673–80.

Imbert-Bismut, F., Ratziu, V., Pieroni, L., Charlotte, F., Benhamou, Y., Poynard, T. (2001), 'Biochemical markers of liver fibrosis in patients with hepatitis C virus infection: a prospective study', *The Lancet* 357: 1069–75.

Lauer, G., Walker, B. D. (2001), 'Hepatitis C virus infection', *New England Journal of Medicine* 345: 41–52.

Lindsay, K., Trepo, C., Heintges, T. et al. (2001), 'A randomised, double blind trial comparing pegylated interferon alfa-2b to interferon alfa-2b as initial treatment for chronic hepatitis C', *Hepatology* 34: 395–403.

Manns, M. P., McHutchison, J. G., Gordon, S. C. et al. (2001), 'PEG-interferon alfa-2b in combination with ribavirin compared to interferon alfa-2b plus ribavirin for initial treatment of chronic hepatitis C', *The Lancet* 358: 958–65.

McHutchison, J. G., Gordon, S. C., Schiff, E. R., Shiffman, M. L., Lee, W. M., Rustgi, V. K., Goodman, Z. D., Ling, M. H., Cort, S., Albrecht, J. K. (1998), 'Interferon alfa-2b alone or in combination with ribavirin as initial treatment for chronic hepatitis C. Hepatitis Interventional Therapy Group', *New England Journal of Medicine* 339: 1485–92.

METAVIR Cooperative Study Group (1994), 'Intraobserver and interobserver variations in liver biopsy interpretation in patients with chronic hepatitis C', *Hepatology* 20: 15–20.

Myers, R. P., Benhamou, Y., Imbert-Bismut, F., Thibault, V., Bochet, M., Charlotte, F., Ratziu, V., Bricaire, F., Katlama, C., Poynard, T. (2003), 'Serum biochemical markers accurately predict liver fibrosis in HIV and hepatitis C virus-coinfected patients', *AIDS* 17: 721–5.

Nishiguchi, S., Kuroki, T., Nakatani, S. et al. (1995), 'Randomised trial of effects of interferon alfa on incidence of hepatocellular carcinoma in chronic active hepatitis C with cirrhosis', *The Lancet* 346: 1051–55.

Pawlotsky, J. M. (2002), 'Use and interpretation of virological tests for hepatitis C', *Hepatology* 36: S65–S73.

Pawlotsky, J. M., Bouvier-Alias, M., Hezode, C., Darthuy, F., Remire, J., Dhumeaux, D. (2000), 'Standardisation of hepatitis C virus RNA quantification', *Hepatology* 32: 654–9.

Poynard, T., Marcellin, P., Lee, S., Niederau, C., Minuk, G. S., Ideo, G., Bain, V., Heathcote, J., Zeuzem, S., Trepo, C., Albrecht, J. (1998a), 'Randomised trial of interferon alpha 2b plus ribavirin for 48 weeks or for 24 weeks versus interferon alpha 2b plus placebo for 48 weeks for treatment of chronic infection with hepatitis C virus. International Hepatitis Interventional Therapy Group', *The Lancet* 352: 1426–32.

Poynard, T., Moussalli, J., Ratziu, V., Thevenot, T., Regimbeau, C., Opolon, P., Horsman, Y. R. B., Closon, M., Fevery, J., Hautekeete, M. (1998b), 'Is antiviral treatment (IFN alpha and/or ribavirin), justified in cirrhosis related to hepatitis C virus?', Societe Royale Belge de Gastroenterologie, *Acta Gastroenterologica Belgica* 61: 431–7.

Poynard, T., Ratziu, V., Bedossa, P. (2000a), 'Appropriateness of liver biopsy', *Canadian Journal of Gastroenterology* 14: 543–8.

Poynard, T., Ratziu, V., Benhamou, Y., Di Martino, V. D., Bedossa, P., Opolon, P. (2000b), 'Fibrosis in patients with chronic hepatitis C: detection and significance', *Seminars in Liver Disease* 20: 47–55.

Poynard, T., McHutchison, J. G., Goodman, Z., Ling, M. H., Albrecht, J. (2000c), 'Is an "à la carte" combination interferon alfa-2b plus ribavirin regimen possible for the first line treatment in patients with chronic hepatitis C?', *Hepatology* 31: 211–8.

Poynard, T., McHutchison, J. G., Davis, G. L. et al. (2000d), 'Impact of interferon alfa-2b and ribavirin on progression of liver fibrosis in patients with chronic hepatitis C', *Hepatology* 32: 1131–7.

Poynard, T., Imbert-Bismut, F., Ratziu, V., Chevret, S., Jardel, C., Moussalli, J., Messous, D., Degos, F. for the Germed cyt04 Group (2002a), 'Biochemical markers of liver fibrosis in patients infected by hepatitis C virus: longitudinal validation in a randomised trial', *Journal of Viral Hepatitis* 9: 128–33

Poynard, T., McHutchison, J. G., Manns, M., Trepo, C., Lindsay, K., Goodman, Z., Ling, M. H., Albrecht, J. (2002b), 'Impact of pegylated interferon alfa-2b and ribavirin on liver fibrosis in patients with chronic hepatitis C', *Gastroenterology* 122: 1303–13.

Poynard, T., McHutchison, J. G., Manns, M., Myers, R. P., Albrecht, J. (2003), 'Biochemical surrogate markers of liver fibrosis and activity in a randomised trial of peginterferon alfa-2b and ribavirin', *Hepatology* 38: 481–92.

Schalm, S. W., Weiland, O., Hansen, B. E. et al. (1999), 'Interferon–ribavirin for chronic hepatitis C with and without cirrhosis: analysis of individual patient data of six controlled trials. Eurohep Study Group for Viral Hepatitis', *Gastroenterology* 117: 408–13.

Shiffman, M. L., Hofmann, C. M., Melissa, J. et al. (1999), 'A randomised, controlled trial of maintenance interferon therapy for patients with chronic hepatitis C virus and persistent viraemia', *Gastroenterology* 117: 1164–72.

Shiratori, Y., Imazeki, F., Moriyama, M. et al. (2000), 'Histologic improvement of fibrosis in patients with hepatitis C who have sustained response to interferon therapy', *Annals of Internal Medicine* 132: 517–24.

Siebert, U., Sroczynski, G., Rossol, S., Wasem, J., Ravens-Sieberer, U., Kurth, B. M., Manns, M. P., McHutchison, J. G., Wong, J. B. (2003), 'Cost-effectiveness of peginterferon alpha-2b plus ribavirin versus interferon alpha-2b plus ribavirin for initial treatment of chronic hepatitis C', *Gut* 52: 425–32.

Sobesky, R., Mathurin, P., Charlotte, F., Moussalli, J., Olivi, M., Vidaud, M., Ratziu, V., Opolon, P., Poynard, T. (1999), 'Modelling the impact of interferon alfa treatment on liver fibrosis progression in chronic hepatitis C: a dynamic view. The Multivirc Group', *Gastroenterology* 116: 378–86.

Takaki, A., Wiese, M., Maertens, G. et al. (2000), 'Cellular immune responses persist and humoral responses decrease two decades after recovery from a single-source outbreak of hepatitis C', *Nature Medicine* 6: 578–82.

Thevenot, T., Regimbeau, C., Ratziu, V., Leroy, V., Opolon, P., Poynard, T. (2001), 'Meta-analysis of interferon randomised trials in the treatment of viral hepatitis C in naive patients: 1999 update', *Journal of Viral Hepatitis* 8: 48–62.

Yoshida, H., Shiratori, Y., Moriyama, M. et al. (1999), 'Interferon therapy reduces the risk for hepatocellular carcinoma: national surveillance program of cirrhotic and non-cirrhotic patients with chronic hepatitis C in Japan', *Annals of Internal Medicine* 131: 174–81.

Zeuzem, S., Feinman, S. V., Rasenack, J. et al. (2000), 'Peginterferon alfa-2a in patients with chronic hepatitis C and cirrhosis', *New England Journal of Medicine* 343: 1666–72.

Zylberberg, H., Benhamou, Y., Lagneaux, J. L. et al. (2000), 'Safety and efficacy of interferon–ribavirin combination therapy in HCV-HIV coinfected subjects: an early report', *Gut* 47: 694–7.

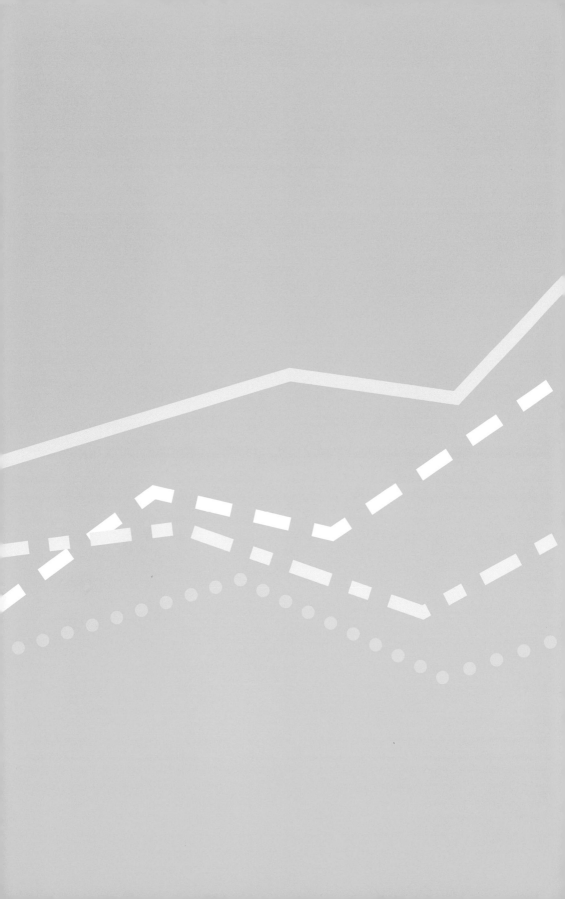

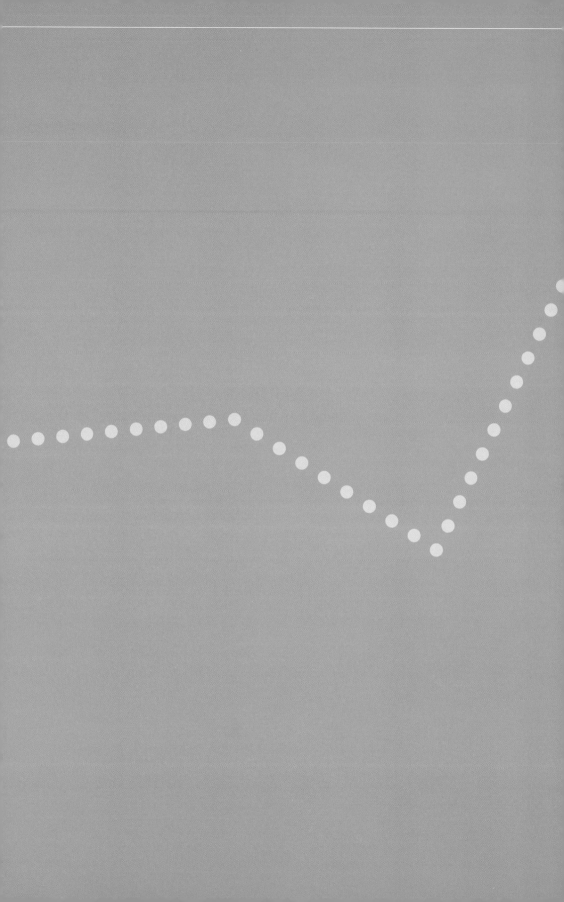

Chapter 3
Hepatitis C and quality of life

Graham Foster

Introduction

HCV is a single-stranded RNA virus that is known to infect hepatocytes (Choo et al., 1989). The virus may also infect other tissues including leucocytes, although this is still controversial (Fornasieri et al., 2000). Following exposure to the virus, some people (around 20 %) eliminate it, but most infected people develop a chronic infection that persists for decades (Alter et al., 1992). In some individuals, this persistent infection causes slowly progressive liver damage that leads, over a period of many decades, to significant liver fibrosis and, eventually, to cirrhosis (Tong et al., 1995). In addition to causing cirrhosis, chronic hepatitis C infection is associated with a variety of other disorders involving a wide range of different tissues (Hadziyannis, 1997). These non-hepatic manifestations of chronic hepatitis C infection are rare, and some, such as cryoglobulinaemia and glomerulonephritis, may be associated with significant renal disease and even renal failure. Thus, chronic hepatitis C infection may lead to end-organ damage in a number of different organ systems and, inevitably, these significant clinical disorders lead to a marked impairment of an individual's quality of life.

In many patients with chronic hepatitis C infection, the liver disease is mild and progressive liver damage is not seen. The majority of these patients do not have any of the non-hepatic manifestations of chronic HCV infection and they are traditionally described as 'asymptomatic'. In many of these patients, it is assumed that their hepatitis C infection is of little consequence and such patients are usually excluded from treatment and reviewed on an irregular basis (NICE, 2000). However, when patients with 'asymptomatic' chronic hepatitis C infection have been studied, it is clear that many such patients are far from 'asymptomatic' and many complain of a variety of different symptoms that lead to a significant reduction in their day-to-day functioning and cause a marked reduction in their quality of life. This impairment in quality of life is seen in patients who do not have any of the classical non-hepatic manifestations of chronic HCV and who do not have significant liver disease. This chapter discusses the symptoms caused by the non-hepatic effects of chronic hepatitis C infection in the absence of other obvious organ involvement.

Quality of life studies — aims and techniques

Over the last decade, there has been increasing interest in the effects of illness on an individual's quality of life. Many studies have attempted to assess the impact of a physical disorder on a patient's well-being and such studies have provided valuable data on the impact of disease on an individual. It is now clear that different individuals experience the effects of a disease in a different way and patients' views of the effects of their illness differ markedly (Nease et al., 1995). When patients' views of their illness are compared with the physicians' views, there are marked discrepancies, suggesting that what patients regard as important may not be the same as what a physician regards as important (Owens et al., 1997). The goal of quality of life studies is to examine the effects of a disease on an individual and to attempt to quantify the impact of a disease on that individual. Such studies deliberately ignore the views of healthcare professionals and concentrate on the affected patient rather than his or her carers.

To analyse the effects of an illness on a subject's quality of life, a large number of different measurement instruments have been developed. All of these are based on questionnaires, which are usually completed by the patient, and which may include visual analogue scales. After completing the questionnaire, the patient's responses are analysed according to a predetermined protocol and compared with normal data from a panel of healthy controls. The questionnaires used differ markedly in their sophistication and quality — the best measurement tools have been developed over many years and have been characterised in very large populations with a variety of different healthcare problems. High-quality questionnaires should be robust (i.e. the same patient should have a similar score if tested on different occasions), sensitive (small changes in quality of life should be detectable), and they must be validated in different patient populations to show that they can assess the impact of different physical and mental disorders. A number of such generic questionnaires have been developed and they include the widely used short form 36 (SF36) scoring system (Ware and Sherbourne, 1992; Jenkinson et al., 1993). This health questionnaire has 36 items which measure eight multi-item variables and generates a series of eight scores. These eight scores (physical function — role, physical, body pain, vitality, general health — and social functioning — role, emotional and mental health) are coded and summed before being transformed into a scale that ranges from 0 (worst) to 100 (best). The eight scores can be summarised further into two scores (physical and mental health summary scales), which facilitates comparisons between different patient groups.

In addition to the generic quality of life questionnaires, a number of disease-specific questionnaires have also been developed. These examine specific symptoms associated with particular disorders. Such questionnaires have the obvious advantage that they examine the effects of a particular disease with great precision, but they have the major disadvantage that they do not allow comparisons of the effects of different illnesses. In general, these specific questionnaires are used in clinical trials for particular disorders.

Quality of life in patients with chronic hepatitis C

Patients with chronic hepatitis C infection often complain of a number of non-specific symptoms. The most common complaints are fatigue, non-refreshing sleep and upper abdominal pain. However, a wide variety of different symptoms are often described by patients with chronic hepatitis C infection and these include arthralgia, chest pain, abdominal bloating, urinary frequency and irritable bowel- and bladder-type symptoms. These vague, non-specific complaints contribute to a feeling of ill health that can be quantified by using appropriate quality of life questionnaires. A number of studies have examined the effects of chronic HCV infection on quality of life and all have shown that many patients have a significant reduction in their health-related quality of life. The reduction in quality of life seen in patients with chronic hepatitis C is clearly a composite score for a variety of different symptoms which are highly individual — in a simplistic sense, all patients with hepatitis C have a series of different, non-specific personal symptoms which contribute to an overall reduction in their sense of well-being. Some of the larger studies are summarised in Table 1.

It is important to note that, although the mean quality of life scores are reduced in patients with chronic hepatitis C, there is a wide variation in the magnitude of the changes. Thus, some patients are truly asymptomatic and have a normal quality of life score, whereas others are incapacitated by their symptoms. The natural history of the symptoms associated with chronic hepatitis C is not yet clear — anecdotal evidence suggests that the severity of the symptoms may increase with time, but no studies have yet addressed this important issue.

Many of the studies that have examined the quality of life changes seen in chronic hepatitis C have used the widely adopted SF36 scoring system, discussed in detail above. One of the major advantages of this system is that it allows comparisons with changes seen in other diseases. These comparisons show that the magnitude of the quality of life changes seen in chronic hepatitis C infection is large and the changes are similar to those seen in other disease states, such as diabetes. Hence,

Table 1: Summary of clinical studies evaluating quality of life (QOL) scores in patients with chronic hepatitis C

Reference	Health questionnaire used	Number of patients	Comments
Davies et al. (1994)	SIP	160	Reduction in QOL scores of general population
Carithers et al. (1996)	Modified SF36	157	Reduction in QOL scores of general population and patients with diabetes and hypertension
Foster et al. (1998)	SF36	72	Reduction in QOL scores of patients with chronic HBV and general population
Desmorat (1998)	SF36	466	Reduction in QOL scores were greater in female patients and those with more advanced disease
Wollschlaeger et al. (1998)	Local QOL scores	51	Reduction in QOL scores of general population
Coughlan et al. (1998)	General health questionnaire and anxiety/depression scores	93	Reduction in QOL scores of patients with antibodies against HCV, no differences between RNA-positive and RNA-negative patients
Hussain et al. (2001)	SF36	220	Reduction in QOL scores of patients with HCV infection was greatest in those with comorbid illness

asymptomatic patients with chronic hepatitis C have a reduction in their quality of life that is similar to that seen in other progressive diseases and the phrase 'asymptomatic hepatitis C' should be avoided.

Patients with chronic hepatitis C infection are usually infected by either injecting drug use or by blood transfusions for a clinical disorder (Alter et al., 1999). It is well established that individuals who inject drugs have a variety of health-related disorders that impair their quality of life (Lipsitz et al., 1994; Kendall et al., 1995). Likewise, patients who have received a blood transfusion in the past clearly have suffered from a significant clinical illness. It is therefore possible that the reduction in quality of life seen in patients with chronic hepatitis C infection is not due to the virus alone, but is also related to other, compounding factors. A number of studies have addressed this issue and studies in patients who have never injected drugs and who have no ongoing health problems show that these patients still have symptoms that lead to a reduction in health-related quality of life (Foster et al., 1998). However, the reduction in quality of life scores that are seen in patients who have never injected drugs are less than the changes seen in those who have used drugs (Foster et al., 1998). Hence, the reduction in quality of life scores seen in patients with chronic hepatitis C is due to a number of different factors including premorbid personality and illicit drug use as well as infection with the virus itself. This view is confirmed by studies (see below) which show that successful therapy for chronic hepatitis C does improve quality of life scores, but in some patients there is a persistent decrease in quality of life scores which is not improved by viral eradication.

Effect of therapy on quality of life in patients with chronic hepatitis C

Therapy with interferon and ribavirin eliminates chronic infection with HCV in up to 40 % of treated patients (Poynard et al., 1998). A number of groups have examined the effects of successful therapy on patients' symptoms and studies that have used a sensitive marker of health-related quality of life have shown that effective therapy does improve patients' quality of life. Some of the key studies in this area are listed in Table 2.

As noted above, the quality of life scores do not always return to normal following successful therapy, suggesting that either hepatitis C infection causes long-lasting symptoms or, more likely, many patients with chronic hepatitis C infection have other healthcare issues that lead to a persistent impairment in quality of life despite elimination of the virus. These issues may include ongoing problems associated with continuing drug use or medical disorders (e.g. haemophilia) requiring blood or blood product transfusion that leads to infection with HCV.

Combination therapy with interferon and ribavirin is unpleasant and is associated with a wide range of different side effects. These include interferon-related fatigue and depression (Fattovich et al., 1996) as well as ribavirin-associated anaemia

Table 2: **Summary of clinical studies evaluating the effects of therapy on health-related quality of life**

Reference	Health questionnaire used	Number of patients	Comments
Ware et al. (1999)	SF36	324	Successful therapy improved QOL scores
Bonkovsky et al. (1999)	SF36	642	Successful therapy improved QOL scores
Bianchi et al. (2000)	SF36 and Nottingham health profile	126	Deterioration in QOL scores during treatment with an improvement post-therapy seen only with the Nottingham health profile
McHutchison et al. (1998)	SF36	912	Successful therapy improved QOL scores

(McHutchison et al., 1998). These side effects are severe in some patients and up to 20 % of treated patients withdraw from therapy because of them (McHutchison et al., 1998). It is therefore clear that therapy for chronic hepatitis C involves a significant, albeit transient, decrease in an individual's quality of life, but the magnitude of this change has not yet been documented in detail. However, it is clear from studies involving interferon alpha monotherapy that patients are aware of the impact of therapy on their quality of life and, indeed, many patients decline therapy because they are concerned about the side effects of treatment (Foster et al., 1997). On the other hand, some patients with very mild hepatitis C demand therapy because they find that the symptoms associated with infection are so severe that they warrant the use of unpleasant therapies (Foster et al., 1997). Hence, patients evaluate the benefits and costs of therapy on the basis of their personal symptoms and attempts to increase the popularity of therapy for chronic hepatitis C must involve an analysis of the patient's perception of therapy and the benefits that it may bring.

Factors that may contribute to the impairment in quality of life

It is not yet known why chronic hepatitis C infection has such a marked impact on patients' quality of life, but a number of factors have been implicated and it is likely that different factors will play a different role in different patients.

Knowledge of the infection

Chronic infection with HCV carries a significant risk of developing chronic liver disease and HCC. Patients who are infected are often concerned about the possibility of transmitting the virus to sexual, or other, partners. Hence, one factor that may contribute to the observed reduction in quality of life scores is knowledge of the diagnosis and its consequences. It is possible that this anxiety plays only a relatively minor role in the hepatitis-C-associated symptoms as comparisons with chronic hepatitis B infection (where the same concerns regarding transmission and outcome are found) have shown that patients with hepatitis B have only a relatively small impairment in quality of life compared with patients with chronic hepatitis C (Foster et al., 1998). However, chronic HBV infection has been recognised by the medical profession for many years and it is possible that patients with this infection receive greater support than patients who are infected with HCV and hence the anxiety associated with chronic HBV infection may be less than that associated with chronic HCV. One Australian study examined patients with chronic hepatitis C infection who did not know their diagnosis at the time that they were questioned (Rodger et al., 1999). This study found that patients who were aware of their diagnosis had a much greater reduction in their quality of life scores than patients who did not know their diagnosis. However, some quality of life scores were reduced in patients who were infected with hepatitis C but were unaware of their infection, suggesting that viraemia itself may play a role in reducing quality of life scores. It is not yet clear which factors contribute to the increase in symptoms seen in patients who are aware of their diagnosis and it will be important to address this area to determine whether appropriate counselling and support can reduce this distressing component of chronic infection.

Cytokine release

Viral infection of the liver leads to the release of a wide range of cytokines including chemokines and inflammatory cytokines (such as tumour necrosis factor, interferon gamma and interleukin-1) as well as the antiviral cytokine interferon alpha. These cytokines may all induce symptoms (e.g. the administration of interferon gamma to patients is associated with a wide range of unpleasant side effects (Riddell et al., 2001)) and it is possible that the symptoms that are observed in patients with chronic hepatitis C are due to the release of these cytokines. Some patients complain that the symptoms of chronic hepatitis C infection are similar to the symptoms experienced during therapeutic interferon, leading to suggestions that release of interferon may be responsible for the symptoms associated with chronic hepatitis C infection. This issue has been addressed by one study that examined the correlation between a number of circulating cytokines and symptoms and found no significant correlation (Gershon et al., 2000). This study did not measure the serum levels of endogenous interferon alpha, but studies from our group have failed to show a correlation between serum levels of interferon alpha and symptoms in patients with chronic hepatitis C (Paterson, M., personal communication). However, further studies examining a wider range of cytokines will be required to determine whether cytokine release plays any role in the symptoms associated with chronic hepatitis C infection.

Cerebral infection

HCV is a flavivirus and the closely related flaviviridae (such as Dengue virus) can infect the central nervous system. One possible explanation for the symptoms associated with chronic hepatitis C infection is that the virus can infect brain tissue. This hypothesis has not yet been directly addressed, but studies using magnetic resonance spectroscopy have shown that patients with chronic hepatitis C infection have altered choline/creatine ratios in the basal ganglia and white matter of their brains (Forton et al., 2001). This altered ratio is also seen in patients with chronic HIV infection where the virus is known to infect cerebral tissue. This observation raises the interesting possibility that HCV may infect brain tissue, but further studies involving a direct analysis of cerebral tissue will be required before this hypothesis can be confirmed.

Conclusion

It is now well established that chronic infection with HCV leads to a symptom complex that includes fatigue, malaise and non-specific aches and pains. These symptoms lead to a significant reduction in an infected individual's quality of life, which may be substantially improved by successful therapy. The factors that lead to this symptom complex are poorly understood, but they include knowledge and concern regarding the diagnosis as well as specific factors that are unique to HCV. Further work will be required to determine how these symptoms should be managed in clinical practice, but for the present the presence of significant symptoms associated with chronic hepatitis C should be regarded as an indication for combination therapy with interferon and ribavirin.

References

Alter, M. J., Margolis, H., Krawczynski, K. et al. (1992), 'The natural history of community acquired hepatitis C in the United States', *New England Journal of Medicine* 327: 1899–905.

Alter, M. J., Kruszon-Moran, D., Nainan, O. V. (1999), 'The prevalence of hepatitis C virus infection in the United States, 1988 through 1994', *New England Journal of Medicine* 341: 556–62.

Choo, Q.-L., Weiner, A., Overby, L., Bradley, D., Houghton, M. (1989), 'Isolation of a cDNA clone derived from a blood-borne non-A, non-B viral hepatitis clone', *Science* 244: 359–61.

Fattovich, G., Giustina, G., Favarato, S., Ruol, A. (1996), 'A survey of adverse events in 11 241 patients with chronic viral hepatitis treated with alfa interferon', *Journal of Hepatology* 24: 38–47.

Fornasieri, A., Bernasconi, P., Ribero, M. L. et al. (2000), 'Hepatitis C virus (HCV) in lymphocyte subsets and in B lymphocytes expressing rheumatoid factor cross-reacting idiotype in type II mixed cryoglobulinaemia', *Clinical and Experimental Immunology* 122(3): 400–3.

Forton, D., Allsop, J. M., Main, J., Foster, G. R., Thomas, H. C., Taylor-Robinson, S. D. (2001), 'Evidence for a cerebral effect of the hepatitis C virus', *The Lancet* 358: 38–39.

Foster, G. R., Goldin, R. D., Main, J., Murray-Lyon, I., Hargreaves, S., Thomas, H. C. (1997), 'Management of chronic hepatitis C: clinical audit of biopsy based management algorithm', *British Medical Journal* 315: 453–8.

Foster, G. R., Goldin, R. D., Thomas, H. C. (1998), 'Chronic hepatitis C virus infection causes a significant reduction in quality of life in the absence of cirrhosis', *Hepatology* 27: 209–12.

Gershon, A. S., Margulies, M., Gorczynski, R. M., Heathcote, E. J. (2000), 'Serum cytokine values and fatigue in chronic hepatitis C infection', *Journal of Viral Hepatitis* 7: 397–402.

Hadziyannis, S. (1997), 'Non-hepatic manifestations of chronic HCV infection', *Journal of Viral Hepatitis* 4: 1–17.

Jenkinson, C., Coulter, A., Wright, L. (1993), 'Short form 36 (SF36) health survey questionnaire: normative data for adults of working age', *British Medical Journal* 306: 1437–40.

Kendall, J., Sherman, M., Bigelow, G. (1995), 'Psychiatric symptoms in polysubstance abusers. Relationship to race, sex and age', *Addictive Behaviour* 20: 685–90.

Lipsitz, J., Williams, J., Rabkin, J. (1994), 'Psychopathology in male and female intravenous drug users with and without HIV infection', *American Journal of Psychiatry* 151: 1662–68.

McHutchison, J. G., Gordon, S. C., Schiff, E. R., Shiffman, M. L., Lee, W. M., Rustgi, V. K., Goodman, Z. D., Ling, M. H., Cort, S., Albrecht, J. K. (1998), 'Interferon alfa-2b alone or in combination with ribavirin as initial treatment for chronic hepatitis C. Hepatitis Interventional Therapy Group', *New England Journal of Medicine* 339: 1485–92.

National Institute for Clinical Excellence (NICE) (2000), 'Guidance on the use of ribavirin and interferon alpha for hepatitis C' (http://www.nice.org.uk).

Nease, R. F., Kneeland, T., O'Connor, G. T. et al. (1995), 'Variation in patient utilities for outcomes of the management of chronic stable angina. Implications for clinical practice guidelines. Ischaemic heart disease patient outcomes research team', *Journal of the American Medical Association* 273: 1185–90.

Owens, D. K., Cardinalli, A. B., Nease, R. F., Jr (1997), 'Physicians' assessments of the utility of health states associated with human immunodeficiency virus (HIV) and hepatitis B virus (HBV) infection', *Quality of Life Research* 6: 77–86.

Poynard, T., Marcellin, P., Lee, S. S., Niederau, C., Minuk, G. S., Ideo, G., Bain, V., Heathcote, J., Zeuzem, S., Trepo, C., Albrecht, J. (1998), 'Randomised trial of interferon alpha 2b plus ribavirin for 48 weeks or for 24 weeks versus interferon alpha 2b plus placebo for 48 weeks for treatment of chronic infection with hepatitis C virus. International Hepatitis Interventional Therapy Group', *The Lancet* 352, 1426–32.

Riddell, L. A., Pinching, A. J., Hill, S. et al. (2001), 'A phase III study of recombinant human interferon gamma to prevent opportunistic infections in advanced HIV disease', *AIDS Research and Human Retroviruses* 17: 789–97.

Rodger, A. J., Jolley, D., Thompson, S. C., Lanigan, A., Crofts, N. (1999), 'The impact of diagnosis of hepatitis C virus on quality of life', *Hepatology* 30: 1299–301.

Tong, M., El-Farrah, N., Reikes, A., Co, R. (1995), 'Clinical outcomes after transfusion associated hepatitis C virus', *New England Journal of Medicine* 332: 1463–66.

Ware, J. E., Jr, Sherbourne, C. D. (1992), 'The MOS 36-item short-form health survey (SF-36). I. Conceptual framework and item selection', *Medical Care* 30: 473–83.

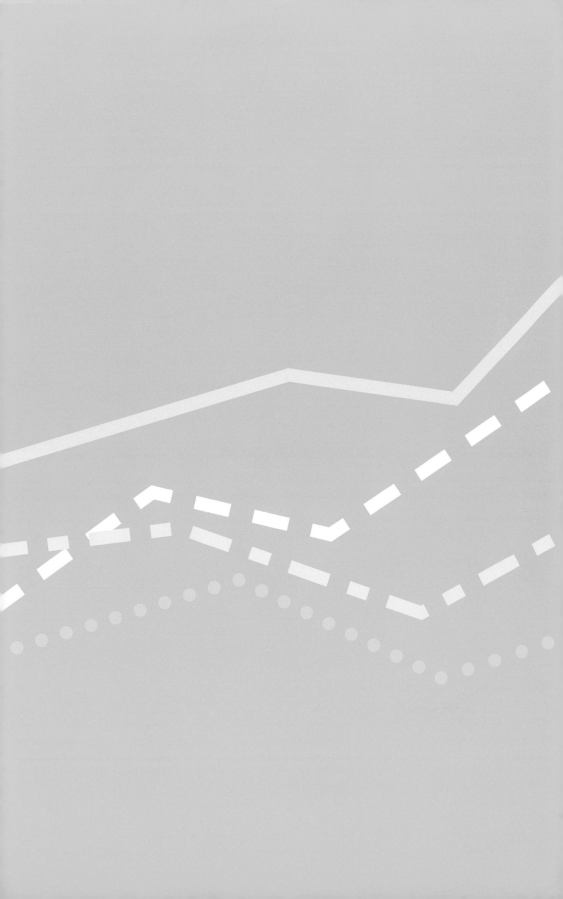

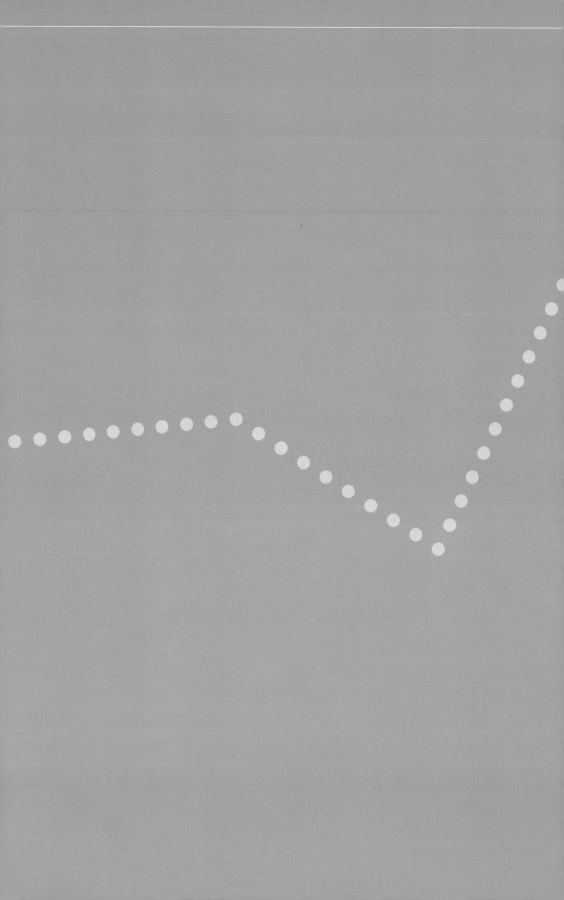

Chapter 4
Surveillance of hepatitis C infection among injecting drug users in the European Union

Lucas Wiessing, Kirsty Roy, David Sapinho, Gordon Hay, Avril Taylor, David Goldberg and Richard Hartnoll, for the EMCDDA Study Group (¹) on Drug-related Infectious Diseases

Introduction

In this chapter, we provide an overview of the available data on HCV prevalence in IDUs. These data are being collected by the EMCDDA in collaboration with national focal points (national coordinating institutions for drugs data) and experts in the EU Member States, with the aim of setting up a specialised surveillance system on blood-borne infections among IDUs. We first provide some background information regarding estimates and trends of injecting drug use and briefly describe the importance of giving increased attention to IDUs in the context of HCV prevention and treatment. As the EU is currently in the process of enlargement, the current analysis of available data still refers to the 15 members of the 'old' EU, in western Europe, while new data from the acceding central and east European countries will only be presented in future publications.

Since other routes of HCV transmission have been effectively prevented, IDUs are the largest risk group for HCV infection in western Europe, currently comprising up to 90 % of hepatitis C notifications in several countries (EMCDDA, 2003). Prevalence of HCV among IDUs has been shown to be extremely high (40 to 100 %) in the early to mid-1990s; however, more recent comprehensive information is unavailable (Matheï et al., 2002; Roy, K. M. et al., 2002). Prevention of HCV infection among IDUs is urgently needed, not only to protect IDUs, but also to prevent possible contamination of other individuals from this remaining large reservoir of infection. Data that are recent, and that demonstrate trends over time, are necessary to track the epidemic and evaluate the impact of prevention efforts.

Because injecting drug use is currently the main determinant of HCV infection, changes in drug injecting practice are likely to influence trends in HCV infection. Although the prevalence of injecting drug use decreased considerably in some

(¹) See Annex 1.

countries during the 1990s (de la Fuente et al., 1997; Welp et al., 2002), this is not the case throughout the EU, and in several countries injecting is still highly prevalent. Rates of injecting among opiate users in drug treatment indicate that trends in drug injecting prevalence vary between countries (Figure 1). While rates are low in some countries (the Netherlands, Portugal, Spain), they may still be coming down from high levels in others (France, Greece), and some decreases may have stopped (UK) or may even be turning into new increases (Finland, Ireland). Estimates of problem drug use, derived from indirect estimations using multiple methods and observable data such as numbers of treated drug users, are not very reliable. However, in general, they indicate levels of problem drug use (defined as 'injecting drug use or long-duration/regular use of opiates, cocaine

Figure 1: Trends in injecting drug use in EU Member States, 1990–2001 (percentage of current injectors among heroin users in treatment)

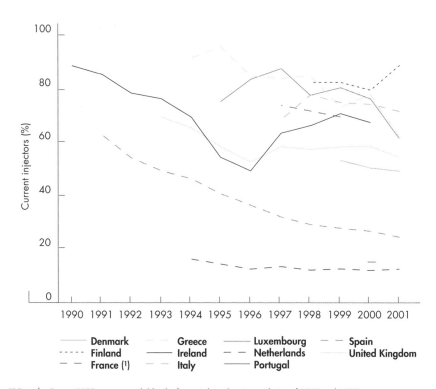

('} Data for France 1998 are not available; the figure is based on interpolation of 1997 and 1999.

Note: Data represent several thousands of cases per country per year and in most countries include almost all treated cases at national level.

Source: National focal points through EMCDDA project: 'Treatment demand indicator' (http://www.emcdda.eu.int/?nnodeid=1420).

and/or amphetamines') of between four and six cases per 1 000 population aged
15 to 64, corresponding to about 1 to 1.5 million problem drug users in the 15
EU Member States (EMCDDA, 2003). Combining these estimates with observed
rates of injecting among opiate users in treatment (the weighted average in the EU
is about 60 %) suggests that there are some 600 000 to 900 000 current injectors.
Estimates based on drug overdose (current injectors) or HIV data (lifetime injectors)
are fewer in number, but show comparable results, with a rate of about two to five
IDUs per 1 000 population aged 15 to 64, or 0.5 to 1.25 million injectors (Figure
2) (EMCDDA, 2003; Kraus et al., 2003).

Hepatitis C infection can lead to severe liver disease over the course of decades,
and ultimately lead to liver cancer and premature death. Recently, estimates of the
proportion of cases progressing to severe liver disease have been adjusted
downwards; however, this probably still occurs in at least some 5 to 10 % of
chronic infections (Freeman et al., 2001). Even in the absence of liver disease,
HCV infection frequently results in serious impairments in daily functioning and
well-being (see Chapters 2 and 3). Taken together, existing data suggest that HCV

Figure 2: Estimates of injecting drug use in EU Member States
(most recent one-year prevalence per 1 000 inhabitants aged 15 to 64)

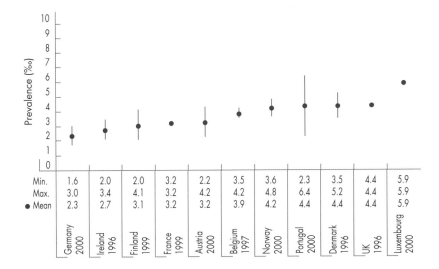

Note: Figures are partly based on different methods and data sources and should be interpreted with caution (see
statistical tables at http://annualreport.emcdda.eu.int for full details).
Source: National focal points through EMCDDA project: 'National prevalence estimates of problem drug use in the
European Union, 1995–2000', CT.00.RTX.23, Lisbon, EMCDDA, 2003. Coordinated by the Institut für
Therapieforschung, Munich.

infections in IDUs will lead to substantial healthcare costs in the near future (see Chapter 8) (Postma et al., 2001).

Prevention of HCV infections in IDUs is difficult, as the virus may be transmitted through the sharing of injecting materials used to prepare drugs as well as through sharing of needles and syringes (Thorpe et al., 2002). This means that standard prevention measures for blood-borne viruses, which have mainly been geared to HIV, need to be intensified. HIV prevention measures such as needle exchange have been widely introduced in western Europe, but coverage of measures varies considerably and may be low in many countries (Wiessing et al., 2001). Specific HCV prevention strategies remain to be implemented in most countries. There are some exceptions (e.g. in the UK and France), where information is widely circulated and sterile injecting paraphernalia other than needles and syringes are being distributed. Given the large numbers of infected IDUs, and the rapidly improving effectiveness of combination therapy, HCV treatment is quickly gaining relevance. Treatment, however, in many countries remains contraindicated for IDUs and in other countries IDUs have less access than other patients to HCV treatment (Edlin et al., 2001; Wiessing, 2001); the recent revisions of existing guidelines for the treatment of hepatitis C may improve matters.

For effective prevention, high-quality surveillance is crucial. Ideally, both HCV infections and prevention efforts should be monitored at a regional or even a local level, in order that trends in both can be compared and the effectiveness of the interventions estimated. It may not be possible to causally link declining HCV incidence to increased HCV prevention effort; however, it is paramount to distinguish regions with high or rising prevalence from those with low or declining prevalence, so that possible explanations for such differences might be explored further. At present, hepatitis C surveillance does not exist at a European level because national systems are not comparable; indeed many are unable to distinguish IDUs from other patients (Nalpas et al., 1998; Eurosurveillance Monthly, 2003).

In the context of this monograph, we have limited this chapter to describing the available HCV data.

Methods

In close collaboration with the EMCDDA, an expert network of country representatives and national focal points collect published and unpublished HCV prevalence data in the EU. Data was sourced from (i) specific epidemiological studies, (ii) HCV-testing laboratories and (iii) settings in which data on named HCV testing among IDUs were collected; these included from drug treatment centres, low-threshold drug services including needle and syringe programmes, prisons, sexually transmitted disease clinics/hospitals, antenatal clinics.

Data have been collected annually since 1996, using a standardised form ('EMCDDA standard reporting table No 9', available on request). For each data source and geographic site, the following information is sought: overall HCV prevalence, and prevalence by gender, age group, years injected, and opiate use. Prevalence rates among young injectors (aged under 25 years) and among new injectors (an injecting history of less than two years) provide proxies for incidence. Numerator and denominator figures for each prevalence estimate are also asked for. Requested background information relating to each prevalence estimate source includes: country, reporting date, definition of injectors, some basic descriptors of the sample (gender, age range and years injecting), geographical coverage of the sample, whether the data can be disaggregated into smaller region, study setting or data source, data collection method (i.e. exhaustive or sampling), sampling method where applicable, periodicity of the data collection, whether the data reflect self-reporting or a confirmed laboratory result, type of specimen tested (serum or oral fluid) and the serological markers tested. Finally, the bibliographic reference of the publication or the name of the person and institution responsible for the data are noted. An additional information section on the standard reporting table gives the data originator (data source) the opportunity to describe any inconspicuous potential biases to assist in interpretation of the data.

In addition to the data collected via the standard tables, each of the national focal points provides an annual national report on the drugs situation to the EMCDDA. These national reports contain a section on new trends and developments, relevant to infectious diseases among IDUs, that provide the drug context in which infection data can be interpreted (http://www.emcdda.eu.int/?nnodeid=400). This qualitative and quantitative information is collated by the EMCDDA which, in collaboration with the national focal points and the country experts, publishes the data in the *Annual report on the state of the drugs problem in the European Union and Norway*, available at http://www.emcdda.eu.int (EMCDDA, 2003). Meetings are held yearly at the national and European level, to discuss data quality and problems and possible improvements (EMCDDA, 2002).

For this chapter, where HCV data were provided both at an aggregate (national) and disaggregated (region) level, the former were excluded. Self-reported test results are reported to the EMCDDA by several countries, but for hepatitis B and C they are not recommended (Thornton et al., 2000; EMCDDA, 2002; Schlicting, 2003) and were also excluded from this analysis.

Prevalence rates are presented with 95 % confidence limits, calculated using the normal approximation of the binomial distribution. Confidence limits around values near to 0 or 1 were calculated using the Poisson distribution. The statistical significance of time trends in prevalence was calculated using the Cochrane–Armitage trend test. The statistical software used was SAS 8.0 (http://www.sas.com), Stata 7.0 (www.stata.com), Microsoft Excel 2002 and SISA (http://home.clara.net/sisa).

Results

Data availability and settings

By September 2002, information from 63 data sources had been obtained covering the period 1996–2002 (three sources could provide data for part of 2002). Including regional breakdowns, data from a total of 111 study sites in 14 countries of the EU are available (no data are available from Sweden) (Table 1 and Figure 3).

Of the 111 sites, 69 were drug treatment centres, 15 were prisons, 16 were providing low-threshold services including NSPs and 4 were of a multiple nature including community-wide settings. Seven countries reported at least one source with national coverage, while in two others (Belgium and the UK), one source covered a large part of the country. The 14 countries reported 233 overall, 67 young injector and 25 new injector prevalence estimates. Time data, available from almost half of the sites (52/111) comprised 174 of the 233 overall estimates (see more detail in Table 1 and Annex 2).

Overall HCV prevalence and trends

As with the pre-1996 data for western Europe and other regions of the world (Crofts et al., 1999; Matheï et al., 2002; Roy, K. M. et al., 2002), HCV prevalence in the 1996–2002 period remains high. Of the 233 prevalence figures, 25 (11 %) were under 40 %, 177 (75 %) were over 50 % and 116 exceeded 65.8 %; a rate which constitutes the unweighted median of reported HCV prevalence in IDUs in the EU over the period 1996–2002. An unweighted median may better account for geographical variability than a weighted median or a weighted mean, given the very large differences in sample size between countries. However, the weighted

Table 1: Summary description of data on HCV prevalence in IDUs (*) by country, 1996–2002

	Total EU-14	Austria	Belgium	Denmark	Finland
Sources with national coverage (^{1})	12	0	0	0	2
Number of study sites (^{2})	111	3	2	2	7
Number of prevalence estimates (^{2})	233	15	6	2	15
Number of estimates within time series (^{2})	174	15	5	0	13
Total sample size 1996 onwards	371 607	924	901	602	2 079
Recent sample size 2000 onwards	186 071	319	536	0	1 642
% data from oral fluid samples (^{3})	5	0	0	0	33
% data from diagnostic testing (^{3})	92	100	72	0	60
% data from drug treatment (^{3}) (^{4})	91–95	67	72	44	0
Unweighted median HCV prevalence (%)	65.8	67.6	38.7	80	43.4
Unweighted quartiles HCV prevalence (%)	50.5–77.4	56.8–73	36–46.4	75–85	33.2–52
Weighted mean HCV prevalence (%)	65.1	65.7	49.7	80.6	36.4

	France	Germany	Greece	Ireland	Italy
Sources with national coverage (^{1})	0	0	4	2	1
Number of study sites (^{2})	2	6	9	5	35
Number of prevalence estimates (^{2})	2	12	18	6	99
Number of estimates within time series (^{2})	0	8	15	2	86
Total sample size 1996 onwards	339	7 499	6 171	1 387	307 441
Recent sample size 2000 onwards	0	301	3 165	0	153 682
% data from oral fluid samples (^{3})	29	0	0	49	0
% data from diagnostic testing (^{3})	0	10	99	34	100
% data from drug treatment (^{3}) (^{4})	0	10	42–60	24	100
Unweighted median HCV prevalence (%)	66.7	84.3	58.8	72.2	68.8
Unweighted quartiles HCV prevalence (%)	53.2–80.1	66.6–91.2	46.3–68.5	62.1–78.8	63.7–78
Weighted mean HCV prevalence (%)	72.3	77.1	56.8	73.5	67.3

Table 1 (continued)

	Luxem-bourg	Nether-lands	Portugal	Spain	UK
Sources with national coverage ([1])	1	0	1	1	0
Number of study sites ([2])	1	2	21	5	11
Number of prevalence estimates ([2])	1	2	31	5	19
Number of estimates within time series ([2])	0	0	18	0	12
Total sample size 1996 onwards	116	487	24 143 ([5])	2 597	16 921
Recent sample size 2000 onwards	0	199	19 839	0	6 388
% data from oral fluid samples ([3])	100	0	1	0	90
% data from diagnostic testing ([3])	0	0	93	61	0
% data from drug treatment ([3]) ([4])	0	0–100	95	91	0–81
Unweighted median HCV prevalence (%)	37	60.3	65.9	71.1	44
Unweighted quartiles HCV prevalence (%)	—	47.2–73.3	48.7–82	66–83.2	30.9–56.4
Weighted mean HCV prevalence (%)	37	62.6	56.7 ([5])	79.7	35.7

(*) Data from Italy (EMCDDA, 2003) are estimated to contain 5–10 % non-IDUs; data from Portugal, where IDU status is not known, are reported to relate mainly to IDUs. The proportion of non-IDUs included may, however, change by geographic region and over time and reduce comparability of data.
([1]) In Belgium, full coverage exists for the Flemish Community; in the UK, two sources together provide almost national coverage.
([2]) Excluding national aggregates of regional data to prevent double counting (Italy, Portugal, UK).
([3]) Weighted by sample size.
([4]) Where a range is given, the lower value is the percentage of data exclusively from treatment, and the higher value is the percentage when including mixed sources that contain treatment data.
([5]) One estimate where sample size is missing not included.

median (68.4 %) and the unweighted and weighted means (63.9 and 65.1 %, respectively) were near to this value.

Trends are available from a total of 52 time series (22 are from Italy), of which 21 (40 %; 9 of which are from Italy) show a statistically significant decrease over time and 7 (13 %; 5 from Italy) an increase (Annex 2). In some countries (e.g. Greece, Portugal, Italy), different sources or regions show different trends, demonstrating the importance of collecting region-specific data and not relying on national-level aggregates only. In Finland, important decreases in prevalence among needle

Figure 3: Prevalence of HCV among injecting drug users in the European Union, 1996–2002, by country and study setting

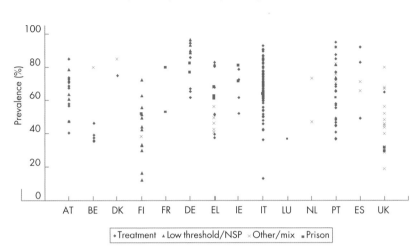

Note: Comparisons between countries should be done with caution, as data are from different study settings and study methods.

exchange attendees are observed, both in studies involving the use of oral fluid samples and in the examination of results from diagnostic tests on serum samples. In London, UK, data from multiple settings indicate a non-significant decrease in overall prevalence (52.2–45.8 %, $p = 0.08$, 1998–2001) while, elsewhere in England and Wales, overall prevalence remains low and stable. However, during the same years, an increase is observed in prevalence among young injectors (see below), while, more recently (data not available), a very high incidence is again provisionally reported in London (approximately 38 cases per 100 person-years per annum; CI 26–56) (Judd et al., 2003a). (For full detail, see Annex 2, Table A1.)

Prevalence in young injectors

Overall, prevalence also appears to be very high among young IDUs, with an unweighted median of reported prevalence in these IDUs of 30.8 % (weighted median 13.9 %, weighted mean 23.5 %; note that weighted figures are strongly influenced by large sample sizes from England and Wales) (Table 2 and Figure 4).

Variation in prevalence also appears, however, to be larger among samples of young IDUs. Of the 67 prevalence values obtained, 39 (58 %) are below 40 % and 18 (27 %) are over 60 %. Some time trends are available for young IDUs,

Figure 4: HCV prevalence data from injecting drug users under age 25

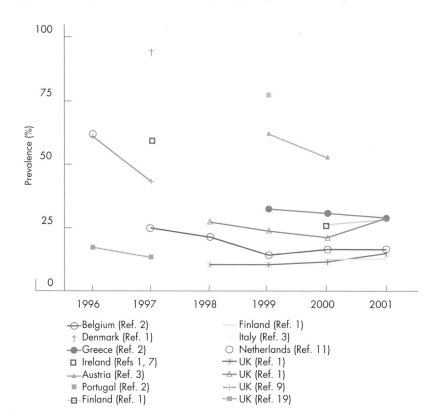

Note: See Annex 2, Table A2 for references.
Comparisons between countries should be done with caution, as data are from different study settings and study methods. Only longest samples and/or trends data per country are shown.

suggesting some decreases in several countries, but sample sizes are in general too small for trends to become statistically significant. However, in the UK, opposing statistically significant (p < 0.01) trends are observed between different regions and time-frames; in the Greater Glasgow area, a major decrease from 61 % in 1996 to 43 % in 1997 was observed; in more recent years this decline has halted (Hutchinson et al., 2002) (data from public health laboratories, more recent data not reported), while, since 1998, a small but steady increase in HCV prevalence is visible among large samples of young IDUs in England and Wales outside London (from 10.1 % in 1998 to 14.2 % in 2001, data from unlinked anonymous surveys). (For full detail, see Annex 2, Table A2.)

Table 2: Summary description of data on HCV prevalence in young and new IDUs (*) by country, 1996–2002

	Total EU-14	Austria	Belgium	Denmark	Finland
Young IDUs (age < 25 years)					
Number of prevalence estimates ([1])	67	11	6	2	9
Number of estimates within time series ([1])	51	11	5	0	7
Total sample size	11 314	219	274	29	748
% data from drug treatment ([2])	20–81	50	98–100	0–100	0
Unweighted median HCV young IDUs (%)	30.8	53	18.9	82.5	25.8
Unweighted quartiles HCV young IDUs (%)	16.4–61.8	44.4–67	16.3–24.6	75–90	13.3–29.3
New IDUs (injecting history < 2 years)					
Number of prevalence estimates ([1])	25	6	3	0	0
Number of estimates within time series ([1])	18	6	3	0	0
Total sample size	1 613	94	142	0	0
% data from drug treatment ([2])	65–83	100	100	0	0
Unweighted median HCV new IDUs (%)	47.6	42.0	45.7	—	—
Unweighted quartiles HCV new IDUs (%)	35.8–55.6	33.3–47.6	37.5–53.1	—	—

Country	France	Germany	Greece	Ireland	Italy
Young IDUs (age < 25 years)					
Number of prevalence estimates ([1])	0	0	10	1	1
Number of estimates within time series ([1])	0	0	7	0	0
Total sample size	0	0	1 471	535	644
% data from drug treatment ([2])	0	0	40–61	100	100
Unweighted median HCV young IDUs (%)	—	—	32.2	59.3	60.2
Unweighted quartiles HCV young IDUs (%)	—	—	30.6–39	—	—

Table 2 (continued)

Country	France	Germany	Greece	Ireland	Italy
New IDUs (injecting history < 2 years)					
Number of prevalence estimates (¹)	0	0	1	1	1
Number of estimates within time series (¹)	0	0	0	0	0
Total sample size	0	0	115	499	178
% data from drug treatment (²)	0	0	0–100	100	100
Unweighted median HCV new IDUs (%)	—	—	24.3	53.1	44.4
Unweighted quartiles HCV new IDUs (%)	—	—	—	—	—

Country	Luxem-bourg	Nether-lands	Portugal	Spain	UK
Young IDUs (age < 25 years)					
Number of prevalence estimates (¹)	0	1	8	0	18
Number of estimates within time series (¹)	0	0	5	0	16
Total sample size	0	21	170	0	7 203
% data from drug treatment (²)	0	0–100	100	0	0–90
Unweighted median HCV young IDUs (%)	—	61.8	71.2	—	14.6
Unweighted quartiles HCV young IDUs (%)	—	—	62.7–84.3	—	11.1–24.2
New IDUs (injecting history < 2 years)					
Number of prevalence estimates (¹)	0	0	3	7	3
Number of estimates within time series (¹)	0	0	2	7	0
Total sample size	0	0	133	158	294
% data from drug treatment (²)	0	0	100	0	0–59
Unweighted median HCV new IDUs (%)	—	—	65.1	55.6	14.3
Unweighted quartiles HCV new IDUs (%)	—	—	60.7–100	50–68.8	1.9–35.8

(*) Data from Italy (EMCDDA, 2003) are estimated to contain 5–10 % non-IDUs; data from Portugal, where IDU status is not known, are reported to relate mainly to IDUs. The proportion non-IDUs included may, however, change by geographic region and over time and reduce comparability of data.
(¹) Excluding national aggregates of regional data to prevent double counting (Italy, Portugal, UK).
(²) Weighted by sample size. Where a range is given, the lower value is the percentage of data exclusively from treatment, and the higher value is the percentage when including mixed sources that contain treatment data.

Prevalence in new injectors

Prevalence data for new injectors (injecting less than two years) are available from only a few sources and countries (Table 2 and Figure 5). Of 25 prevalence figures obtained, 9 are under 40 % and 12 are over 50 %. The lowest reported prevalence was 1.9 % among new injectors in England and Wales outside of London (CI 0.2–6.7 %) during 1998, suggesting very low transmission in that region. High prevalences are seen in new injectors in Dublin, Ireland (53.1 %), Coimbra, Portugal (60.7–65.1 %), and Glasgow, UK (35.8 %). Other data (from Austria, Belgium, Greece, Italy and Spain) suffer from small sample sizes but suggest that incidence may be high in those areas too. For new injectors, only four time series are available, none of them showing significant trends. (For full details, see Annex 2, Table A3.)

Potential confounding factors

Prevalence may be associated with the study type, specimen type or study setting (Table 3 and Figures 6 to 8); however, our aggregate-level data do not allow for strong inferences. The data from drug treatment, prisons or low-threshold services are on average associated with higher prevalence (unweighted medians 67.7,

Figure 5: HCV prevalence in IDUs injecting less than two years (error bars show 95 % confidence interval)

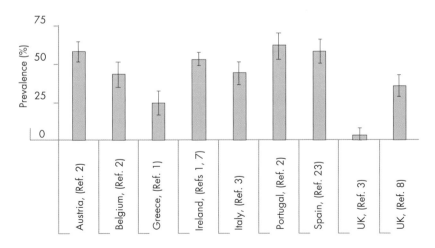

Note: See Annex 2, Table A3, for references.
Comparisons should be done with caution, as data are from different study settings and study methods.

63.1 and 61.0 % respectively) than data from other or mixed settings (unweighted median 49.6 %), but the variance per setting is also large and the interquartile intervals overlap strongly, indicating that the distributions are not statistically different. Because the study setting is highly associated with country (Figure 3), intercountry differences may reflect methodological rather than time variations. Similarly, prevalence may be associated with specimen type. Prevalence figures based on the testing of oral fluid samples are lower than those based on serum samples (47 % versus 68 %); this is likely, in part, to be due to the higher sensitivity of HCV antibody tests in saliva. Study type (data from diagnostic testing or special studies) also has an association with prevalence, with unweighted medians of 66.0 and 52.0 %, respectively, but again interquartile intervals overlap strongly and these study methods are correlated with country.

Table 3: Prevalence of HCV in IDUs by data type, specimen and setting

| | Study sites | Prevalence estimates | Total sample size | Unweighted | | | |
				Mean	Median	First quartile	Third quartile
Study type							
DT	72	178	341 591	64.5	66.0	52.1	76.3
SP	24	34	19 186	52.4	52.0	37.0	68.5
DT/SP	2	4	1 409	58.0	56.0	42.0	74.0
Unknown	13	17	9 421	81.9	85.2	76.0	92.0
Specimen type							
Serum	74	181	347 418	64.2	67.1	51.7	76.3
Saliva	16	25	17 244	46.4	45.8	31.9	55.9
Unknown	21	27	6 945	78.2	82.0	65.8	90.3
Setting							
Treatment	67	161	337 469	66.8	67.7	58.1	77.7
Low-threshold/NSP	9	24	2 911	59.3	58.5	43.1	80.5
Prison	14	15	9 300	61.0	63.1	52.0	77.0
Other/mixed	21	33	21 927	54.7	49.6	41.2	70.4

Abbreviations: DT = diagnostic testing, SP = special study, NSP= needle and syringe programme.

Figure 6: Prevalence of HCV among injecting drug users in the EU by study setting

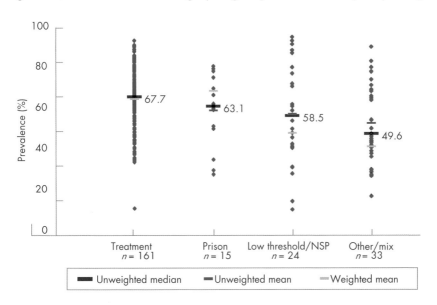

Note: Study setting is correlated with country and other study methods; therefore, this comparison reflects to an unknown extent geographic differences in prevalence or differences related to the other methodological aspects.

Figure 7: Prevalence of HCV among injecting drug users in the EU by specimen type

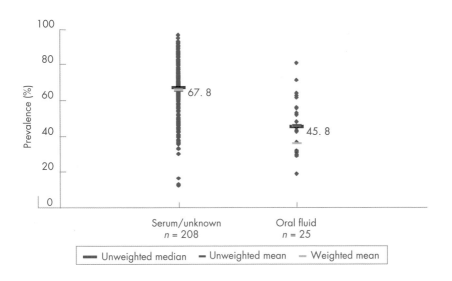

Note: Specimen type used is correlated with country and other study methods; therefore, this comparison reflects to an unknown extent geographic differences in prevalence or differences related to the other methodological aspects.

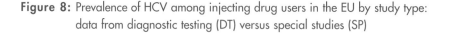

Figure 8: Prevalence of HCV among injecting drug users in the EU by study type: data from diagnostic testing (DT) versus special studies (SP)

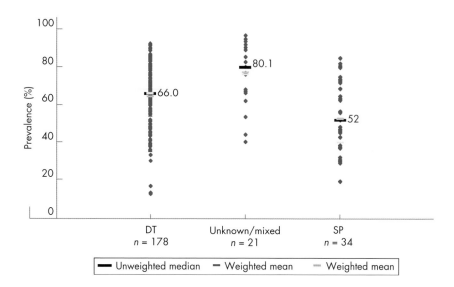

Note: Study type is correlated with country and other study methods; therefore, this comparison reflects to an unknown extent geographic differences in prevalence or differences related to the other methodological aspects.

Discussion

We are routinely collecting data on HCV prevalence in IDUs in the EU from a range of settings. Available data are mainly sourced through the diagnostic testing of IDUs in drug treatment; other settings remain to be further exploited. Data quality, consistency and coverage can still be much improved, and this is one of the aims of the recently established EMCDDA Study Group on Drug-related Infectious Diseases (EMCDDA, 2002).

Despite their limitations, the results suggest that HCV prevalence in IDUs tested during the period 1996–2002 in the EU continued to be extremely high, with an overall unweighted median of 65.8 %. However, a large variation is observed both within and between countries. Prevalence figures may be confounded by study setting, specimen type and whether or not data are from routine diagnostic testing, and these data should therefore be interpreted with caution. On the other hand, in some regions, lower prevalence is consistently found over time, or between different samples and study methods, therefore possibly reflecting real geographic differences in prevalence. Where a region's prevalence figures are generated through the same methods, any such difference or similarity in prevalence could be related to the average length of injecting history of IDU populations, other demographic factors, differing levels of injecting risk behaviour (which, in turn, can be related to changing patterns of drug use such as increased cocaine injecting (Tyndall et al., 2003)) and 'mixing patterns' (see Chapter 5) between subgroups of IDUs.

Important evidence of continuing high HCV transmission is provided by the high prevalence among young and new injectors (unweighted medians 30.8 and 47.6 %, respectively, data from different sample selections). New injectors are defined as having less than two years of injecting experience. For young injectors, the career duration is not defined, but if the average age of initiation of IDU is around 18 to 19 years (Doherty et al., 2000; Roy, E. et al., 2002), then the average duration of injecting in a typical sample of IDUs aged under 25 would be just over three years ((25 − 18.5)/2). Large variation in incidence has been found in local cohort studies, ranging from 4.2 per 100 person-years of injecting in Switzerland (Broers et al., 1998), 10.0 in Chicago, US (Thorpe et al., 2002), 10.7 in Victoria, Australia (Crofts and Aitken, 1997), 13 in New Zealand (Brunton et al., 2000), 16.7 in Seattle, US (Hagan et al., 2001), 20.9 in Sydney, Australia (van Beek et al., 1998), 26.3 in Malmö, Sweden (Mansson et al., 2000), 28.4 (CI 15.7–51.2) in Glasgow, Scotland (Roy et al., 2001), 29.1 (CI 22.3–37.3) in Vancouver, Canada (Patrick et al., 2001) and up to 75.6 per 100 person-years in IDUs under age 20 in Sydney (van Beek et al., 1998).

Observed trends, as opposed to single-point/period prevalence data, may provide evidence to gauge intra- and interregional performance apropos interventions to prevent HCV among IDUs. Our data suggest appreciable changes in prevalence among tested IDUs in about half of the time series available. In all, 21 of the 52 time series (40 %) show a statistically significant downward trend and 7 (13 %) an upward trend, suggesting that, at present, decreases in HCV prevalence and incidence among tested IDUs may be more widespread than increases (see Annex 2). In some instances, however, these findings might partly reflect changes in testing practice (Desenclos, 2003). For example, in some cases (e.g. in Greece and Portugal), the changes in reported prevalence are so abrupt that they seem implausible. To aid data interpretation, more complete data about changes in testing practice need to be sought from participating countries.

Whether some of the declines in prevalence or the lower prevalence figures could be the effect of interventions remains unclear. As mentioned earlier, observed decreases since the early 1990s have been attributed to the introduction of harm reduction measures in Scotland (Taylor et al., 2000; Goldberg et al., 2001), but in Spain, where HIV prevention measures for IDUs were widely implemented during the 1990s (Pesesud, 1998; Rinken and Romero Vallecillos, 2002), HCV prevalence has not declined (Hernandez-Aguado et al., 2001).

The strong north–south gradient observed in HIV prevalence and AIDS incidence in western Europe (Hamers et al., 1997; EMCDDA, 2003) is not seen for HCV. HCV is many times more infectious than HIV (Weusten et al., 2002) and levels of risk behaviour in IDUs, particularly those in the late 1980s and 1990s (Hunter et al., 1995), may have been sufficient for HCV, but not for HIV, to establish a high prevalence generally. For example, in Barcelona, a strong decrease has been recorded in needle sharing, but residual risk behaviour such as front- and backloading (sharing drugs with a common syringe), which in some studies is still reported by 80 % of respondents, might be sufficient to support ongoing HCV transmission (Ceescat, 2001).

Despite the opportunities provided by these data for large-scale monitoring of HCV spread in IDUs, they are subject to important limitations. These include differences in study method, including recruitment setting, sample size, eligibility for inclusion, biological specimen used, and, in some cases, unclear case definitions; the data were not originally collected using an agreed standard protocol. On a European scale, this has not been feasible until now, and promoting the establishment of comparable pan-European sentinel studies is an important additional objective to the aggregate data collection described here (EMCDDA, 2002).

With regard to the study setting, prevalence data estimated from drug treatment centres, prisons and low threshold services are higher than those from other or mixed settings (public health laboratories, STD clinics, community-recruited studies and combinations). While this suggests that study setting may have an influence on prevalence, the aggregate nature of the data does not allow for strong inferences. Furthermore, even apparently similar settings such as prisons or drug treatment centres are not necessarily comparable across countries, since they are organised in different ways and can lead to different selections of IDUs. For example, in some countries with limited drug treatment capacity (Greece, Portugal), the selective referral of IDUs with health problems, such as HIV infection, potentially causing important upward bias. Also, from some treatment centres, a lack of testing criteria is reported and decisions for testing seem not to be based on a systematic approach (Raes, 2002). Nevertheless, different settings may lead to an overestimate or underestimate of the actual prevalence in the IDU population of the same geographic area or country (Haw et al., 1992; Lampinen et al., 1992). These data should therefore be treated with some circumspection.

Apart from study setting, the type of biological specimen used can have a significant effect on prevalence. Several studies that reported lower HCV prevalence figures (e.g. in the UK and Finland) are based on antibody tests using oral fluid. These underestimate HCV antibody seroprevalence due to their lower sensitivity (around 80–85 %: in Ireland, a 95 % CI of test sensitivity is reported of 70.2–87.7, see Annex 2), thereby reducing comparability with serum-based studies. Accordingly, this warns that comparisons between the results from studies using oral fluid and serum samples should be undertaken with care, for example by specifying the type of specimen or calculating a prevalence adjusted for test sensitivity. This problem may diminish in the future, as higher test sensitivities, of 92 to 96 %, have recently been reported from the UK (EMCDDA, 2002; Judd et al., 2003b). It remains important that oral fluid HCV antibody tests are always well validated (Bello et al., 1998; Elsana et al., 2001; van Doornum et al., 2001; EMCDDA, 2002; Judd et al., 2003b).

In conclusion, recent data on HCV prevalence in IDUs from a variety of sources are available from most EU Member States. Despite methodological limitations, these data show continued high prevalence of HCV infection among IDUs in the EU over the period 1996–2002, as well as region-specific trends over time. High HCV prevalence figures in young and new IDUs provides evidence of high recent transmission. These data may constitute a simple and cost-effective indicator of incidence, as infections among young and new IDUs will, on average, have occurred more recently and therefore better reflect recent changes in transmission. Since HCV prevalence in IDUs reflects injecting risk behaviour, its relevance extends beyond HCV to other blood-borne diseases such as HIV and HBV. Ongoing efforts are in place to improve the quality, comparability and availability of the data.

References

Bello, P. Y., Pasquier, C., Gourney, P., Puel, J., Izopet, J. (1998), 'Assessment of a hepatitis C virus antibody assay in saliva for epidemiological studies', *European Journal of Clinical Microbiology and Infectious Diseases* 17: 570–2.

Broers, B., Junet, C., Bourquin, M., Deglon, J. J., Perrin, L., Hirschel, B. (1998), 'Prevalence and incidence rate of HIV, hepatitis B and C among drug users on methadone maintenance treatment in Geneva between 1988 and 1995', *AIDS* 12: 2059–66.

Brunton, C., Kemp, R., Raynel, P., Harte, D., Baker, M. (2000), 'Cumulative incidence of hepatitis C seroconversion in a cohort of seronegative injecting drug users', New Zealand Medical Journal 113: 98–101.

Centre d'Estudis Epidemiològics sobre la Sida de Catalunya (Ceescat) (Spain) (2001), 'Sistema integrat de vigilància epidemiològica de l'HIV/sida a Catalunya (SIVES): informe anual 2000. [13]', Generalitat de Catalunya, Departament de Sanitat i Seguretat Social, Document Tècnic Ceescat, Barcelona.

Crofts, N., Aitken, C. K. (1997), 'Incidence of bloodborne virus infection and risk behaviours in a cohort of injecting drug users in Victoria, 1990–1995', Medical Journal of Australia 167: 17–20.

Crofts, N., Thompson, S., Kaldor, J. (1999), Epidemiology of the hepatitis C virus, Communicable Diseases Network Australia and New Zealand, Technical Report Series No 3, Commonwealth Department of Health and Aged Care, Canberra.

de la Fuente, L., Barrio, G., Royuela, L., Bravo, M. J. (1997), 'The transition from injecting to smoking heroin in three Spanish cities', The Spanish group for the study of the route of heroin administration, Addiction 92: 1749–63.

Desenclos, J. C. (2003), 'The challenge of hepatitis C surveillance in Europe', Eurosurveillance 8: 99–100.

Doherty, M. C., Garfein. R. S., Monterroso, E., Latkin, C., Vlahov, D. (2000), 'Gender differences in the initiation of injection drug use among young adults', Journal of Urban Health 77: 396–414.

Edlin, B. R., Seal, K. H., Lorvick, J., Kral, A. H., Ciccarone, D. H., Moore, L. D., Lo, B. (2001), 'Is it justifiable to withhold treatment for hepatitis C from illicit drug users?', New England Journal of Medicine 345: 211–5.

Elsana, S., Sikuler, E., Yaari, A., Shemer-Avni, Y., Margalith, M. (2001), 'Salivary HCV-antibodies: a follow-up cohort study of liver disease patients', Clinical Laboratory 47: 335–8.

European Monitoring Centre for Drugs and Drug Addiction (EMCDDA) (2002), Expert meeting: 'Surveillance of drug-related infectious diseases in the European Union: routine data and seroprevalence studies', Lisbon, 29 November to 1 December 2001, Final meeting report, EMCDDA (http://www.emcdda.eu.int/situation/themes/infectious_diseases.shtml).

European Monitoring Centre for Drugs and Drug Addiction (EMCDDA) (2003), Annual report on the state of the drugs problem in the European Union, EMCDDA, Lisbon (http://annualreport.emcdda.eu.int/).

Eurosurveillance Monthly (2003), 'Hepatitis C', Eurosurveillance 8: 99–118 (http://www.eurosurveillance.org/index-02.asp).

Fisker, N., Christensen, P. B. (2001), 'Vacunación frente a hepatitis B en usuarios de drogas inyectadas en prisiones y centros de tratamiento de drogadicción: pauta corta versus standard', Revista Española de Sanidad Penitenciaria 3(1): 42–51.

Freeman, A. J., Dore, G. J., Law, M. G., Thorpe, M., von Overbeck, J., Lloyd, A. R., Marinos, G., Kaldor, J. M. (2001), 'Estimating progression to cirrhosis in chronic hepatitis C virus infection', Hepatology 34: 809–16.

Garfein, R. S., Vlahov, D., Galai, N., Doherty, M. C., Nelson, K. E. (1996), 'Viral infections in short-term injection drug users: the prevalence of the hepatitis C, hepatitis B, human immunodeficiency, and human T-lymphotropic viruses', American Journal of Public Health 86: 655–61.

Goldberg, D., Burns, S., Taylor, A., Cameron, S., Hargreaves, D., Hutchinson, S. (2001), 'Trends in HCV prevalence among injecting drug users in Glasgow and Edinburgh during the era of needle/syringe exchange', Scandinavian Journal of Infectious Diseases 33: 457–61.

Hagan, H., Thiede, H., Weiss, N. S., Hopkins, S. G., Duchin, J. S., Alexander, E. R. (2001), 'Sharing of drug preparation equipment as a risk factor for hepatitis C', *American Journal of Public Health* 91: 42–6.

Hamers, F. F., Batter, V., Downs, A. M., Alix, J., Cazein, F., Brunet, J. B. (1997), 'The HIV epidemic associated with injecting drug use in Europe: geographic and time trends', *AIDS* 11: 1365–74.

Haw, S., Frischer, M., Donoghoe, M., Green, S., Crosier, A., Hunter, G., Finlay, A., Covell, R., Ettmore, B., Bloor, M. et al. (1992), 'The importance of multisite sampling in determining the prevalence of HIV among drug injectors in Glasgow and London', *AIDS* 6: 517–8.

Hernandez-Aguado, I., Ramos-Rincon, J. M., Avinio, M. J., Gonzalez-Aracil, J., Perez-Hoyos, S., de la Hera, M. G. (2001), 'Measures to reduce HIV infection have not been successful to reduce the prevalence of HCV in intravenous drug users', *European Journal of Epidemiology* 17: 539–44.

Hope, V. D., Judd, A., Hickman, M., Lamagni, T., Hunter, G., Stimson, G. V., Jones, S., Donovan, L., Parry, J. V., Gill, O. N. (2001), 'Prevalence of hepatitis C virus in current injecting drug users in England and Wales: is harm reduction working?', *American Journal of Public Health* 91: 38–42.

Hunter, G. M., Donoghoe, M. C., Stimson, G. V., Rhodes, T., Chalmers, C. P. (1995), 'Changes in the injecting risk behaviour of injecting drug users in London, 1990–1993', *AIDS* 9: 493–501.

Hutchinson, S. J., McIntyre, P. G., Molyneaux, P., Cameron, S., Burns, S., Taylor, A., Goldberg, D. J. (2002), 'Prevalence of hepatitis C among injectors in Scotland 1989–2000: declining trends among young injectors halt in the late 1990s', *Epidemiology of Infection* 128: 473–7.

Judd, A., Hickman, M., Jones, S., Parry, J. V. (2003a), 'Prevalence and incidence of hepatitis C and HIV among injecting drug users in London — evidence for increasing transmission', 14th International Conference on the Reduction of Drug-related Harm, Chaing Mai, 2003.

Judd, A., Parry, J. V., Hickman, M. et al. (2003b), 'Evaluation of a modified commercial assay in detecting antibody to hepatitis C virus in oral fluids and dried blood spots', *Journal of Medical Virology* 71: 49–55.

Kraus, L., Augustin, R., Frischer, M., Kümmler, P., Uhl, A., Wiessing, L. (2003), 'Estimating prevalence of problem drug use at national level in countries of the European Union and Norway', *Addiction* 98: 471–85.

Lampinen, T. M., Joo, E., Seweryn, S., Hershow, R. C., Wiebel, W. (1992), 'HIV seropositivity in community-recruited and drug treatment samples of injecting drug users', *AIDS* 6: 123–6.

Mansson, A. S., Moestrup, T., Nordenfelt, E., Widell, A. (2000), 'Continued transmission of hepatitis B and C viruses, but no transmission of human immunodeficiency virus among intravenous drug users participating in a syringe/needle exchange program', *Scandinavian Journal of Infectious Diseases* 32: 253–8.

Matheï, C., Buntinx, F., van Damme, P. (2002), 'Seroprevalence of hepatitis C markers among intravenous drug users in western European countries: a systematic review', *Journal of Viral Hepatitis* 9: 157–73.

Nalpas, B., Desenclos, J. C., Delarocque-Astagneau, E., Drucker, J. (1998), 'State of epidemiological knowledge and national management of hepatitis C virus infection in the European Community, 1996', *European Journal of Public Health* 8: 305–12.

Parsons, J., Hickman, M., Turnbull, P. J., McSweeney, T., Stimson, G. V., Judd, A., Roberts, K. (2002), 'Over a decade of syringe exchange: results from 1997 UK survey', *Addiction* 97: 845–50.

Patrick, D. M., Tyndall, M. W., Cornelisse, P. G., Li, K., Sherlock, C. H., Rekart, M. L., Strathdee, S. A., Currie, S. L., Schechter, M. T., O'Shaughnessy, M. V. (2001), 'Incidence of hepatitis C virus infection among injection drug users during an outbreak of HIV infection', *Canadian Medical Association Journal* 165: 889–95.

Postma, M. J., Wiessing, L. G., Jager, J. C. (2001), 'Pharmaco-economics of drug addiction: estimating the costs of hepatitis C virus, hepatitis B virus and human immunodeficiency virus infection among injecting drug users in Member States of the European Union', UN Bulletin of Narcotics 53 (1, 2): 79–89.

Programas Échange Seringues Europa Sud (Pesesud) (1998), Syringe exchange programmes for HIV prevention in southern European countries, Final report to the European Commission, Ceescat, Barcelona.

Raes, V. (2002), Written communication of 12 December 2002 from the head of scientific research and quality, Drug Service De Sleutel, Merelbeke, Belgium.

Rinken, S., Romero Vallecillos, M. (2002), 'The evolution of Spanish HIV prevention policy targeted at opiate users: a review', Drugs Education, Prevention and Policy 9: 45–56.

Roy, K. M., Goldberg, D., Taylor, A., Hutchinson, S. J., MacDonald, L., Wilson, K. S., Cameron, S. O. (2001), 'A method to detect the incidence of hepatitis C infection among injecting drug users in Glasgow 1993–98', Journal of Infection 43: 200–5.

Roy, K. M., Hay, G., Andragetti, R., Taylor, A., Goldberg, D., Wiessing, L. (2002), 'Monitoring hepatitis C virus infection among injecting drug users in the European Union: a review of the literature', Epidemiology and Infection 129: 577–85.

Roy, E., Haley, N., Leclerc, P., Cedras, L., Boivin, J. F. (2002), 'Drug injection among street youth: the first time', Addiction 97: 1003–9.

Schlicting, E. G., Johnson, M. E., Brems, C., Wells, R. S., Fisher, D. G., Reynolds, G. (2003), 'Validity of injecting drug users' self report of hepatitis A, B, and C', Clinical Laboratory Science 16: 99–106.

Taylor, A., Goldberg, D., Hutchinson, S., Cameron, S., Gore, S. M., McMenamin, J., Green, S., Pithie, A., Fox, R. (2000), 'Prevalence of hepatitis C among injecting drug users in Glasgow 1990–1996: are current harm reduction policies working?', Journal of Infection 40: 176–83.

Thornton, L., Barry, J., Long, J., Allwright, S., Bradley, F., Parry, J. V. (2000), 'Comparison between self-reported hepatitis B, hepatitis C, and HIV antibody status and oral fluid assay results in Irish prisoners', Community Disease and Public Health 3: 253–5.

Thorpe, L. E., Ouellet, L. J., Hershow, R., Bailey, S. L., Williams, I. T., Williamson, J., Monterroso, E. R., Garfein, R. S. (2002), 'Risk of hepatitis C virus infection among young adult injection drug users who share injection equipment', American Journal of Epidemiology 155: 645–53.

Tyndall, M. W., Currie, S., Spittal, P., Li, K., Wood, E., O'Shaughnessy, M. V., Schechter, M. T. (2003), 'Intensive injection cocaine use as the primary risk factor in the Vancouver HIV-1 epidemic', AIDS 17: 887–93.

van Beek, I., Dwyer, R., Dore, G. J., Luo, K., Kaldor, J. M. (1998), 'Infection with HIV and hepatitis C virus among injecting drug users in a prevention setting: retrospective cohort study', British Medical Journal 317: 433–7.

van Doornum, G. J., Lodder, A., Buimer, M., van Ameijden, E. J., Bruisten, S. (2001), 'Evaluation of hepatitis C antibody testing in saliva specimens collected by two different systems in comparison with HCV antibody and HCV RNA in serum', Journal of Medical Virology 64: 13–20.

Welp, E. A., Lodder, A. C., Langendam, M. W., Coutinho, R. A., van Ameijden, E. J. (2002), 'HIV prevalence and risk behaviour in young drug users in Amsterdam', AIDS 16: 1279–84.

Weusten, J. J., van Drimmelen, H. A., Lelie, P. N. (2002), 'Mathematic modeling of the risk of HBV, HCV, and HIV transmission by window-phase donations not detected by NAT', *Transfusion* 42: 537–48.

Wiessing, L. (2001), 'The access of injecting drug users to hepatitis C treatment is low and should be improved', *Eurosurveillance Weekly* 5: 010802 (http://www.eurosurv.org/2001/010802.html).

Wiessing, L. G., Denis, B., Guttormsson, U. et al. (2001), 'Estimating coverage of harm reduction measures for injection drug users in the European Union', *Proceedings of 2000 global research network meeting on HIV prevention in drug using populations*, Third annual meeting, Durban, South Africa, 5 to 7 July 2000, National Institute on Drug Abuse, National Institutes of Health, US Department of Health and Human Services (available at http://www.emcdda.eu.int/?nnodeid=1375).

Annex 1: Study group participants and acknowledgements

EMCDDA Study Group on Drug-related Infectious Diseases (as at end of 2002)

(fp = focal point representative, ne = representative of national expert group):

Austria: Martin Busch fp, Sabina Haas fp, Franz Riedl ne. Belgium: Fabienne Hariga, Catharina Matheï, Veerle Raes, Francis Sartor, Sophie Quoilin, Denise Walckiers ne/fp. Denmark: Peer Christensen ne, Kari Grasaasen fp, Else Smith ne. Finland: Henrikki Brummer-Korvenkontio, Pekka Holmström ne, Pauli Leinikki, Airi Partanen fp. France: Pierre-Yves Bello ne/fp, Françoise Hamers. Germany: Osamah Hamouda ne, Roland Simon fp, Hedwig Spegel fp, Klaus Stark ne, Caren Weilandt ne. Greece: Manina Terzidou ne/fp, Katerina Kontogeorgiou fp, Maria Spiropoulou fp. Ireland: Lucy Dillon fp, Jean Long fp, Hamish Sinclair ne/fp. Italy: Carla Rossi, Giuseppe Salamina ne, Giuseppe Schinaia, Silvia Zanone fp. Luxembourg: Henri Goedertz, Alain Origer ne/fp. The Netherlands: Erik van Ameijden, Roelien Beuker ne, Eline Op de Coul ne, Margriet van Laar fp, Marita van de Laar, Gerrit van Santen, Esther Welp. Portugal: Manuel Cardoso, António Maia ne, Paula Marques, Maria Moreira fp, Teresa Paixão, Jorge Ribeiro ne Rui Susano. Spain: Francisco Javier Alvarez, Gregorio Barrio fp, Ferrán Bolao, Jordi Casabona, Luis de la Fuente, Esther García Usieto, Robert Muga, Catherine Pérez, Juan Carlos Valderrama ne. Sweden: Kajsa Mickelsson fp, Linnea Rask fp, Daniel Svensson, Staffan Sylvan ne. United Kingdom: Roberta Andraghetti, Sheila Cameron, Leah De Souza, Noël Gill, David Goldberg, Gordon Hay, Vivian Hope, Ali Judd ne, Fortune Ncube, Kirsty Roy, Avril Taylor. EMCDDA: Norbert Frost, Richard Hartnoll, Dagmar Hedrich, Paul Griffiths, Linda Montanari, David Sapinho, Colin Taylor, Lucas Wiessing.

Acknowledgements:

The authors wish to thank the EMCDDA national expert representatives, national expert groups and national focal points, and especially the staff of the reporting agencies for their ongoing efforts to collect and improve the data reported in this article. Dr Nick Crofts and Prof. Roel Coutinho provided important comments on an early version of this text. Participants from EU acceding countries are participating in the study group from 2003 onwards. We thank Barbara Broers (Switzerland), Olga Gridassova (Russia), Margaret MacDonald (†) (Australia), Eszter Ujhelyi (Hungary) and Tomas Zabransky (Czech Republic) for their contribution to this work.

Annex 2

In the tables in Annex 2, countries appear in alphabetical order according to their respective languages. This order is: Belgium, Denmark, Germany, Greece, Spain, France, Ireland, Italy, Luxembourg, the Netherlands, Austria, Portugal, Finland, Sweden and the UK.

(†) Deceased.

Table A1: Prevalence of hepatitis C infection (%) among injecting drug users in the EU (sample sizes in parentheses)

HCV — total Country, region/city	1996	1997	1998	1999	2000	2001	2002	P trend (1)	DT/SP (2)	Setting/comments	Ref. (3)
Belgium, Flemish Community		39.5 (114)	46.4 (56)	37.9 (195)	36.0 (164)	35.8 (120)		0.3079	DT	Drug treatment centres; screening serum	2
Belgium, Flemish Community — Antwerp						79.8 [252]			SP	Drug treatment centres, low-threshold services; screening serum	8
Denmark, Funen		85 (338)							SP	Prison, drug treatment centres; screening serum	1
Denmark, Copenhagen		75 (264)							SP	Drug treatment centres; screening serum	2
Germany, Frankfurt	88.9 (90)	95.0 (60)	96.8 (63)	(75)	93.3 (72)	90.3		0.8797	n.a.	Low-threshold services	2
Germany, Munich		61.9 (181)	67.3 (171)	65.7 (140)				0.4391	DT	Inpatient treatment	4
Germany, Lohr	65.8 (120)								DT	Inpatient treatment; data 1995–97	5
Germany, Hamburg		86.0 (171)							DT	Inpatient treatment	6
Germany, Hamburg		77 (6 202)							n.a.	Prisons; screening serum	18
Germany, Berlin					82.5 (154)				n.a.	Syringe exchange in two prisons; data 1998–2001	7
Greece, Northern region		80.5 (297)		81.6 (174)	82.9 (41)			0.6674	DT	Methadone, drug treatment centres; screening serum; data 1997 is 1996–98	5
Greece, Athens			49.6 (409)	41.2 (393)	42.8 (650)			0.0454	DT	Public health laboratories; screening serum	6

Table A1 (continued)

HCV — total Country, region/city	1996	1997	1998	1999	2000	2001	2002	P trend (1)	DT/SP (2)	Setting/comments	Ref. (3)
Greece, National			61.3 (253)	63.1 (130)				0.7295	DT	Prisons; screening serum	10
Greece, National				51.7 (286)	40.1 (439)	37.9 (398)		0.0005	DT	Drug treatment centres; screening serum	2
Greece, Athens		68.0 (693)							DT	Methadone treatment; screening serum; data 1996–98	7
Greece, Athens				56.2 (317)	46.3 (281)			0.0157	DT	STD clinics; screening serum	8
Greece, National					52 (131)	80.9 (131)		0.0001	DT	Drug treatment centres; screening serum	9
Greece, National						67.9 (1 094)			DT	Drug treatment centres, low-threshold services, public health laboratories, STD clinics; screening serum	1
Greece, Thessaloniki	68.5 (54)								SP	Prison; screening serum	14
Spain, National, excluding Galicia	83.2 (993)								DT	Survey of drug treatment centres	3
Spain, Fuenlabrada y Leganés (Madrid)		49.3 (233)							DT	Drug treatment centres, first and tertiary care centres	8
Spain, El Prat de Llobregat (Barcelona)	71.1 (355)								DT	Drug treatment, hospital; screening serum; data 1995–96	15
Spain, Seville		92.0 (789)							n.a.	Drug treatment centres	20

HCV — total Country, region/city	1996	1997	1998	1999	2000	2001	2002	P trend (1)	DT/SP (2)	Setting/comments	Ref. (3)
Spain, Barcelona				66.0 (227)					n.a.	Two hospitals; screening serum; data 1996–2002; IDUs who started injecting after 1994	23
France, Grasse, Argentan	80.1 (241)	53.2 (98)							n.a.	Marseille 1996–97: three prisons; screening saliva	5
France, Lille	52.5 (118)	62.1 (116)							n.a.	Prison; data 1995 and 1996	6
Ireland, Dublin								0.1288	SP	Drug treatment centre Trinity Court, first attendees 1992–97; ever-IDUs; screening serum	1, 7
Ireland, National			81.3 (509)						SP	Prison inmates; screening saliva (test sensitivity 80 %, 95 % CI 70.2–87.7)	4
Ireland, National				71.7 (173)					SP	Prison entrants; screening saliva (test sensitivity 80 %, 95 % CI 70.2–87.7)	2
Ireland, Eastern Regional Health Authority				72.6 (372)					DT	Survey GPs: methadone clients, laboratory reports or clinical notes; 13.6 % (78/571) non-IDUs, 35 % (199/571) missing HCV status	5
Ireland, Dublin		78.8 (99)							DT	Five drug treatment centres: methadone clients, laboratory reports or clinical notes; serum; may include non-IDUs	6
Italy, National	67.1 (65 911)		67.6 (72 336)	67.0 (73 512)	67.4 (74 771)	66.3 (79 096)		0.0005	DT	Drug treatment centres; screening serum; 5–10 % non-IDUs	1
Italy, Calabria, Campania, Emilia-Romagna, Friuli, Lazio, Liguria, Marche, Piedmont, Trento, Apulia, Sardinia, Sicily, Tuscany				78.6 (5 436)					DT	Drug treatment centres; study in 13 regions; data are for 1998–2000; screening serum	3

Table A1 (continued)

HCV – total Country, region/city	1996	1997	1998	1999	2000	2001	2002	P trend (¹)	DT/SP (²)	Setting/comments	Ref. (³)
Italy, Piedmont			68.8 (7 402)	67.7 (7 050)	76.3 (6 949)	76.3 (5 998)		0.0001	DT	Drug treatment centres; screening serum; 5–10 % non-IDUs	1
Italy, Piedmont				85.2 (1 402)					DT	Drug treatment centres; study in 13 regions; data are for 1998–2000; screening serum	3
Italy, Valle d'Aosta			86.9 (176)	43.0 (142)	13.2 (68)	36.7 (60)		0.0001	DT	Drug treatment centres; screening serum; 5–10 % non-IDUs	1
Italy, Lombardy			71.3 (15 064)	70.6 (15 401)	71.0 (14 965)	70.9 (15 331)		0.6317	DT	Drug treatment centres; screening serum; 5–10 % non-IDUs	1
Italy, Trentino			82.9 (742)	87.2 (782)	89.7 (1 005)	85.7 (677)		0.0288	DT	Drug treatment centres; screening serum; 5–10 % non-IDUs	1
Italy, Trento				85.2 (508)	86.7 (525)	84.3 (529)		0.6642	DT	Drug treatment centres; screening serum; 5–10 % non-IDUs	1
Italy, Bolzano				90.9 (274)	92.9 (480)	90.5 (148)		0.8836	DT	Drug treatment centres; screening serum; 5–10 % non-IDUs	1
Italy, Veneto			69.5 (4 797)	72.5 (5 355)	64.3 (3 915)	68.6 (4 465)		0.0004	DT	Drug treatment centres; screening serum; 5–10 % non-IDUs	1
Italy, Friuli			79.9 (1 295)	77.8 (1 295)	77.5 (1 403)	75.9 (1 474)		0.0137	DT	Drug treatment centres; screening serum; 5–10 % non-IDUs	1
Italy, Friuli				82.4 (170)					DT	Drug treatment centres; study in 13 regions; data are for 1998–2000; screening serum	3
Italy, Liguria			77.4 (1 586)	84.9 (1 664)	77.7 (1 696)	67.1 (3 422)		0.0001	DT	Drug treatment centres; screening serum; 5–10 % non-IDUs	1
Italy, Liguria				67.9 (159)					DT	Drug treatment centres; study in 13 regions; data are for 1998–2000; screening serum	3

HCV – total Country, region/city	1996	1997	1998	1999	2000	2001	2002	P trend (1)	DT/SP (2)	Setting/comments	Ref. (3)
Italy, Emilia-Romagna			79.8 (4 968)	82.1 (5 333)	85.7 (5 159)	85.2 (5 261)		0.0001	DT	Drug treatment centres; screening serum; 5-10 % non-IDUs	1
Italy, Emilia-Romagna				90.5 (304)					DT	Drug treatment centres; study in 13 regions; data are for 1998–2000; screening serum	3
Italy, Tuscany			73.5 (4 600)	70.3 (4 802)	63.7 (5 544)	68.4 (5 019)		0.0001	DT	Drug treatment centres; screening serum; 5-10 % non-IDUs	1
Italy, Tuscany				64.0 (442)					DT	Drug treatment centres; study in 13 regions; data are for 1998–2000; screening serum	3
Italy, Umbria			75.8 (1 354)	64.0 (902)	62.4 (975)	52.1 (1 030)		0.0001	DT	Drug treatment centres; screening serum; 5-10 % non-IDUs	1
Italy, Marche			65.4 (1 821)	67.8 (1 871)	69.9 (2 197)	65.3 (1 508)		0.4748	DT	Drug treatment centres; screening serum; 5-10 % non-IDUs	1
Italy, Marche				74.4 (238)					DT	Drug treatment centres; study in 13 regions; data are for 1998–2000; screening serum	3
Italy, Lazio			65.2 (4 187)	65.0 (4 250)	65.5 (4 054)	65.4 (4 000)		0.7462	DT	Drug treatment centres; screening serum; 5-10 % non-IDUs	1
Italy, Lazio				80.7 (789)					DT	Drug treatment centres; study in 13 regions; data are for 1998–2000; screening serum	3
Italy, Abruzzi			54.0 (1 669)	50.6 (1 329)	50.5 (1 662)	48.4 (2 328)		0.0009	DT	Drug treatment centres; screening serum; 5-10 % non-IDUs	1
Italy, Molise			69.2 (295)	66.5 (319)	70.7 (266)	59.9 (207)		0.1205	DT	Drug treatment centres; screening serum; 5-10 % non-IDUs	1
Italy, Campania			50.3 (7 017)	42.3 (8 044)	46.3 (8 354)	46.1 (9 421)		0.0049	DT	Drug treatment centres; screening serum; 5-10 % non-IDUs	1
Italy, Campania				64.1 (357)					DT	Drug treatment centres; study in 13 regions; data are for 1998–2000; screening serum	3

Table A1 (continued)

HCV — total Country, region/city	1996	1997	1998	1999	2000	2001	2002	P trend (1)	DT/SP (2)	Setting/comments	Ref. (3)
Italy, Apulia			60.3 (7 939)	63.8 (6 494)	63.2 (7 202)	62.9 (6 741)		0.0020	DT	Drug treatment centres; screening serum; 5–10 % non-IDUs	1
Italy, Apulia				71.0 (131)					DT	Drug treatment centres; study in 13 regions; data are for 1998–2000; screening serum	3
Italy, Basilicata			66.0 (456)	67.4 (488)	77.6 (424)	64.5 (541)		0.7759	DT	Drug treatment centres; screening serum; 5–10 % non-IDUs	1
Italy, Calabria			58.6 (2 401)	61.2 (1 821)	56.1 (1 724)	54.6 (2 117)		0.0007	DT	Drug treatment centres; screening serum; 5–10 % non-IDUs	1
Italy, Calabria				61.4 (202)					DT	Drug treatment centres; study in 13 regions; data are for 1998–2000; screening serum	3
Italy, Sicily			65.0 (3 557)	60.9 (3 821)	63.9 (4 601)	61.9 (5 086)		0.0721	DT	Drug treatment centres; screening serum; 5–10 % non-IDUs	1
Italy, Sicily				74.9 (545)					DT	Drug treatment centres; study in 13 regions; data are for 1998–2000; screening serum	3
Italy, Sardinia			72.0 (2 539)	83.2 (2 349)	83.1 (2 608)	78.0 (2 543)		0.0001	DT	Drug treatment centres; screening serum; 5–10 % non-IDUs	1
Italy, Sardinia				86.6 (696)					DT	Drug treatment centres; study in 13 regions; data are for 1998–2000; screening serum	3
Italy, Brescia-Mombello, Monza, Milan-Opera				64.2 (165)					SP	Three prisons, screening saliva	7
Luxembourg, National			37.0 (116)						SP	Prison study; screening saliva	4

HCV — total Country, region/city	1996	1997	1998	1999	2000	2001	2002	P trend (1)	DT/SP (2)	Setting/comments	Ref. (3)
Netherlands, Limburg, Heerlen/Maastricht	73.3 (288)								SP	Drug treatment centres, needle exchanges, low-threshold services; screening serum	11
Netherlands, The Hague					47.2 (199)				SP	Drug treatment centres, needle exchanges, low-threshold services; screening serum	9
Austria, Vienna			79.0 (19)	64.0 (92)	61.0 (88)	47.7 (107)		0.0026	DT	Needle exchanges, low-threshold services; screening serum	3
Austria, Vienna, Lower Austria	85.0 (79)	73.0 (99)	74.0 (107)	72.0 (68)	71.0 (65)			0.0765	DT	Drug treatment centres; screening serum	4
Austria, Vorarlberg	56.8 (37)	40.7 (27)	58.3 (48)	69.0 (29)	48.0 (25)	67.6 (34)		0.6745	DT	Drug treatment centres; screening serum	2
Portugal, National				55.7 (n.a.)	48.8 (5 765)	44.7 (2 603)		0.0005	DT	Drug treatment centres; IDU status unknown, prevalence may be too low; screening serum	10
Portugal, National					68.6 (3 280)	57.5 (2 806)		0.0001	DT	Drug treatment centres, detoxification units; IDU status unknown, prevalence may be too low; screening serum	10
Portugal, National					48.8 (3 367)	50.9 (3 980)		0.0719	DT	Drug treatment centres, therapeutic communities; IDU status unknown, prevalence may be too low; screening serum	10
Portugal, Lisbon					77.29 (502)	48.7 (726)		0.0001	DT	Drug treatment centres; IDU status unknown, prevalence may be too low; screening serum	10
Portugal, Lisbon-Xabregas			70.0 (203)	72.8 (180)	45.3 (106)			0.0002	DT	Drug treatment centres; screening serum	1
Portugal, Lisbon-Xabregas				65.8 (407)					DT	Drug treatment centre; IDU status unknown, prevalence may be too low	18

Table A1 (continued)

HCV – total Country, region/city	1996	1997	1998	1999	2000	2001	2002	P trend (1)	DT/SP (2)	Setting/comments	Ref. (3)
Portugal, Lisbon-Taipas				65.9 (320)					DT	Drug treatment centre; IDU status unknown, prevalence may be too low	18
Portugal, Lisbon-Casal Ventoso				82 (194)					SP	Low-threshold services in high-problem area; IDU status unknown, prevalence may be too low	9, 20
Portugal, Lisbon-Casal Ventoso				74 (252)					SP	Low-threshold services in high-problem area, data 1998–99; IDU status unknown, prevalence may be too low; screening serum	4
Portugal, North					44.9 (775)	49.3 (817)		0.0772	DT	Drug treatment centres; IDU status unknown, prevalence may be too low; screening serum	10
Portugal, Oporto		87.6 (443)							DT	Drug treatment centres; screening serum	8
Portugal, Oporto				58.1 (415)					DT	Drug treatment centre; IDU status unknown, prevalence may be too low	18
Portugal, Oporto-Boavista		87.8 (443)							DT	Drug treatment centre; IDU status unknown, prevalence may be too low	21
Portugal, Central					37.0 (883)	37.5 (890)		0.8293	DT	Drug treatment centres; IDU status unknown, prevalence may be too low; screening serum	10
Portugal, Coimbra				70.4 (227)	82.0 (106)			0.0244	DT	Drug treatment centres, public health laboratory, pregnant IDUs; screening serum	2
Portugal, Santarém					92.4 (66)				DT	Drug treatment centres; screening serum	7
Portugal, Region n.a.				76 (448)					n.a.	Setting n.a.	9
Portugal, Algarve					46.8 (380)	41 (134)		0.2464	DT	Drug treatment centres; IDU status unknown, prevalence may be too low; screening serum	10

HCV – total Country, region/city	1996	1997	1998	1999	2000	2001	2002	P trend (1)	DT/SP (2)	Setting/comments	Ref. (3)
Portugal, Lisbon-Leiria-Oporto		61.9 (181)							n.a.	Three prisons, screening saliva	15
Portugal, Setúbal				92 (238)					n.a.	Setting n.a.	9
Portugal, Setúbal			95.1 (123)						n.a.	Drug treatment centre; IDU status unknown, prevalence may be too low	19
Portugal, Setúbal-Almada	85.2 (230)								n.a.	Drug treatment centre; data 1995–96	17
Finland, Helsinki			63 (135)			55.9 (59)	52.0 (199)	0.0437	SP	Needle exchanges, screening saliva	1, 6
Finland, Helsinki				72.7 (22)	33.5 (194)	33.2 (274)		0.0288	DT	Needle exchanges, screening serum	1
Finland, Vantaa					50 (20)	44.6 (92)	30.2 (149)	0.0119	DT	Needle exchanges, screening serum	1
Finland, Vantaa						43.4 (83)	42.7 (82)	0.9286	SP	Needle exchanges, screening saliva	1
Finland, Tampere					12.6 (261)	16.6 (229)		0.2152	DT	Needle exchanges, screening serum	1
Finland, National				38.4 (146)					SP	Overdose deaths, screening serum	1
Finland, National				52.0 (134)					SP	Prisons; screening saliva	1
UK, England and Wales, excluding London			30.9 (2 711)	29.0 (2 940)	29.7 (2 866)	32.2 (2 448)		0.2946	SP	Drug treatment centres, needle exchanges, low-threshold services, primary care and outreach; screening saliva	1

Table A1 (continued)

HCV — total Country, region/city	1996	1997	1998	1999	2000	2001	2002	P trend (1)	DT/SP (2)	Setting/comments	Ref. (3)
UK, England and Wales, excluding London			19.1 (514)						SP	Community surveys; current IDUs, screening saliva	3
UK, England and Wales			35.1 (3 366)	32.4 (3 731)	32.7 (3 425)	34.6 (2 963)		0.6909	SP	Drug treatment centres, needle exchanges, low-threshold services, primary care and outreach; screening saliva	1
UK, England			29.8 (805)						SP	Prisons; ever IDUs, screening saliva	4
UK, England		65.3 (72)							DT	Drug treatment; ever injectors; data 1996 and 1997	12
UK, London			52.2 (655)	45.1 (791)	48.3 (559)	45.8 (515)		0.0846	SP	Drug treatment centres, needle exchanges, low-threshold services; screening saliva	1
UK, London			31.9 (226)						SP	Community surveys; current IDUs, screening saliva	3
UK, Glasgow	56.4 (195)								SP	Drug treatment centres, needle exchanges, street, screening saliva	8
UK, Greater Glasgow	80 (312)	68 (463)						0.0019	DT/SP	Public health laboratories; serum taken for named HIV testing	19
UK, Lothian	44 (307)	40 (327)						0.0001	DT/SP	Public health laboratories; serum taken for named HIV testing	19
UK, Liverpool	67 (130)								n.a.	Hospital inpatients	17
UK, Lowmoss	31.8 (85)								SP	Prison; ever injectors; screening saliva	16

(1) Statistical significance of time trend using the Cochrane–Armitage trend test.
(2) Abbreviations: DT = diagnostic testing; SP = specific prevalence study.
(3) See Annex 3 for references.

Notes:

1. Sample size is the number of positive plus negative tests (total valid tests). Prevalence is the number of positive tests divided by total valid tests, excluding missing values. Prevalence from sample size under 50 is not reliable.

2. Self-reported test results for HCV may be unreliable. Prevalence is the number reporting a positive test result divided by the number reporting a positive or negative result.

3. Saliva tests for hepatitis C antibodies underestimate prevalence. If test sensitivity is known, then figures can be adjusted upwards by dividing prevalence by test sensitivity. Test sensitivity is around 70–90 % in older studies and may be up to 90–95 % in some recent studies. Figures have not been adjusted.

4. Having health problems is one selection criterion for admission to drug treatment in some countries or cities (Greece, Portugal, Rome), due to long waiting lists or special programmes for infected IDUs, this may result in upward bias of prevalence. Prevalence from treatment data should therefore be interpreted in combination with non-treatment data.

5. Data sources with no information on injecting status were excluded as far as possible, as such prevalence can severely underestimate prevalence among injectors in the same source. Some such sources were, however, included if samples were large or they provided trends over time, in which case it is indicated that injecting status is unknown and prevalence among injectors may be underestimated.

Part of these data were taken from two literature reviews on HCV prevalence in Europe; most figures were subsequently checked by the national focal points. These reviews are:

- Mathei, C., Buntinx, F., van Damme, P. (2002), 'Seroprevalence of hepatitis C markers among intravenous drug users in western European countries: a systematic review', *Journal of Viral Hepatitis* 9: 157–73.
- Roy, K., Hay, G., Andragetti, R., Taylor, A., Goldberg, D., Wiessing, L. (2002), 'Monitoring hepatitis C virus infection among injecting drug users in the European Union: a review of the literature', *Epidemiology and Infection* 129: 577–85.

Table A2: Prevalence of hepatitis C infection (%) among injecting drug users under age 25 in the EU (sample sizes in parentheses)

HCV — young IDUs Country, region/city	1996	1997	1998	1999	2000	2001	P trend [1]	DT/SP [2]	Setting/comments	Ref. [3]
Belgium, Flemish Community		24.6 (65)	21.4 (14)	13.9 (79)	16.4 (67)	16.3 (43)	0.1811	DT	Drug treatment centres; screening serum	2
Belgium, Flemish Community — Antwerp							83 (6)	SP	Drug treatment centres, low-threshold services; screening serum	8
Denmark, Copenhagen		75 (n.a.)						SP	Drug treatment centres; screening serum	2
Denmark, Funen		90 (29)						SP	Prison, drug treatment centres; screening serum	1
Greece, Athens					25.9 (324)			DT	Public health laboratory; screening serum	6
Greece, National			61.1 (36)	33.3 (12)			0.0944	DT	Prisons; screening serum	10
Greece, National				32.2 (115)	30.6 (248)	28.6 (189)	0.4940	DT	Drug treatment centres; screening serum	2
Greece, Athens				32.1 (78)	30.7 (127)		0.8404	DT	STD clinics; screening serum	8
Greece, National						84.4 (32)		DT	Drug treatment centres; screening serum	9
Greece, National						39.0 (310)		DT	Drug treatment centres, low-threshold services, public health laboratories, STD clinics; screening serum	1
Ireland, Dublin		59.3 (535)						SP	Drug treatment centre Trinity Court, first attendees 1992–97; ever-IDUs; screening serum	1,7

HCV — young IDUs Country, region/city	1996	1997	1998	1999	2000	2001	P trend [1]	DT/SP [2]	Setting/comments	Ref. [3]
Italy, Calabria, Campania, Emilia-Romagna, Friuli, Lazio, Liguria, Marche, Piedmont Trento, Apulia, Sardinia, Sicily, Tuscany				60.2 (644)				DT	Drug treatment centres; study in 13 regions; data are for 1998–2000; screening serum	3
Netherlands, Limburg, Heerlen/Maastricht	61.8 (21)							SP	Drug treatment centres, needle exchanges, low-threshold services; screening serum	11
Austria, Vienna			67 (9)	62 (50)	53 (51)		0.2934	DT	Low-threshold services; screening serum	3
Austria, Vorarlberg	44.4 (18)	40.0 (10)	47.1 (17)	63.6 (11)	30.0 (10)	50.0 (12)	0.8642	DT	Drug treatment centres; screening serum	2
Austria, Lower Austria				67 (n.a.)	67 (31)			DT	Drug treatment centres; screening serum	4
Portugal, Lisbon			58.6 (29)	68.4 (19)	66.7 (12)		0.5422	DT	Drug treatment centres; screening serum	1
Portugal, Oporto		89.5 (19)						DT	Drug treatment centres; screening serum	8
Portugal, Coimbra				79.0 (43)	74.0 (27)		0.6280	DT	Drug treatment centres; includes data from public health laboratory and pregnant IDUs; screening serum	2
Portugal, Santarém					93 (14)			DT	Drug treatment centres; screening serum	7
Portugal, Évora					57.1 (7)			DT	Drug treatment centres; screening serum	6
Finland, Helsinki				75 (8)	25.8 (97)	28.1 (174)	0.2650	DT	Needle exchanges; screening serum	1
Finland, Helsinki						13.3 (15)		SP	Needle exchanges, screening saliva	1

Table A2 (continued)

HCV — young IDUs Country, region/city	1996	1997	1998	1999	2000	2001	P trend (1)	DT/SP (2)	Setting/comments	Ref. (3)
Finland, Vantaa					22.2 (9)	29.3 (58)	0.6607	DT	Needle exchanges; screening serum	1
Finland, Vantaa						30.8 (39)		SP	Needle exchanges; screening saliva	1
Finland, Tampere					12.2 (188)	12.5 (160)	0.9401	DT	Needle exchanges; screening serum	1
UK, England and Wales excluding London			10.1 (784)	10.1 (843)	11.1 (754)	14.2 (614)	0.0160	SP	Drug treatment centres, needle exchanges, low-threshold services; screening saliva	1
UK, England and Wales excluding London			8.6 (210)					SP	Community surveys, prisons; current IDUs; screening saliva	3
UK, England and Wales			11.1 (835)	11.5 (938)	11.9 (815)	15.4 (669)	0.0183	SP	Drug treatment centres, needle exchanges, low-threshold services; screening saliva	1
UK, London			27.5 (51)	24.2 (95)	21.3 (61)	29.1 (55)	0.9150	SP	Drug treatment centres, needle exchanges, low-threshold services; screening saliva	1
UK, London			15 (20)					SP	Community surveys, prisons; current IDUs; screening saliva	2, 3
UK, Greater Glasgow	61 (97)	43 (136)					0.0062	DT/SP	Public health laboratories; serum taken for named HIV testing	9
UK, Lothian	17 (114)	13 (112)						DT/SP	Public health laboratories; serum taken for named HIV testing	19

(1) Statistical significance of time trend using the Cochrane–Armitage trend test.
(2) Abbreviations: DT = diagnostic testing; SP = specific prevalence study.
(3) See Annex 3 for references.

Note: See notes to Table A1.

Table A3: Prevalence of hepatitis C infection (%) among new injecting drug users (injecting less than two years) in the EU (sample sizes in parentheses)

HCV – New IDUs Country, region/city	1996	1997	1998	1999	2000	2001	2002	P trend (1)	DT/SP (2)	Setting/comments	Ref. (3)
Belgium, Flemish Community			45.7 (46)	53.1 (32)				0.2660	DT	Drug treatment centres; screening serum	2
Greece, National						24.3 (115)			DT	Drug treatment centres, low-threshold, public health laboratories, STD clinics; screening serum	1
Spain, Barcelona	55.6 (27)	68.8 (32)	54.5 (33)	85.7 (14)	55.6 (27)	50.0 (18)	28.6 (7)	0.2542	n.a.	Two hospitals; screening serum	23
Ireland, Dublin		53.1 (499)							SP	Drug treatment centre Trinity Court, first attendees 1992–97; ever-IDUs; screening serum	1, 7
Italy, Calabria, Campania, Emilia-Romagna, Friuli, Lazio, Liguria, Marche, Piedmont, Trento, Apulia, Sardinia, Sicily, Tuscany				44.4 (178)					DT	Drug treatment centres; study in 13 regions; data are for 1998–2000; screening serum	3
Austria, Vorarlberg	47.6 (21)	15.4 (13)	46.4 (28)	57.1 (7)	37.5 (16)	33.3 (9)		0.8514	DT	Drug treatment centres; screening serum	2
Portugal, Coimbra				60.7 (84)	65.1 (43)			0.6283	DT	Drug treatment centres; includes data from public health laboratory and pregnant IDUs; screening serum	2
Portugal, Santarém					100 (6)				DT	Drug treatment centres; screening serum	7
UK, England and Wales, excluding London			1.9 (107)						SP	Community surveys, prisons; screening saliva	3

Table A3 (continued)

HCV – New IDUs Country, region/city	1996	1997	1998	1999	2000	2001	2002	P trend [1]	DT/SP [2]	Setting/comments	Ref. [3]
UK, London			14.3 (14)						SP	Community surveys, prisons; screening saliva	3
UK, Glasgow	35.8 (173)								SP	Drug treatment centres, needle exchanges, street; screening saliva	8

(1) Statistical significance of time trend using the Cochrane–Armitage trend test.
(2) Abbreviations: DT = diagnostic testing; SP = specific prevalence study.
(3) See Annex 3 for references.

Note: See notes to Table A1.

Annex 3: References (*) for Annex 2

Belgium

2   Raes, V., De Sleutel, Dienst Wetenschappelijk Onderzoek, Jaarverslag 1999, Merelbeke, July 2000.

8   Matheï, C., Free Clinic, Van Arteveldestraat 64, Antwerp, Belgium, unpublished data.

Denmark

1   Christensen, P. B., Krarup, H. B., Niesters, H. G. M. et al. (2000), 'Prevalence and incidence of blood-borne viral infections among Danish prisoners', European Journal of Epidemiology 16: 1043–9;

    and

    Christensen, P. B., Krarup, H. B., Niesters, H. G. M. et al. (2001), 'Outbreak of hepatitis B among injecting drug users in Denmark', Journal of Clinical Virology 22: 133–41;

    and

    Christensen, P. B., Engle, R. E., Jacobsen, S. E. H. et al. (2002), 'High prevalence of hepatitis E antibodies among Danish prisoners and drug users', Journal of Medical Virology 66: 49–55.

2   Fuglsang, T., Fouchard, J. R., Ege, P. P. (2000), 'Prevalence of HIV, hepatitis C and B among drug users in the city of Copenhagen', Ugeskrift for Læger 162: 3860–4.

Germany

2   Jugendberatung und Jugendhilfe (eV), Frankfurt, 1998, unpublished data.

4   Backmund, M., Meyer, K., von Zielonka, M. (2001), 'Prävalenzdaten zu Hepatitis B und C bei Drogenabhängigen in München', Suchtmedizin 3(1): 21–4.

5   Holbach, M., Frösner, G., Donnerbauer, E. et al. (1998), 'Prävalenz von Hepatitismarkern der Typen A, B, C und assoziiertes Risikoverhalten unter Patienten nach intravenösem Drogenkonsum', Sucht 44(6): 390–8.

6   Brack, J. (2002), 'Hepatitis B and C in drug dependent patients: an epidemiological study', Suchttherapie (Suppl. 3): S3–S10.11.

7   Stark, K., Herrmann, U., Ehrhardt, S., Bienzle, U. (submitted), 'Provision of syringes for injecting drug users in prison. Results of a three-year programme in Berlin'.

18 Heinemann, A., Püschel, K. (1999), 'Drogenkonsum und Infektionen im Strafvollzug', Drogen in der Metropole, Hg: Krausz, Raschke, Lambertus, Freiburg.

Greece

1   Greek Reitox focal point (EKTEPN), University Mental Health Research Institute.

2   Therapy Centre for Dependent Individuals (Kethea), unpublished data.

(*) The numbering of references is consistent with the EMCDDA full database on HIV and hepatitis B and C and is therefore not always consecutive. Countries appear in alphabetical order according to the respective languages. This order is: Belgium, Denmark, Germany, Greece, Spain, France, Ireland, Italy, Luxembourg, the Netherlands, Austria, Portugal, Finland, Sweden and the UK.

5   Organisation against Drugs (OKANA), Methadone substitution programme — Salonica units, unpublished data.

6   National School of Public Health — Reference Centre of AIDS, Epidemiology and Biostatistics Unit, Athens, unpublished data.

7   Organisation against Drugs (OKANA), Methadone substitution programme — Athens units, unpublished data.

8   Centre of STDs and AIDS, A. Syngros Hospital, unpublished data.

9   Psychiatric Hospital of Attica — Unit 18 ANO, unpublished data.

10 Mr Papadourakis, Ministry of Justice, unpublished data.

14 Pavlitou, K., Polidorou, F., Pastore, F. et al. (1998), 'Prevalence of hepatitis B and C markers in prisoners', *Acta Microbiologica Hellenica* 43: 271–5.

Spain

3   Delegación del Gobierno para Plan Nacional Sobre Drogas (DGPNSD), Encuesta sobre Consumidores de Heroina en Tratamiento (ECHT), 1996 report, DGPNSD, Madrid, 1997.

8   Delgado-Iribarren, A., Calvo, M., Perez, A. et al. (2000), 'Intravenous drug user serologic control: what may be prevented?', *Enferm. Infecc. Microbiol. Clin.* 18(1): 2–5.

15 Jiménez, X., Caraballo, A., Batalla, C. et al. (1999), 'Prevalència de la infecctió por los vírus de la hepatitis B, C e inmudeficiencia humana en usuarios de drogas', *Atención Primaria* 24: 368–71.

20 Munoz-Perez, M. A., Rodriguez-Pichardo, A., Camacho, F., Colmenero, M. A. (1999), 'Hepatitis C virus infection in a cohort of 1 161 HIV-infected patients', *International Journal of Sexually Transmitted Diseases and AIDS* 10: 69–70.

23 Bolao, F., Sanvisens, A., Egea, J. M. et al. (2002), 'HIV-1 and hepatitis C virus infections among recent injecting drug users in Spain', XIVth International Conference on AIDS, Barcelona, 7 to 12 July 2002, Abstract MoPeC3380.

France

5   Rotily, M., Weilandt, C., Bird, S. M. et al., 'Surveillance of HIV infection and related risk behaviour in European prisons — a multicentre pilot study';

    and

    Weilandt, C., Rotily, M. (1998), *European Network on HIV/AIDS and Hepatitis Prevention in Prisons — Second annual report*, ORS/Wiad, Marseille/Bonn.

6   Hedouin, V., Gosset, D. (1998), 'Infection par les virus de l'hepatite C en milieu carceral. Étude prospective realisee a Loos-lez-Lille' (Infection with hepatitis C virus in a prison environment. A prospective study in Loos-lez-Lille, France), *Gastroenterol. Clin. Biol. 1998*, 22: 55–8.

Ireland

1   Smyth, B., Keenan, E., O'Connor, J. J. (1998), 'Blood-borne viral infection in Irish injecting drug users', *Addiction* 93: 1649–56.

2   Long, J., Allwright, S., Barry, J. et al. (2001), 'Hepatitis B, hepatitis C and HIV antibodies prevalence and risk factors in entrants to Irish prisons: a national survey', British Medical Journal 323: 1209–13.

4   Allwright, S., Bradley, F., Long, J. et al. (2000), 'Prevalence of antibodies to hepatitis B, hepatitis C and HIV and risk factors in Irish prisoners: results of a national cross-sectional survey', British Medical Journal 321: 78–82.

5   Cullen, W., Bury, G., Barry, J., O'Kelly, F. (2000), 'Drug users attending general practice in the Eastern Regional Health Authority (ERHA) area', Irish Medical Journal 93: 214–17.

6   Fitzgerald, M., Barry, J., O'Sullivan, P., Thornton, L. (2001), 'Blood-borne infections in Dublin's opiate users', Irish Journal of Medical Science 170: 32–4.

7   Smyth, B., Keenan, E., O'Connor, J. J. (1999), 'Evaluation of the impact of Dublin's expanded harm reduction programme on prevalence of hepatitis C among short-term injecting drug users', Journal of Epidemiology and Community Health 53: 434–5.

Italy

1   Rilevazione Attività nel Settore Tossicodipendenze — Anno 2001, Ministero della Salute, Sistema Informativo Sanitario, Direzione Generale della Prevenzione, Ufficio Dipendenze da Farmaci e Sostanze d'Abuso e AIDS.

3   Vedette study — 'IDUs entering drug treatment' (unpublished data).

7   Rotily, M., Weilandt, C., Bird, S. M. et al., 'Surveillance of HIV infection and related risk behaviour in European prisons — a multicentre pilot study';

and

Weilandt, C., Rotily, M. (1998), European Network on HIV/AIDS and Hepatitis Prevention in Prisons — Second annual report, ORS/Wiad, Marseille/Bonn.

Luxembourg

4   Schlink, J. (2000), Étude épidémiologique des infections HIV et à l'hépatite virale C dans les prisons luxembourgeoises, CPL, Luxembourg.

Netherlands

9   Beuker, R. J., Berns, M. P. H., Watzeels, J. C. M. et al. (2001), Surveillance of HIV infection among injecting drug users in the Netherlands: results. The Hague 2000 (in Dutch), Report No 441100015, Rijksinstituut voor Volksgezondheid en Milieu (RIVM), Bilthoven.

11   Carsauw, H. H. C., van Rozendaal, C. M., Scheepens, J. M. F. A. et al. (1997), Infections with HIV, HBV and HCV among injecting drug users in Heerlen/Maastricht (in the Netherlands) (in Dutch), Report No 441100006, Rijksinstituut voor Volksgezondheid en Milieu (RIVM), Bilthoven.

Austria

2   Inpatient treatment centre, Lukasfeld, Vorarlberg, unpublished data.

3   Verein Wiener Sozialprojekte, low-threshold facility, Ganslwirt, Vienna, unpublished data.

4   Inpatient treatment centre, Anton Proksch Institut Mödling, Vienna, unpublished data.

Portugal

1   Centros de Atendimento a Toxicodependentes (CAT), Serviço de Prevenção e Tratamento da
    Toxicodependência (SPTT), Xabregas Lisbon, unpublished data.

2   Monteiro Carvalho, C., Centros de Atendimento a Toxicodependentes (CAT), Serviço de Prevenção e
    Tratamento da Toxicodependência (SPTT), DR Centro Coimbra, unpublished data.

4   Valle, H., Rodrigues, L., Coutinho, R. et al. (1999), 'HIV, HCV and HBV infection in a group of drug
    addicts from Lisbon', Seventh European Conference on Clinical Aspects and Treatment of HIV Infection,
    Lisbon, 1999 (Abstract 866).

7   Direcção Regional de Lisboa e Vale do Tejo (CAT de Sintra), unpublished data.

8   Viegas, E., Drug treatment centre, CAT Boavista — SPTT, Oporto, unpublished data.

9   Marinho, R. T., Moura, M. C., Giria, J. A., Ferrinho, P. (2001), 'Epidemiological aspects of hepatitis C in
    Portugal', Journal of Gastroenterology and Hepatology 16: 1076–9.

10 Maia, A., SPTT, Lisbon, unpublished data.

15 Rotily, M., Weilandt, C., Bird, S. M. et al., 'Surveillance of HIV infection and related risk behaviour in
    European prisons — a multicentre pilot study';

    and

    Weilandt, C., Rotily, M. (1998), European Network on HIV/AIDS and Hepatitis Prevention in Prisons —
    Second annual report, ORS/Wiad, Marseille/Bonn.

17 Godinho, J., Costa, H., Padre-Santo, D., Rato, C. (1999), 'Infecção pelo HIV, hepatite C e hepatite B.
    Dados epidemiológicos, características sócio-demográficas e factores de risco', Toxicodependências 3:
    55–60;

    and

    Godinho, J. (1999) op. cit.; CAT Coimbra (2000) op. cit.; CAT Xabregas (2000) op. cit.; CAT Taipas
    (2000) op. cit.; CAT Cedofeita (2000) op. cit.;

    and

    Godinho, J., Costa, H., Costa, C. (1996), 'Comportamentos de risco de doenças infecciosas',
    Toxicodependências 3: 55–60.

18 Portuguese national report to the EMCDDA, IPDT 2000.

19 Padre-Santo, D., Banza, R., Silva, A. et al. (1999), 'Estudo evolutivo do programa de substituição
    opiácea no CAT de Setúbal', Toxicodependências 3: 61–8.

20 Silva, E. (2000), 'Experiência de apoios a toxicodependentes de rua', Colectânea de Textos das Taipas
    XII: 90–7.

21 Viegas, E., Viana, L., 'Estudo dos doentes em tratamento com metadona no CAT da Boavista: análise da
    regularidade na frequência à consulta e resultados dos metabolitos urinários', Toxicodependências 1:
    49–60.

Finland

1   National Public Health Institute (KTL), Department of Infectious Diseases Epidemiology, Helsinki, unpublished data.

6   Liitsola, W., Ristola, M., Holström, D. et al. (2000), 'An outbreak of the circulating recombinant form AECMZ40 HIV-1 in the Finnish IDU population [letter], *AIDS* 14: 2613–9.

United Kingdom

1   Unlinked Anonymous Surveys Steering Group (2000), 'Prevalence of HIV and hepatitis infections in the United Kingdom', Department of Health, London.

3   Hope, V. D., Judd, A., Hickman, M. et al. (2001), 'Prevalence of hepatitis C virus in current injecting drug users in England and Wales: is harm reduction working?', *American Journal of Public Health* 91: 38–42.

4   Weild, A. R., Gill, O. N., Bennett, D. et al. (2000), 'Prevalence of HIV, hepatitis B and hepatitis C antibodies in prisoners in England and Wales: a national survey', *Communicable Disease and Public Health* 3: 121–6.

8   Taylor, A., Goldberg, D, Hutchinson, S. et al. (2000), 'Prevalence of hepatitis C virus infection among injecting drug users in Glasgow 1990–1996: are current harm reduction strategies working?', *Journal of Infection* 40: 176–83.

12   Edeh, J., Spalding, P. (2000), 'Screening for HIV, HBV and HCV markers among drug users in treatment in rural south-east England', *Journal of Public Health Medicine* 22: 531–9.

16   Gore, S. M., Bird, A. G., Cameron, S. O. et al. (1999), 'Prevalence of hepatitis C in prisons: WASH-C surveillance linked to self-reported risk behaviours', *Quarterly Journal of Medicine* 92: 25–32.

17   Kennedy, N., Tong, C. Y., Beeching, N. J. et al. (1998), 'Hepatitis G virus infection in drug users in Liverpool', *Journal of Infection* 37: 140–7.

19   Goldberg, D. et al. (2001), *Scandinavian Journal of Infectious Diseases* 33: 457–61.

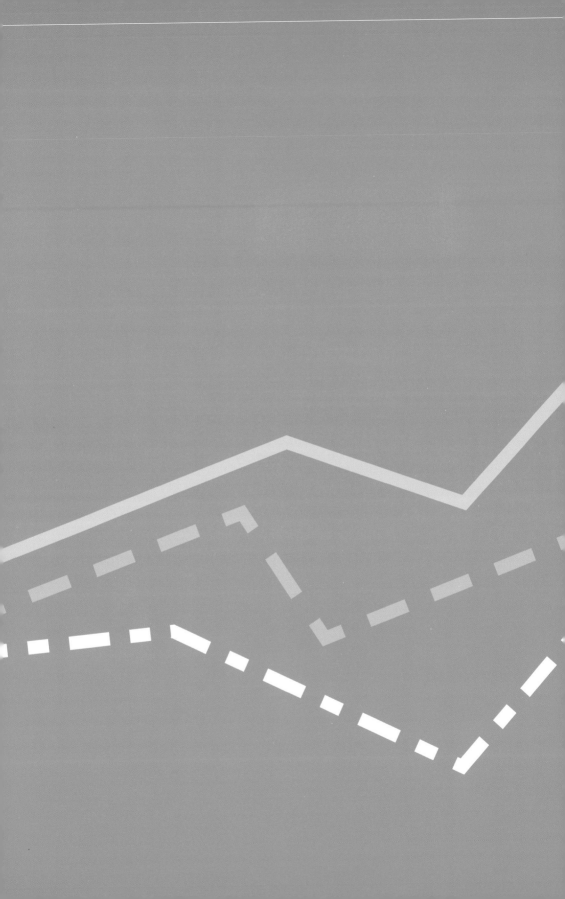

Models of
hepatitis C,
injecting drug
use and policy
options

PART II

Introduction

In 1990, a pilot NSP was implemented in New Haven, Connecticut, US, to fight the spread of HIV among IDUs. Because a permanent implementation of an NSP was met by resistance among state legislators, there was funding for the pilot programme to be evaluated. Kaplan and O'Keefe (1993) evaluated the programme by using an ingenious syringe tracking and testing system in combination with a mathematical model of disease transmission. The idea behind the model was elegant and simple: injecting needles were considered as the vector that transports infection from one drug user to another. By measuring the prevalence of HIV infection among exchanged needles as an outcome variable and using this information in the model, Kaplan and O'Keefe showed that needle and syringe exchange could reduce the incidence of HIV among IDUs by about 33 % within one year. The evaluation of the pilot programme was so successful that the Connecticut legislature decided to continue the funding of the programme and to extend it to other cities. New NSPs were also developed in other states, partially as a result of Kaplan and O'Keefe's work. This shows, in an exemplary way, how mathematical modelling can support policy-making. The model in this case served two functions. One was to provide a new and original way of thinking about the dynamic process of needle and syringe exchange and disease transmission, while the other was to provide a tool for an exploration of the parameters that determine the process and the information needed to evaluate an intervention measure. This is not the only example of the success of mathematical modelling in supporting policy-making, as is convincingly demonstrated in a recent paper by Rauner and Brandeau (2001), which reviews AIDS policy-modelling over the last two decades and discusses future issues in the field.

While a lot of work has been done in the field of AIDS modelling and policy-making, in other areas we are still at the beginning. To better understand the complex dynamics of injecting drug use and of hepatitis C transmission, we need to develop new mathematical models that take the specific characteristics of those processes into account. Considering the rising incidence of injecting drug use in eastern Europe (UNODCCP, 2002) and the extremely high prevalence of hepatitis C in almost all populations of IDUs (see Chapter 4), it is clear that the problem is only going to become more pressing in the years to come and good policy decisions are urgently required. In this part of the monograph, some first steps in the development of those models are presented. In Chapter 5, a simple model for hepatitis C transmission is introduced, and the information that is necessary to estimate the model parameters is reviewed. Possible extensions of the basic model structure are discussed. Risk behaviour of IDUs is incorporated by defining a core group of high-risk users. In Chapter 6, a model is introduced that describes the typical stages of a drug using career with transitions between high- and low-risk behaviour, and whether or not an IDU is a client of healthcare services. The model therefore describes the epidemic of injecting drug use, but can be extended to also include transmission of an infectious disease.

In Chapter 7, a model is developed that enables the determination of an optimal combination of control strategies like prevention, treatment and law enforcement. It was developed in an attempt to answer a fundamental question in drug policy, namely how to allocate scarce resources among different control strategies. The author draws tentative conclusions as to which strategies to apply at various stages of a drug use epidemic and to which strategies resources should best be allocated. The model is flexible enough to incorporate the spread of blood-borne diseases such as hepatitis C in IDUs.

Once a model structure is formulated that incorporates the essential mechanisms of injecting risk behaviour and transmission of infection, we want to use it to identify the key parameters that drive the dynamics of the epidemic, identify the gaps in currently available information, and compare various prevention and intervention strategies in their effectiveness in reducing the incidence of injecting drug use and hepatitis C infection and the prevalence of hepatitis C carriers within the IDU population. Those prevention and intervention measures could then also be evaluated in a cost-effectiveness analysis, where the dynamic epidemic models are combined with cost models as described in Parts III, IV and V of this monograph.

Mirjam Kretzschmar

References

Kaplan, E. H., O'Keefe, E. (1993), 'Let the needles do the talking! Evaluating the New Haven needle exchange', *Interfaces* 23: 7–26.

Rauner, M. S., Brandeau, M. L. (2001), 'AIDS policy modelling for the 21st century: an overview of key issues', *Health Care Management Science* 4: 165–80.

United Nations Office for Drug Control and Crime Prevention (UNODCCP) (2002), 'Global illicit drug trends', United Nations (www.unodc.org).

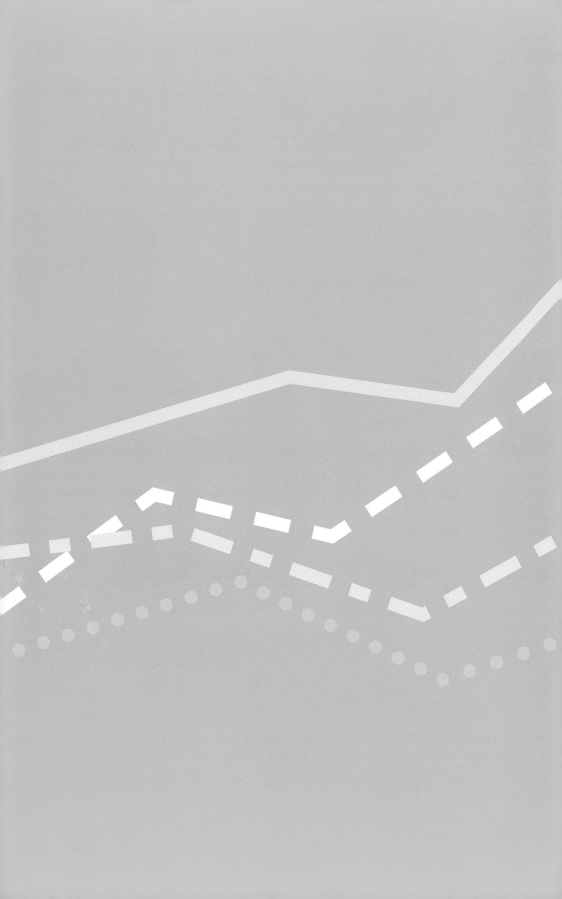

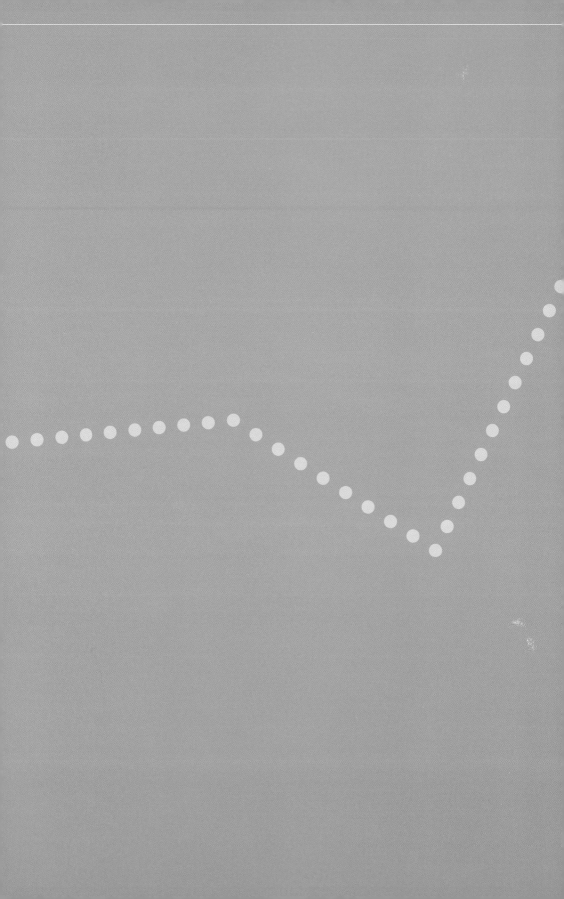

Chapter 5
Modelling the transmission of hepatitis C in injecting drug users

Mirjam Kretzschmar and Lucas Wiessing

Based on literature about the natural history of hepatitis C infections, we discuss the issues that one has to deal with when developing a mathematical model for hepatitis C transmission dynamics. We introduce a model that takes into account the most important stages of infection (acute infection, chronic carrier) and the heterogeneity in behaviour among drug users (high and low frequencies of needle sharing). For this model, we derive an explicit expression for the basic reproduction number R_0. This can be used to investigate the sensitivity of R_0 for changes in the parameter values, and therefore for an estimation of the prevention effort needed to substantially reduce hepatitis C transmission or even interrupt the virus circulation. We then use the model to simulate the effects of various prevention and intervention strategies on the prevalence and incidence of hepatitis C. We do not aim to describe the situation in a specific population or country, but use plausible parameter values to describe a hypothetical, but not unrealistic, situation. The objective of such an approach is to identify which data are needed to provide parameters for the model of a specific population.

Background

In 1989, HCV was identified and the possibility of screening blood products for contamination with hepatitis C arose. Unfortunately, the virus had by that time already spread through large parts of the world's population, and had established itself as a leading cause of severe liver disease (Di Bisceglie, 1998). The features of hepatitis C infection that make it hard to combat are that a large fraction of all acute infections are asymptomatic, that a large fraction of all infected individuals become chronic carriers of the virus, and that severe disease only manifests many years after infection (Alter and Seeff, 2000). The strict screening procedures for blood products have succeeded in reducing the number of new infections in the developed world. But there remain groups in the population that are at higher risk of contracting the infection, most notably IDUs, currently the largest risk group for hepatitis C infection in the US and Europe. In that group, transmission occurs via sharing injecting equipment, and transmission is efficient enough to ensure a high prevalence of hepatitis C infections in many populations of IDUs in Europe (EMCDDA, 2002; Matheï et al., 2002; Roy et al., 2002).

IDUs as a group present specific difficulties for healthcare intervention. Often, they are not easily reached by conventional healthcare, and there are often a number of simultaneous health problems. To make decisions about how best to approach the problem of prevention and intervention in that risk group, one needs to have a deeper understanding of how different factors that lead to transmission act together, and which factors are the most influential for continued incidence and high prevalence. For example, in the group of IDUs, behavioural factors that determine the frequency of sharing of injecting equipment play an important role. But also biological factors, such as the probability of becoming a carrier after infection, are important determinants of prevalence. Some biological factors are amenable to prevention; for example, by treating chronic infections, one can reduce the duration of the infectious period, and, by treating acutely infected persons, one may reduce the fraction of infected persons that become carriers (Jaeckel et al., 2001). What effects on prevalence can we expect as a result of treatment of acute or chronic infections?

To answer these questions, it is often useful to employ a mathematical model of the transmission process. Such a model summarises, in an abstract and simplified way, the mechanisms that lead to transmission of infection and can therefore be used as a tool to explore the effects of changes in those factors on the outcome of transmission, namely incidence and prevalence. While for other diseases, such as HIV and AIDS, modelling has been an accepted tool in designing prevention programmes for many years, the application of mathematical modelling in the epidemiology of hepatitis C infection is only just beginning. Mathematical models have been used to describe the within-host dynamics of the virus interacting with the immune system and to assess the effects of interferon therapy on the viral load (Blower and Ganem, 1998; Neumann et al., 1998; Perelson, 1999). In Deuffic et al. (1999), Freeman et al. (2001) and Griffiths and Nix (2002), models are used to describe the natural history of hepatitis C infection and its sequelae. Deuffic et al. then estimate HCV incidence from epidemiological and mortality data using a back-calculation method. Decision models to determine best treatment and screening strategies have been discussed in Bennett et al. (1996) and Lapane et al. (1998). A microsimulation model for the spread of hepatitis C among IDUs was used by Mather and Crofts (1999).

In developing mathematical models for the transmission of hepatitis C in a population of IDUs, we have to build on work already done in related areas. In modelling the spread of HIV, much research has been devoted to investigating the effects of contact patterns on the spread of the epidemic (e.g. Koopman et al., 1988; Morris and Kretzschmar, 1997; Ghani and Garnett, 2000), and some models have focused specifically on the spread of HIV among IDUs (Blower and Medley, 1992; Greenhalgh and Hay, 1996; Kretzschmar and Wiessing, 1998). Regarding hepatitis B, the focus of modelling has been to assess the impact of vaccination programmes on the prevalence of carriers, and to analyse the cost-effectiveness of vaccination programmes (Williams et al., 1996a, b; Kretzschmar et al., 2002). Here, we want to discuss the type of information needed and the main features that should be included in a model for hepatitis C among IDUs. By no means do we intend to present a full model analysis, but we want to indicate the direction in which a modelling analysis should go and outline the steps that need to be taken.

Information needed for a transmission model of hepatitis C

Demographic information

A mathematical model describes the spread of an infectious disease in a well-defined population. New individuals can enter the population by birth or recruitment and they can leave the population by death or emigration. Therefore, if we want to formulate a model for the population of IDUs, we have to specify the population size, the recruitment rate and the per capita death rate or rate of leaving the population. Some estimates of European IDU population sizes and mortality rates can be found in EMCDDA (2002) and Wiessing et al. (2001). The rate at which new injectors are recruited determines the supply of susceptibles in the population and is therefore an important factor in determining the incidence of new infections. The recruitment rate may display large changes over time, possibly due to factors such as changes in the type of heroin on the market (de la Fuente et al., 1997). It might also be influenced by prevention, if one succeeds in reducing the rate at which drug users start injecting (Hunt et al., 1998). The rate of leaving the population can be influenced by healthcare (decreasing mortality) or by increasing the rate at which IDUs stop injecting and take part in treatment programmes. For example, methadone programmes have been shown to be effective in getting drug users to reduce or stop injecting (Drucker et al., 1998). It has been estimated that the sojourn time in the IDU population is around 8 to 10 years (Frischer et al., 1993; Marks, 1990).

Risk behaviour and transmission

For the population of IDUs that we intend to describe in the model, we need information on the frequency of needle sharing or, in other words, how often used needles are borrowed from others, and from how many different persons. Ideally, to get information about mixing, one would like to know whether persons who borrow needles frequently borrow from others who also borrow frequently, but, realistically, we will have to make some assumptions about the mixing patterns. In Hunter et al. (2000), it was found that between 52 and 78 % (depending on the definition of sharing) of IDUs had shared injecting equipment in the last four weeks with a median number of sharing partners of two. This fraction is higher than that found in earlier studies, where the fraction of IDUs that had shared equipment was around 20 % (van Ameijden et al., 1999), and could partly be a consequence of the interviewing technique, and partly due to real geographic/temporal differences. IDUs under treatment were found to have a lower sharing frequency — between 30 and 43 % (Hunter et al., 2000).

It would also be very useful to have information on changes in the risk behaviour of individuals over time. There is some evidence that new IDUs start with a high frequency of sharing, and at a later point in their drug using career switch to low-risk behaviour (Fennema et al., 1997). With prevention, one would like to influence those transitions of risk behaviour, for example by shifting reductions in risk behaviour to an earlier time in a drug using career, or even to prevent the initial high-risk period.

Natural course of infection

We need estimates for the duration of those disease stages that matter for further transmission. These are the stages of primary acute infection, chronic carrier, recovered from acute infection and, possibly, the stage of secondary acute infection. For each of the infectious states, we need estimates of the probability of transmission in the event that a needle is borrowed from an individual in that state. Furthermore, we need to know the fraction of acutely infected individuals who become chronic carriers, and the rate at which previously infected individuals become reinfected (Mehta et al., 2002).

The duration of the acute phase of infection is estimated at around two months (Clemens et al., 1992). It is estimated that the fraction of acutely infected persons who become chronic carriers is around 80 % (Alter and Seeff, 2000). The rate of spontaneous recovery from chronic infection is very low (Kiyosawa et al., 1994).

The frequency of infection after needle-stick injuries with hepatitis C is at least 10 times higher than with HIV (where it is estimated at 0.3 %) (Villano et al., 1997). For HIV, there are estimates for the infectivity in the different stages of infection (Leynaert et al., 1998). Depending on what one assumes about the duration of the first stage, infectivity in the first stage of infection is about 10 times higher than in the second, asymptomatic stage. Therefore, in the numeric examples presented later in this chapter, we assumed that the transmission probability per contact was 3 % if the infectious individual was a chronic carrier, and 30 % if the infection was in its acute stage.

The natural history of hepatitis C infection could possibly be influenced by a coinfection with HIV or hepatitis B (Herrero Martinez, 2001; Di Martino et al., 2001). As those coinfections occur frequently in some IDU populations, the effects of coinfections on the natural course of an infection with hepatitis C should be taken into account. We will, however, neglect that aspect in our further considerations.

Treatment

We need information on the percentage of chronic carriers who are treated with interferon and what the average reduction of the infectious period is due to treatment. It is assumed that, at present, the fraction of IDUs treated for HCV infection is very low (Wiessing, 2001). This is because it is usually required that a drug user first receives treatment for drug use and, only after that has successfully been completed, receives treatment for hepatitis C infection. One argument being used is the high probability of reinfection of a treated drug user if he or she continues his or her risky behaviour (Davis and Rodrigue, 2001). However, this policy of not treating IDUs is under dispute (Edlin et al., 2001; Wiessing, 2001).

A first step in designing a model

Stages of disease

The most important stages of a hepatitis C infection are acute infection, chronic carrier state, and recovery (viral clearance). It seems that there is no complete lasting immunity for those who were able to clear the virus, but that individuals may contract subsequent infections. These are, on average, of shorter duration than the primary infection, and the viral loads are lower. Usually, secondary infections are then also cleared by the immune system (Thomas et al., 2000; Crabb, 2001; Mehta et al., 2002). As not much is known yet about those secondary infections and their possible impact on disease dynamics, we do not consider them here. This suggests the flow chart of a simple hepatitis C model as shown in Figure 1.

We denote the number of susceptibles by 'S', the number of acutely infected individuals by 'A', the number of chronic carriers by 'C', and the number recovered by 'R'. The demography of the population is determined by recruitment

Figure 1: Flow chart of a simple hepatitis C model

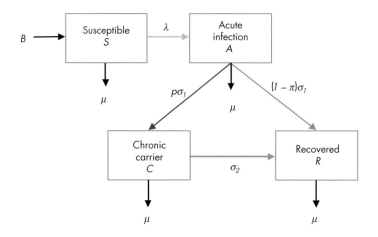

(B), and the mortality rate (μ). Transmission is described by the force of infection (λ), which depends on the rate of borrowing injecting equipment (κ), and the transmission probability. The latter is given by b_a if the susceptible person borrowed from someone with a primary acute infection, and b_c if the infectious person is a chronic carrier. An individual with primary acute infection moves out of that state with rate σ_1, with a fraction 'p' becoming chronic carriers and the remaining fraction, $1 - p$, recovering completely. Those who are chronic carriers can still clear the virus with rate σ_2 and move into the 'recovered' compartment. Finally, by 'N' we denote the total population size: $N(t) = S(t) + A(t) + C(t) + R(t)$.

The model is described by the set of differential equations:

$$\frac{dS(t)}{dt} = B - \lambda S(t) - \mu(t)S(t)$$

$$\frac{dA(t)}{dt} = \lambda S(t) - \sigma_1 A(t) - \mu A(t)$$

$$\frac{dC(t)}{dt} = p\sigma_1 A(t) - \sigma_2 C(t) - \mu C(t)$$

$$\frac{dR(t)}{dt} = (1-p)\sigma_1 A(t) + \sigma_2 C(t) - \mu R(t)$$

with the force of infection:

$$\lambda(t) = \kappa\left(b_a \frac{A(t)}{N(t)} + b_c \frac{C(t)}{N(t)} \right).$$

For this model, one can now compute the basic reproduction number, R_0, which is the number of secondary cases that one index case causes, on average, in a wholly susceptible population (see Diekmann and Heesterbeek, 2000):

$$R_0 = \kappa\left(\frac{b_a}{\mu + \sigma_1} + \frac{b_c p \sigma_1}{(\mu + \sigma_1)(\mu + \sigma_2)} \right).$$

In an equilibrium situation, we have $N = B/\mu$, and one can compute the endemic prevalence. The prevalence of acute infections, i.e. the fraction of the population that is acutely infected in endemic equilibrium, is denoted by a_{end} and can be computed as:

$$a_{end} = \frac{\mu(R_0 - 1)}{(\mu + \sigma_1)R_0}$$

and the prevalence of carriers c_{end} is:

$$c_{end} = \frac{\mu p \sigma_1 (R_0 - 1)}{(\mu + \sigma_1)(\mu + \sigma_2)R_0} = \frac{p \sigma_1}{\mu + \sigma_2} a_{end}.$$

The fraction of the population who has been infected but succeeded in clearing the virus is given by r_{end}:

$$r_{end} = \frac{(R_0 - 1)}{R_0} \frac{\sigma_1}{(\mu + \sigma_1)} \left(1 - p + \frac{p \sigma_2}{\mu + \sigma_2} \right).$$

We can now investigate how the prevalence changes when we apply certain prevention measures. For example, if we succeed in changing the frequency of sharing injection equipment, the rate of contacts κ will decrease. If κ falls below a threshold value, R_0 will become smaller than one and the incidence of new infections will eventually go to zero. Similarly, by treatment of chronic carriers, the duration of the infectious period is decreased, which amounts to increasing σ_2. In Figure 2, it is shown how the endemic prevalence depends on those two parameters, if all other parameters remain constant.

Figure 2: Prevalence of carriers in the population as a function of (a) sharing frequency κ and (b) the rate of leaving the carrier state σ_2

(a) Sharing frequency κ (b) Rate of leaving the carrier state σ_2

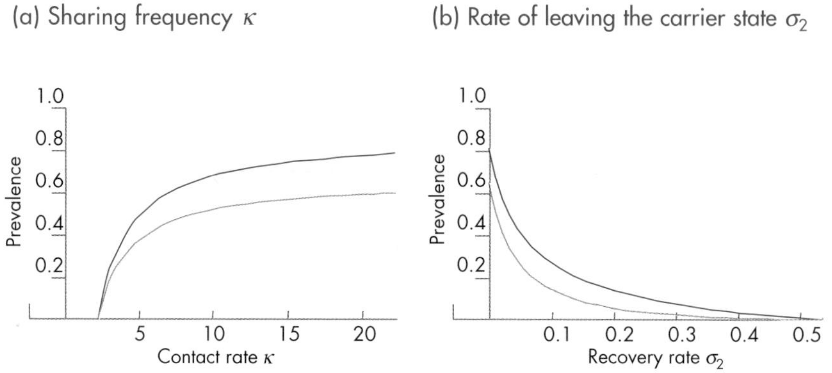

Note: $1/(\sigma_2 + \mu)$ is the average duration of the carrier state, which can be reduced by treatment thus increasing σ_2. The other parameter values used in this figure are $\mu = 0.05$, $p = 0.8$, $\sigma_1 = 5.0$, $b_a = 0.3$, and $b_c = 0.03$. For $\sigma_2 = 0.01$ and $\kappa = 10.0$, we get $R_0 = 4.6$. In (a) the value of σ_2 is chosen as 0.01, while κ is varied, and in (b) the value of κ is 10.0 and σ_2 is varied. The light blue line shows the prevalence of chronic carriers C, the dark blue line the fraction of the population that is seropositive for HCV, i.e. chronic carriers plus those that have cleared the infection and are now recovered $(C + R)$.

One observes that, with the parameters chosen, there is a very steep increase in the prevalence of carriers once the sharing frequency is higher than a critical value (where R_0 crosses the threshold, 1). Once the sharing frequency is above 10 per year, the prevalence of carriers no longer changes much. This also means that, if we have a population of IDUs with a high average sharing frequency and we want to reduce risk behaviour, we need to reach a substantial reduction before any effect on the prevalence of carriers can be seen. On the other hand, Figure 2b shows that reduction of the duration of the period spent as a carrier can be very effective in reducing the prevalence.

A heterogeneous population

In IDUs, it is well known that behaviour is very heterogeneous (Hunter et al., 2000). There are IDUs who hardly ever share injecting equipment and others who share very frequently. Therefore, one would like to take that heterogeneity into account in the model and explore its consequences.

We extend the above model by assuming that there are two subgroups in the population, one with a high and one with a low average rate of needle sharing. We assume that the two subpopulations differ in their behaviour and in their mortalities, but not in the disease-specific parameters. Furthermore, we assume that a fraction, v, of all persons entering the population belong to the low-risk group and the remaining $(1 - v)$ to the high-risk group. Individuals stay in that risk group during their entire drug using career. Mortalities can differ between low- and high-risk groups, i.e. we have parameters μ^1 and μ^2 for the low- and high-risk groups, respectively. When the demographic process is at equilibrium, a constant fraction of the population is in group i, determined by B, v, and μ_i. We find:

$$N = v\frac{V}{\mu_1} + (1-v)\frac{B}{\mu_2}$$

The fraction g_i of the population that belongs to group i can then be computed as:

$$g_1 = \frac{v\mu_2}{\left((1-v)\mu_1 + v\mu_2\right)} \quad \text{and} \quad g_2 = \frac{(1-v)\mu_1}{\left((1-v)\mu_1 + v\mu_2\right)}$$

We now formulate the model in terms of the possible states S_i, A_i, C_i, and R_i for $i = 1$ or 2, where the index, i, denotes the behavioural subgroup. This means that we will have to describe the mixing patterns of the two subgroups: what fraction of needle sharing takes place within a group, and what fraction is borrowed from members of the other group? For each of the two groups, we define mixing parameters, m_{ij}, denoting the fraction of needles that members of group i borrow from members of group j. This implies that $m_{i1} + m_{i2} = 1$ for $i = 1$, 2. As before, κ_i denotes the rate with which a member of group i borrows needles.

The force of infection λ_i, that a member of group i experiences when borrowing a needle, is given by:

$$\lambda_1 = \frac{\kappa_i m_{i1}}{g_1 N}\left(b_a A_1 + b_c C_1\right) + \frac{\kappa_i m_{i2}}{g_2 N}\left(b_a A_2 + b_c C_2\right).$$

For this two-group model, we do not give an explicit formula for the endemic equilibrium, but it is easy to compute it numerically for a given set of parameters.

The basic reproduction number, R_0

For the model we have just formulated, an explicit formula for R_0 can be derived (for mathematical details see Diekmann and Heesterbeek, 2000). We first have to determine the number of secondary cases that an index case of group i causes in group j for all pairs (i,j). An index case in group i can either be acutely infected or be a chronic carrier. The duration of the acute infection is on average $1/(\sigma_1 + \mu_i)$ and during that time the individual causes $b_f \kappa_i m_{ji} g_i / g_i$ new infections in group j.

Similarly, as a chronic carrier, an individual in group i causes $(b_c p \sigma_1 / (\mu_i + \sigma_1)(\mu_i + \sigma_2))$ $k_i m_{ji} g_i / g_i$ secondary cases. So, in total, an index case in group i causes

$$k_{ij} = \kappa_i m_{ji} \frac{g_i}{g_i} \left(\frac{b_a}{\mu_i + \sigma_1} + \frac{b_c p \sigma_1}{(\mu_i + \sigma_1)(\mu_i + \sigma_2)} \right)$$

secondary cases. The k_{ij} form the so-called 'next-generation' matrix, whose dominant eigenvalue is the basic reproduction number:

$$R_0 = \frac{1}{2}(k_{11} + k_{22}) + \frac{1}{2}\sqrt{(k_{11} + k_{22})^2 - 4(k_{11}k_{22} - k_{12}k_{21})}.$$

If we have estimates for the model parameters, we can now look at how R_0 depends on the mixing patterns in the population (vary the m_{ij}), what the effect is of behaviour change (vary κ_i), or what the effect is of treating chronic carriers (increase of σ_2). In Figure 3, it is shown for a typical set of parameter values how R_0 depends on σ_2 and on m_{22}. In Figure 3a, we see, as before, that treating chronic carriers and therefore shortening their infectious period can have a large effect on the basic reproduction number and therefore also on the endemic prevalence. The influence of treatment is large, because of the large fraction of all individuals who become chronic carriers and stay infectious for a very long time. In Figure 3b we see the importance of the group of IDUs with a large sharing frequency on the overall dynamics of hepatitis C transmission. If this high-risk group is a group that mainly mixes among itself, it will ensure the continuing persistence of hepatitis C in the population and will make it difficult to gain an effect with preventive measures. On the other hand, if it is possible to target prevention measures specifically at the high-risk group of persons who frequently share injecting equipment, it might be possible to have a disproportionally large effect on incidence and prevalence.

Time since beginning injecting

In following these steps, one may want to include the time since beginning injecting as a structure variable in the model, especially if some of the parameters (e.g. risk behaviour) clearly depend on it. Then one can investigate the effects of changing behaviour in the course of a drug using career. In formulating the model, one has to express the model equations in terms of partial differential equations with an additional independent variable describing the time since beginning of injecting. Technically, such a model resembles an age-structured model.

In Figure 4, some results are shown for such a model with time since the start of injecting as a variable, but no dependence on that variable in the parameters. In

Figure 3: Basic reproduction number for the model with heterogeneity in behaviour depends on (a) the model parameters σ_2 and (b) the fraction of contacts that high-risk individuals have within their own group

(a) Model parameters σ_2

(b) Fraction of contacts that high-risk individuals have within their own group

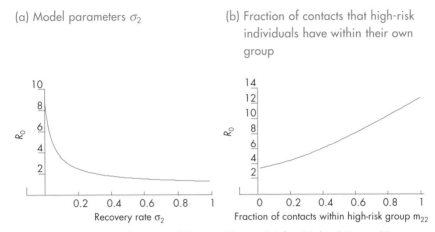

Note: The parameter values were chosen as $v = 0.85$, $m_{11} = 0.5$, $m_{22} = 0.5$, $b_a = 0.3$, $b_c = 0.03$, $\sigma_1 = 5.0$, $\sigma_2 = 0.01$, $p = 0.8$, $\mu_1 = 0.04$, $\mu_2 = 0.05$, $\kappa_1 = 3.0$, and $\kappa_2 = 30.0$. With those parameter values, one gets an R_0 value of 7.6. In endemic equilibrium, 40.7 % of the population is susceptible, 0.5 % has an acute infection, 37.9 % are carriers, and 20.9 % have recovered from infection. This implies that 58.8 % of the population are seropositive for HCV. In (a) m_{22} is varied between 0 and 1, and in (b) σ_2 is increased from 0 to 1.

Figure 4: Average time after entering the IDU population until an individual becomes infected and becomes a carrier — using a model with time since the start of injecting as an independent variable: (a) total population; (b) fractions shown separately for high- and low-risk groups

(a) Total population

(b) Fractions shown separately for high- and low-risk groups

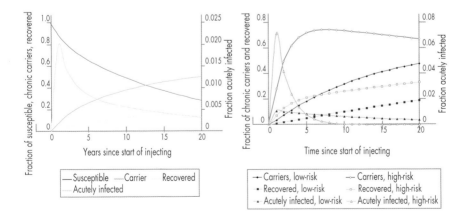

the first three years after entering the population, a large fraction of all individuals go through an acute infection. About five years after entering the population, around 26 % of all IDUs are carriers of hepatitis C, and 33 % are seropositive. Looking at the high- and low-risk groups separately, one can see how transmission dynamics differ in the two groups. While in the high-risk group, more than 70 % of the group are chronic carriers and the prevalence of carriers no longer rises after five years, in the low-risk group, prevalence of carriage continues to rise during the entire time since starting injecting.

When using parameter values as used in Figure 3, but with a proportional mixing of the two subgroups, one observes that a large proportion of new infections takes place in the first three years after individuals start injecting. Figure 4a shows that, in the total population, after five years, around 26 % of the new injectors are chronic carriers of hepatitis C, and almost 34 % have been infected with HCV. In Figure 4b, most of all infections in the high-risk group take place in the first three years after the start of injecting, and more than 70 % of all high-risk injectors are chronic carriers after five years. In contrast, in the low-risk group, new infections continue to occur long after individuals started injecting, and therefore also the fraction of carriers rises until it reaches a level of 30 % after 10 years of injecting, and 47 % after 20 years of injecting.

For prevention, one can draw the conclusions that: (a) prevention should aim at behavioural change before drug users start injecting; (b) behavioural change of high-risk IDUs might be too late to protect those high-risk individuals from becoming infected, but it might have the effect of reducing the force of infection for low-risk individuals; and (c) behavioural change of low-risk individuals can protect those individuals from becoming infected, but can do little to reduce the overall prevalence of hepatitis C carriage.

Possible model extensions

We have now formulated a simple model framework that describes some features of the transmission of hepatitis C in a population of IDUs. With specific questions, it might be necessary to change or extend this model structure. For example, if one wants to investigate the importance of waning immunity and secondary infections on the transmission dynamics, one might think of including an additional infected state into the model. Individuals can move into that state from the immune class by a repeated infection, and they can then contribute to further transmission. Also, if one wants to investigate the consequence of HIV coinfection on the transmission dynamics of hepatitis C, one would have to include a variable distinguishing HIV-infected, and non-infected, persons.

Discussion

In this chapter, we focused on only one type of model, namely a deterministic compartmental model. We started with the simplest situation of describing the spread of hepatitis C in a homogeneous population, where the infection was characterised by the disease stages of acute infections and carriers. When an infection is cleared, we assumed that a permanent immune state would be reached. We extended the model to describe heterogeneity in sharing frequency, and the mixing between population subgroups with different risk behaviour. This type of model can be refined further by increasing the number of subgroups in the model. Finally, we discussed an extension of the model by including the time since starting injecting as an additional model variable.

A model that takes heterogeneity in behaviour into account, even if it only describes two subgroups of the population — a high- and a low-risk group — requires quite detailed data about risk behaviour to estimate the parameters. Not only do we need to know average sharing frequencies for the different subgroups, but we also need to know whether the borrowing takes place within their own risk group or with individuals from another risk group. In other words, we need information about the risk behaviour of those individuals from whom IDUs borrow the injecting equipment. This type of data is usually very hard to collect.

Also, we need information on the relative sizes of the subgroups. These can be estimated if we know the recruitment rates, i.e. how many new IDUs enter the population per year, how the new IDUs are distributed across the risk groups, and their sojourn times in the IDU population. The last is determined by mortality and other rates of leaving the population. In our model formulation above, we assumed that an IDU who entered the population in the high-risk group would stay there during his or her entire injecting career. One might think about refining the model in the sense that transitions from high- to low-risk groups and vice versa are allowed. In a model that takes the time since beginning injecting into account, it might make sense to make the transition rate between risk groups dependent on the time since beginning injecting. Again, one would need detailed data about life histories of drug injecting behaviour to provide parameters for such a model.

An interesting question, which could be studied using a model similar to that introduced here, is the influence of partial immunity and secondary infections on the overall transmission dynamics of hepatitis C (Mehta et al., 2002). Even though the possibility of the occurrence of secondary infections would not change R_0, one would expect that the endemic prevalence is even higher than predicted in a model with lifelong immunity. Also, the loss of immunity and the possibility of acquiring a secondary infection would have an impact on the effort needed for a successful intervention programme. The effort required to reduce the prevalence of carriers would be greater, and the effect of treatment on prevalence would be less pronounced, than in a situation without loss of immunity. Also, the influence of different mixing patterns between low- and high-risk groups on the effect of treatment on prevalence should be investigated in more detail.

Besides the deterministic approach that we described here, it is possible to use a stochastic, individual-based approach to modelling the transmission of infectious diseases in IDUs. The advantage is that contact networks within which risk behaviour takes place can be described in more detail. For example, in a deterministic model, it is always implicitly assumed that there are no longer lasting relationships with repeated contacts between two individuals. Rather, in those models, the assumption is that every contact is with a new individual. In a stochastic network approach as introduced earlier (Peterson et al., 1990; Kretzschmar and Wiessing, 1998), longer-lasting relationships can be described and the importance of sharing with strangers versus sharing with friends/partners can be investigated. The disadvantages of the individual-based model are that they require even more detailed data about sharing behaviour and mixing, and that very computer-intensive simulation methods are needed.

Using mathematical models to describe the transmission dynamics of hepatitis C in populations of IDUs can help to identify those parameters and pieces of information that are needed to understand the epidemiology of hepatitis C and to evaluate the effectiveness of various prevention strategies in reducing the prevalence of hepatitis C carriers. Mathematical models that describe the epidemiology of hepatitis C can then be combined with cost-effectiveness analyses to evaluate the costs and benefits of different prevention strategies and in this way guide policy-makers in their decisions about the best way to counteract the hepatitis C epidemic.

References

Alter, H. J., Seeff, L. B. (2000), 'Recovery, persistence, and sequelae in hepatitis C virus infection: a perspective on long-term outcome', Seminars in Liver Disease 20: 17–35.

Bennett, W. G., Pauker, S. G., Davis, G. L., Wong, J. B. (1996), 'Modelling therapeutic benefit in the midst of uncertainty: therapy for hepatitis C', Digestive Diseases and Sciences 41 (December 1996 Supplement): 56S–62S.

Blower, S. M., Ganem, D. (1998), 'Mathematicians turn their attention to hepatitis C', *Nature Medicine* 4: 1233–4.

Blower, S. M., Medley, G. (1992), 'Epidemiology, HIV and drugs: mathematical models and data', *British Journal of Addiction* 87: 371–9.

Clemens, J. M., Taskar, S., Chau, K., Vallari, D., Shih, J. W., Alter, H. J., Schleicher, J. B., Mimms, L. T. (1992), 'IgM antibody response in acute hepatitis C viral infection', *Blood* 79: 169–72.

Crabb, C. (2001), 'Hard-won advances spark excitement about hepatitis C', *Science* 294: 506–7.

Davis, G. L., Rodrigue, J. R. (2001), 'Treatment of chronic hepatitis C in active drug users', *New England Journal of Medicine* 345: 215–7.

De la Fuente, L., Barrio, G., Royuela, L., Bravo, M. J. (1997), 'The transition from injecting to smoking heroin in three Spanish cities. The Spanish group for the study of the route of heroin administration', *Addiction* 92: 1749–63.

Deuffic, S., Buffat, L., Poynard, T., Valleron, A.-J. (1999), 'Modelling the hepatitis C virus epidemic in France', *Hepatology* 29: 1596–1601.

Di Bisceglie, A. M. (1998), 'Hepatitis C', *The Lancet* 351: 351–5.

Di Martino, V. D., Rufat, P., Boyer, N., Renard, P., Degos, F., Martinot-Peignoux, M., Matheron, S., Le Moing, V., Vachon, F., Degott, C., Valla, D., Marcellin, P. (2001), 'The influence of human immunodeficiency virus coinfection on chronic hepatitis C in injection drug users: a long-term retrospective cohort study', *Hepatology* 34: 1193-9.

Diekmann, O., Heesterbeek, J. A. P. (2000), 'Mathematical epidemiology of infectious diseases', Wiley, Chichester.

Drucker, E., Lurie, P., Wodak, A., Alcabes, P. (1998), 'Measuring harm reduction: the effects of needle and syringe exchange programs and methadone maintenance on the ecology of HIV', *AIDS* 12 (Suppl. A): S217–30.

Edlin, B. R., Seal, K. H., Lorvick, J., Kral, A. H., Ciccarone, D. H., Moore, L. D., Lo, B. (2001), 'Is it justifiable to withhold treatment for hepatitis C from illicit-drug users?', *New England Journal of Medicine* 345, 211–5.

European Monitoring Centre for Drugs and Drug Addiction (EMCDDA) (2002), *Annual report on the state of the drugs problem in the European Union 2002*, EMCDDA, Lisbon (available at http://ar2002.emcdda.eu.int).

Fennema, J. S., van Ameijden, E. J., van den Hoek, J. A. R., Coutinho, R. A. (1997), 'Young and recent onset injecting drug users are at higher risk of HIV', *Addiction* 92: 1457–65.

Freeman, A. J., Dore, G. J., Law, M. G., Thorpe, M., von Overbeck, J., Lloyd, A. R., Marinos, G., Kaldor, J. M. (2001), 'Estimating progression to cirrhosis in chronic hepatitis C virus infection', *Hepatology* 34: 809–16.

Frischer, M., Leyland, A., Cormack, R., Goldberg, D., Bloor, M., Green, S. T., Taylor, A., Covell, R., McKeganey, N., Platt, S. (1993), 'Estimating the population prevalence of injection drug use and infection with human immunodeficiency virus among injection drug users in Glasgow, Scotland', *American Journal of Epidemiology* 138: 170–81.

Ghani, A. C., Garnett, G. P. (2000), 'Risks of acquiring and transmitting sexually transmitted diseases in sexual partner networks', *Sexually Transmitted Diseases* 27: 579–87.

Greenhalgh, D., Hay, G. (1996), 'Mathematical modelling of the spread of HIV/AIDS amongst injecting drug users', *IMA Journal of Mathematics applied in Medicine and Biology* 14: 1–28.

Griffiths, J., Nix, B. (2002), 'Modelling the hepatitis C virus epidemic in France using the temporal pattern of hepatocellular carcinoma deaths', *Hepatology* 35: 709–15.

Herrero Martinez, E. (2001), 'Hepatitis B and hepatitis C coinfection in patients with HIV', *Reviews in Medical Virology* 11: 253–70.

Hunt, N., Stillwell, G., Taylor, C., Griffiths, P. (1998), 'Evaluation of a brief intervention to prevent initiation into injecting', *Drugs Education, Prevention and Policy* 5: 185–94.

Hunter, G. M., Stimson, G. V., Judd, A., Jones, S., Hickman, M. (2000), 'Measuring injecting risk behaviour in the second decade of harm reduction: a survey of injecting drug users in England', *Addiction* 95: 1351–61.

Jaeckel, E., Cornberg, M., Wedemeyer, H., Santantonio, T., Mayer, J., Zankel, M., Pastore, G., Dietrich, M., Trautwein, C., Manns, M. P., German Acute Hepatitis C Therapy Group (2001), 'Treatment of acute hepatitis C with interferon Alfa-2b', *New England Journal of Medicine* 345: 1452–7.

Kiyosawa, K., Tanaka, E., Sodeyama, T., Furuta, S. (1994), 'Natural history of hepatitis C', *Intervirology* 37: 101–7.

Koopman, J., Simon, C., Jacquez, J., Joseph, J., Sattenspiel, L., Park, T. (1988), 'Sexual partner selectiveness effects on homosexual HIV transmission dynamics', *Journal of Acquired Immune Deficiency Syndrome and Human Retrovirology* 1: 486–504.

Kretzschmar, M., Wiessing, L. G. (1998), 'Modelling the spread of HIV in social networks of injecting drug users', *AIDS* 12: 801–11.

Kretzschmar, M., de Wit, G. A., Smits, L. J. M., van de Laar, M. J. W. (2002), 'Vaccination against hepatitis B in low endemic countries', *Epidemiology and Infection* 128: 229–44.

Lapane, K. L., Jakiche, A. F., Sugano, D., Weng, C. S. W., Carey, W. D. (1998), 'Hepatitis C infection risk analysis: who would be screened?', *American Journal of Gastroenterology* 93: 591–6.

Leynaert, B., Downs, A. M., De Vincenzi, I. (1998), 'Heterosexual transmission of human immunodeficiency virus', *American Journal of Epidemiology* 148: 88–96.

Marks, J. A. (1990), 'Staatlich abgegebene Drogen: Eine absurde Politik?' ('State-issued drugs: an absurd policy?'), in Ladewig, D. (ed.), *Drogen und Alkohol*, ISPA-Press, Lausanne, 108–28.

Matheï, C., Buntinx, F., van Damme, P. (2002), 'Seroprevalence of hepatitis C markers among intravenous drug users in western European countries: a systematic review', *Journal of Viral Hepatitis* 9: 157–73.

Mather, D., Crofts, N. (1999), 'A computer model of the spread of hepatitis C virus among injecting drug users', *European Journal of Epidemiology* 15: 5–10.

Mehta, S. H., Cox, A., Hoover, D. R., Wang, X. H., Mao, Q., Ray, S., Strathdee, S. A., Vlakov, D., Thomas, D. L. (2002), 'Protection against persistence of hepatitis C', *The Lancet*, 359: 1478–83.

Morris, M., Kretzschmar, M. (1997), 'Concurrent partnerships and the spread of HIV', *AIDS* 11: 641–8.

Neumann, A. U., Lam, N. P., Dahari, H., Gretch, D. R., Wiley, T. E., Layden, T. J., Perelson, A. S. (1998), 'Hepatitis C viral dynamics in vivo and the antiviral efficacy of interferon-α therapy', *Science* 282: 103–7.

Perelson, A. (1999), 'Viral kinetics and mathematical models', *American Journal of Medicine* 107, 6B: 49S–52S.

Peterson, D., Willard, K., Altmann, M., Gatewood, L., Davidson, G. (1990), 'Monte Carlo simulation of HIV infection in an intravenous drug user community', *Journal of AIDS* 3: 1086–95.

Roy, K., Hay, G., Andragetti, R., Taylor, A., Goldberg, D., Wiessing L. (2002), 'Monitoring hepatitis C virus infection among injecting drug users in the European Union: a review of the literature', *Epidemiology and Infection* 129: 577–85.

Thomas, D. L., Astemborski, J., Rai, R. M., Anania, F. A., Schaeffer, M., Galai, N. et al. (2000), 'The natural history of hepatitis C infection', *Journal of the American Medical Association* 284: 450–6.

van Ameijden, E. J., Langendam, M. W., Notenboom, J., Coutinho, R. A. (1999), 'Continuing injecting risk behaviour: results from the Amsterdam cohort study of drug users', *Addiction* 94: 1051–61.

Villano, S. A., Vlahov, D., Nelson, K. E., Lyles, C. M., Cohn, S., Thomas, D. L. (1997), 'Incidence and risk factors for hepatitis C among injection drug users in Baltimore, Maryland', *Journal of Clinical Microbiology* 35: 3274–7.

Wiessing, L. G. (2001), 'The access of injecting drug users to hepatitis C treatment is low and should be improved', *Eurosurveillance Weekly* 5: 010802 (available at http://www.eurosurv.org/2001/010802.html).

Wiessing, L. G., Denis, B., Guttormsson, U. et al. (2001), 'Estimating coverage of harm reduction measures for injection drug users in the European Union', *Proceedings of 2000 global research network meeting on HIV prevention in drug-using populations*, Third annual meeting, Durban, South Africa, 5 to 7 July 2000, National Institute on Drug Abuse, National Institutes of Health, US Department of Health and Human Services (available at http://www.emcdda.eu.int/?nnodeid=1375).

Williams, J. R., Nokes, D. J., Anderson, R. M. (1996a), 'Targeted hepatitis B vaccination — a cost-effective immunisation strategy for the UK?', *Journal of Epidemiology and Community Health* 50: 667–73.

Williams, J. R., Nokes, D. J., Medley, G. F., Anderson, R. M. (1996b), 'The transmission dynamics of hepatitis B in the UK: a mathematical model for evaluating costs and effectiveness of immunisation programmes', *Epidemiology and Infection* 116: 71–89.

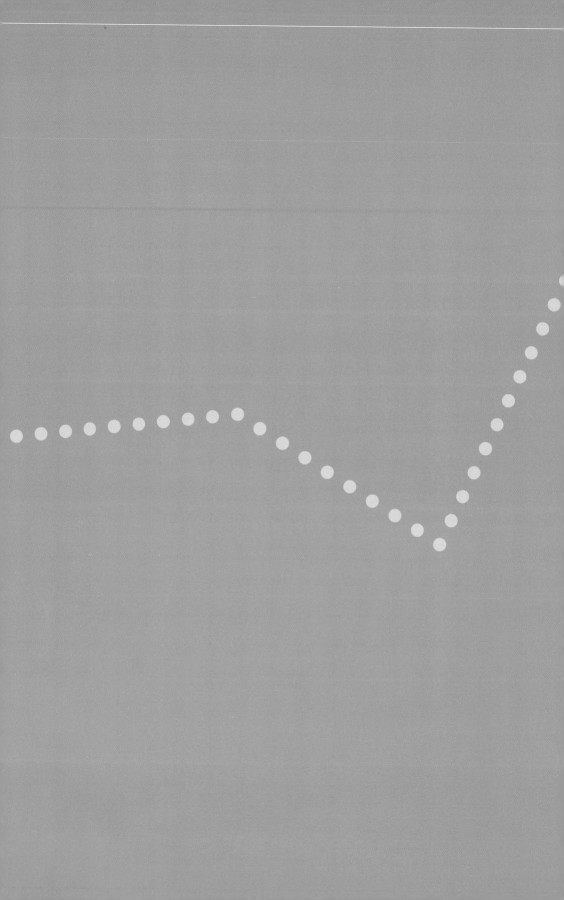

Chapter 6
Modelling injecting drug use and hepatitis C in injecting drug users

Carla Rossi and Nicolino Esposito

Introduction

The illicit use of drugs represents an important social, criminal and public health problem. In particular, injecting is probably the main cause of health damage related to illegal drug use today. It is therefore important for policy-makers not only to examine the possibilities for preventing the further spread of illicit drug use and injecting, but also to think carefully about the most efficient and acceptable approach to meeting the current and future health and social care needs of users and addicts, including those exposed to the risk of becoming infected with HIV, HBV, or HCV. Studying injecting by classical epidemiological methods is no easy task, largely due to its hidden nature and its low prevalence in general population terms. Thus, mathematical modelling can be of major help in performing a qualitative and quantitative evaluation of the costs and possible impact of the various interventions, and to produce forecasts of both injecting drug use and health consequences, such as infectious diseases. On the other hand, epidemiological information on the incidence and prevalence of acquired infections can be useful to estimate, on the basis of suitable models, the size of the hidden population of IDUs (Ravà and Rossi, 1999; Rossi, 1999) and to evaluate the impact of interventions aimed at secondary prevention or harm reduction.

Mathematical models can even help in designing and choosing proper interventions by providing a means of integrating data from different sources, describing a process to increase understanding and simulating policy experiments that are not possible in real life. There is evidence that drug use itself spreads as an infectious disease, i.e. the rate of new cases depends on the number of existing cases and on the number of susceptible cases (De Alarcòn, 1969; Hunt and Chambers, 1976; Mackintosh and Stewart, 1979). Thus, mathematical models developed for epidemiological applications may be of use in this field, although the sociological parameters needed to model drug-related problems may be more transient than the biological parameters used to model the spread of an infectious disease. The length of time that someone remains infectious with a certain disease can be documented and this infectious period would presumably be the same in different countries. This may be different in the drugs field; for example, the reasons for a person in London or Amsterdam to cease using drugs may be different to the reasons for someone living in New York or Sydney, and this may result in different values of some characteristic parameters of the model. In this chapter, the analysis is restricted to compartmental models only.

Compartmental models of epidemics

Compartmental models represent a powerful mathematical tool well established in modelling the spread of diseases in a population (Iannelli, 1992). They provide a framework in which numbers of people in different compartments (each one homogeneous with respect to specific characteristics) and the relationships between the compartments, which model the dynamics of the population, can be described in mathematical terms. Two main types of model have commonly been used to describe the spread of diseases: deterministic models, expressed in terms of systems of differential equations, and stochastic models based on stochastic equations or processes. Both types of model assume that the population can be split into compartments, which can be considered homogeneous with respect to some characteristics. The results from the model usually provide the number of people in a compartment of interest at a specific time (prevalence), or the number of people moving to and/or from a compartment during a specified time interval (incidence). Once the population has been split into relevant compartments, it is an easy task to describe mathematically how the size of these compartments will change over time. This is achieved by means of suitable equations according to the basic hypothesis of the model which describe the dynamics of the population of interest.

A simple general scheme of compartmental models of epidemics is shown in Figure 1.

Transmission and operational models

The spread of an epidemic can be modelled either at the micro or macro level. The first approach gives rise to the development of transmission models, the second to the development of operational models. The main difference between the two kinds of model is the fact that transmission models take into account the dynamic processes at a micro level, modelling the interactions between individuals belonging to different subgroups involved in the epidemic, whereas operational models work on macro-variables or indicators, such as prevalence and incidence.

Figure 1: Scheme of general compartmental models of epidemics

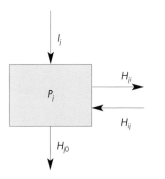

In general, a compartment is represented by a rectangle with the capital letter inside representing the 'level' of the compartment, i.e. a state variable counting the number of individuals or the prevalence in the compartment, normalised if needed.

The arrows represent transitions either from or into the compartment. The inflows can originate either from:

- another compartment (in which case, the order of the subscripts of the transition rate reported near the arrow indicate the originating and the destination compartments),
- or from outside the system (in which case, only one subscript may appear, or the originator is denoted by 0).

The outflow transition rates are similarly denoted.

Two basic types of model can be used: S-I-S and S-I-R.

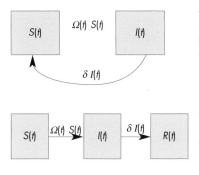

The S-I-S model can be used to represent a situation where individuals pass through a phase of infectivity, recover and again become susceptible.

Further transitions may take into account the possibility of death or other relevant possibilities.

The S-I-R model can be used to represent a situation where individuals pass through a phase of infectivity, recover and become immune.

Further transitions may take into account the possibility of death or other relevant possibilities.

Abbreviations: $S(t)$ = susceptible population at time t; $I(t)$ = infectious population; $\Omega(t)$ = force of the infection — that is the rate at which susceptibles become infectious; $R(t)$ = recovered population.

Thus operational models are appropriate for estimating the size of the phenomenon or monitoring the impact of various interventions, modelled by suitable scenario parameters. Many models of the two types have been developed in the last decade to study the HIV/AIDS epidemic and can also be used, with some modifications, to model the drug use epidemic.

Some examples of transmission models are presented by Dietz (1988), Hadeler (1989), and Kretzschmar and Dietz (1997) for the HIV/AIDS epidemic, and by Billard and Dayananda (1993) and Behrens et al. (1999, 2000) for the drug use epidemic. The complexity of these models is due to the intention of the researchers to introduce into the modelling process a detailed formalisation of the interactions existing, or supposed to exist, between a large number of subjects involved in the epidemic process. This holds true for the analysis of HIV transmission across risk groups, such as drug users and homosexuals, when some specific hypothesis is formulated regarding the contact pattern (Hadeler, 1989; Jacquez et al., 1988). This also holds true when the time during the infectious period at which the contact occurs is supposed to affect somehow the probability of transmission of the infection (Kretzschmar and Dietz, 1997).

A more efficient way of obtaining a simulated epidemic is by using a 'simple' operational model. In contrast to transmission models, simple models do not attempt to include all the possible group or individual interactions in the modelling structure, but summarise the dynamics of the epidemic by some non-linear interaction terms and sum up all the infected individuals in chains of compartments. Most of the parameters controlling the dynamics in such systems are derived from epidemiological studies, external to the model, and their values simply come from specialised studies or from the literature. Only a limited number of 'internal' parameters remain to be estimated by fitting the existing data, or to be used for scenario analyses. Typically, the set of internal parameters includes some form of control of the transmission and of the size of the core group. Other internal parameters may have different origins and interpretations, depending on the design of each single model. The ability of the simple models to describe the epidemic correctly is theoretically much more limited than that of the complex transmission models. However, in general, they turn out to be much more tractable, both because of the limited number of parameters required for their functioning and because of the quality of their output. A main point to stress when introducing an operational model is that it is necessary to consider oversimplified phenomenological situations. Thus, the basic mechanism of interest can be looked at free from the encumbrance of a highly detailed description needing a complex mathematical description, which may hide the essential features of the phenomenon. One of these models for the HIV/AIDS epidemic was proposed at the beginning of the 1990s and has recently been generalised. It allows scenario analyses to be easily obtained (Rossi, 1991; Rossi and Schinaia, 1998). Such a model has also been used for indirectly estimating the prevalence of injecting drug use in Italy (Rossi, 1999) and a modified version of this model was set up to mirror the drug use epidemic (Rossi, 2001). The model is briefly presented in the following section to show how it can be used to support decision-making in the drug policy field.

The operational model for the problem drug use epidemic in the EU

Figure 2 describes the main features of the proposed model. The model is a Mover–Stayer type of model and allows for heterogeneous risk behaviour among the susceptibles. Such a model considers the susceptible population as subdivided into two groups: the group of stayers consisting of individuals who, due to their 'prudent' behaviour, are considered not to be at risk of 'infection' (these models are suitable to make scenario analyses in order to assess the impact of various proportions of vaccinated persons on the probability of extinction of a given epidemic), and the group of movers consisting of individuals who are at risk of infection. Due to interactions between infectious individuals (for our problem, we can imagine these are problem drug users who are also pushers ([2])) and susceptibles, or due to the pressure of the black market on susceptibles, some of them may pass to the drug user compartments and begin a 'drug user career'. In Figure 2, there are two kinds of connection between various compartments: arrows and lines. The lines show that the connections are interactions (non-linear epidemic terms in the equations), whereas the arrows are transitions (linear terms) that occur in a particular direction. Similarly to the model proposed by Behrens et al. (1999),

Figure 2: The simple Mover–Stayer model for problem drug use epidemic

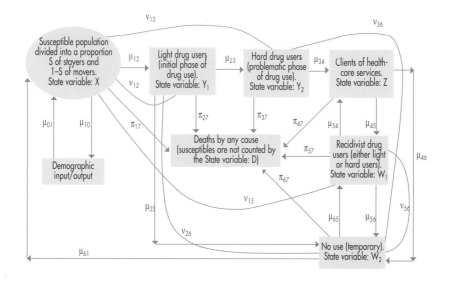

([2]) In surveys conducted among military conscripts — as reported by the national focal point in its 1999 annual report on the state of the drugs problem in Italy — the most frequently mentioned reasons for drug use were curiosity (more than 40 %) and peer group pressure (more than 30 %).

the present model comprises two different stages of hidden drug use. The first (light use) stage is the initial (or non-problematic) stage of drug use; from there, light drug users can either stop using drugs or pass to hard drug use (or death). The other arrows in the figure represent all other possible transitions in a drug user's career. The lines connecting the drug use (infectives) compartments and the susceptible (or temporary no use) compartments indicate the possible interactions which may produce transitions from susceptibles (or temporary no use) to infectives. The other possible transitions from susceptibles (or temporary no use) to infectives are induced by the pressure of the black market and are supposed to be represented by linear terms in the equations ([3]).

From Figure 2, it is straightforward to write the equations of the model either in the form of deterministic (continuous or discrete) equations or in the form of stochastic (continuous or discrete) equations. The discrete stochastic equations are reported elsewhere (Rossi, 2003); only the very general features of the model are considered in this chapter. The state variables used in the model (with the exception of $S(t)$, which is the proportion of stayers at time t) represent prevalences per million inhabitants.

The equation for the proportion of stayers (S) is derived under the hypothesis (Rossi, 1991) that the new entries in the susceptible compartment are divided into stayers and movers according to the constant proportions S_0 and $1 - S_0$ (stationarity), with $0 < S_0 < 1$, even if other hypotheses can be trivially included in the model. It can be observed that the model is a mixture of an S-I-S and an S-I-R model, with the second dominating the first. This follows from the hypothesis of stationarity, which implies that recovered individuals re-enter the compartment of susceptibles according to the proportions S_0 (immune or stayers) and $1 - S_0$ (movers), and, as $S_0 > 0.5$, usually being between 0.95 and 0.99, the S-I-R behaviour of the model is dominant. Thus, the general theory (Lannelli, 1992) allows us to say that an epidemic phase, followed by an endemic phase, is always obtained, as is shown by the simulation results reported in Figure 3.

The qualitative analysis can be conducted by the method used in Rossi (1991) and is comprehensively presented elsewhere (Rossi, 2003). The qualitative characteristics of the model are graphically presented in Figure 3 on the basis of the numerical results obtained by the simulation runs related to the various

---

([3]) The term $\Omega(t)S(t)$ in the S-I-S and S-I-R models represents the non-linear term, whereas the term $\delta I(t)$ is a linear term.

Figure 3: Incidence and prevalence curves and macro indicators of the
Mover–Stayer model

(a) Incidence curve for the transition from   (b) Prevalence curve of light users
susceptibles to light users

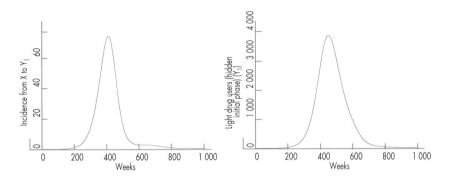

(c) Incidence curve of the transition from   (d) Prevalence curve of hard users
light users to hard users

(e) Epidemic/endemic   (f) Expected impact of a   (g) Expected impact of a
indicator   primary prevention   secondary prevention
                                      intervention   intervention

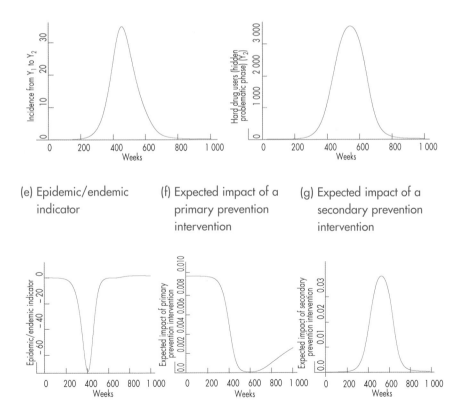

scenarios (Rossi, 2001, 2003) using the available parameter estimates ([4]). The parameters μ and π represent transition rates per person of the origin compartment per unit time, the v parameters are rates per unit time per pair. All the parameters are assumed to be constant

Using the simulation procedure (Rossi, 2001), impact analysis can be conducted to evaluate the influence of the scenario parameters on the course of the epidemic. It is also possible to use scenario analyses for numerical evaluation of the impact of various kinds of interventions (primary and secondary prevention, harm reduction). From the results of various scenario analyses (Rossi, 2001), it can be concluded that the bigger the core group (the lower S_0) the faster the spread of the epidemic and the greater the prevalence and incidence curves. The influence of the parameter representing the pressure of the black market, namely μ_{12}, appears to be less important.

It must be stressed that, although the model presented in Figure 3 has been developed to mirror the problem drug use epidemic in the EU, the same model can be used more specifically to mirror the injecting drug use epidemic. As a matter of fact, it is sufficient to modify the value of some transition parameters to get the corresponding model for an injecting drug use epidemic, whereas all the qualitative considerations related to the general characteristics of the model remain unchanged.

Some general qualitative results

Some scenarios regarding these parameters have been constructed on the basis of various hypotheses (Rossi, 2001, 2003). The numerical results presented in Figure 3 allow the presentation of the main qualitative features of the model, which, in general, are independent of the kind of epidemic described. These results have been obtained on the basis of the values of the various parameters estimated for Italy (Rossi, 2001, 2003).

([4]) As to the parameters and the distributions of the lengths of stay, some of them are already available from the study of the latency period (EMCDDA, 1999a). Others can be derived from therapy data already available at some sites. The demographic parameters regulating the dynamics of the susceptible population, namely μ_{01}, μ_{10} and π_{17}, are supposed to be known and are country specific. The other parameters, π, can be externally estimated using information from mortality studies among drug users which are available for most countries in the EU (EMCDDA, 1999b). The parameters μ_{23} and μ_{34} (natural history parameters) can be estimated on the basis of data available for the study of the latency period. The parameters μ_{45}, μ_{46}, μ_{54}, μ_{56}, μ_{65} and μ_{61} (therapy parameters) can be obtained, at least concerning their order of magnitude, from therapy data available in most countries. The values of all these parameters for Italy (order of magnitude) are reported in a table presented in Rossi (2001, 2003). All the other parameters, namely μ_{12}, μ_{26}, v_{12}, v_{13}, v_{15}, v_{26}, v_{36}, v_{56} and the parameter 'initial proportion of stayers', S_0, can be used as scenario parameters.

As can be seen by the graphs in Figure 3, the first 'epidemic wave' (Figure 3a) relates to the incidence of light use which generates the prevalence of light use (Figure 3b) by a transformation producing a deformed, translated wave. The second incidence wave (Figure 3c) generates the second prevalence wave (Figure 3d; hard drug use), and so on for the following compartments (therapy, recidivist use, etc.), which are not presented in the graphs. The last three curves, representing the behaviours of macro indicators of interest, allow for considerations that may be useful for policy-makers. In Figure 3e, the behaviour of the epidemic/endemic indicator shows that the epidemic spreads fast and that after about seven years the endemic phase sets in. Figure 3f shows that the impact of primary prevention interventions on the epidemic is largest at the beginning, decreasing thereafter, but rising slightly again in the endemic phase. In Figure 3g, the impact of secondary prevention interventions is higher when the prevalence of drug use is higher, decreasing during the endemic phase.

These qualitative considerations may be extended to any epidemic model similar to the one presented, independent of the disease spread it should mirror. Thus, the same applies to any infection spread by sharing needles and by sexual intercourse such as HIV, HBV and HCV.

The simulation procedure used to obtain scenario analyses is written in S-plus for PC programming language. All the parameters can be modified at the beginning of each run. It is possible to choose the total simulation time, which is measured in weeks. The standard output comprises graphs of the prevalence curves in each compartment and of the incidence curves of major interest. The output also comprises the curves representing the main macro indicators, such as the epidemic/endemic indicator that is a function of time which allows qualitative analysis, in particular concerning the incidence of the new use of drugs. In fact, if it is negative, then the epidemic is spreading and going towards the endemic phase, whereas, if it is positive, the endemic phase is ongoing.

Moreover, the impact indicators in the outputs related to primary prevention interventions directed towards susceptibles, to secondary prevention interventions, and to harm reduction directed towards users. These measure the expected difference of the onset incidence (transitions from X to Y_1) when the intervention is applied with respect to the basic situation (no intervention).

The 'nested epidemics' model for the spread of infectious diseases among drug users

The use of suitable markers (marked processes) might allow the incorporation of further descriptions of each individual involved. Thus, a marker may take into account the number of imprisonments, or the number of failed therapy interventions, or the number of non-fatal overdoses. The transition parameters of the model should then depend on the value of the marker. The incorporation of information related to possible infectious diseases can also be obtained by using proper markers. The example concerning HCV is briefly outlined. This is of particular interest as, since the introduction of measures to prevent HCV transmission through blood products, injecting drug use has accounted for the majority of new HCV infections in the EU, with prevalence rates among IDUs of between 50 and 90 % and incidence rates between 10 and 20 % per year (Judd et al., 1999). To model the spread of a disease (HCV) among IDUs, that is a population that is increasing epidemically, all the compartments of the 'external epidemic' (injecting drug use) should be subdivided into two subcompartments: the first comprising individuals unaffected by HCV and the second comprising affected individuals. The two compartments may be identified by a dichotomous variable taking, for example, the value 1 for affected individuals and 0 for the others. Then the transitions within any compartment may be properly modelled allowing individuals to pass from subcompartment 0 to subcompartment 1 according to some epidemic behaviour. A preliminary 'simple' graphical representation of what may be defined as the 'two epidemics' or rather the 'nested epidemics' model is presented in Figure 4. It should be noted that this model is a Mover–Stayer model in relation to the 'external epidemic' (injecting drug use) but is a homogeneous epidemic model in relation to HCV (all individuals are at equal risk of HCV). The corresponding equations can easily be written and a suitable simulation programme can produce numerical results that are highly valuable for policy-making. However, it must be stressed that this model is much more complex than the one previously analysed and that the number of parameters to estimate is much higher. A summary table (Table 1) reports the functions, parameters and variables of the model. Some preliminary qualitative considerations can be made on the basis of the results shown above (Figure 3).

Let us first consider the effect of harm reduction interventions on the external (drug use) and on the internal (HCV) epidemic. In order to do so, we must first recall briefly what is generally intended by harm reduction interventions. Harm reduction is a public health approach, which gives priority to reducing the adverse consequences of drug use for the individual, the community and society, rather

Table 1: Functions, parameters and variables of the 'nested epidemics' model

	Description	Type
μ_{ij}	Transition rates	Constant
π_{ij}	Mortality rates	Constant
v_{ij}	Interaction rates	Constant
$X(t)$	Population of susceptibles	Prevalence
$S(t)$	Proportion of stayers	Proportion
$M(t)$	Proportion of movers/measure of primary prevention interventions	Proportion/function
$Y_1(t)$	Light drug users	Prevalence
$Y_2(t)$	Hard drug users	Prevalence
$PAXY_1(t)$	Incidence of transition from susceptibles to light drug users	Incidence
$PAY_1Y_2(t)$	Incidence of transition from light drug users to hard drug users	Incidence
$Z(t)$	Clients of healthcare services	Prevalence
$PAY_2Z(t)$	Incidence of transition from hard drug users to clients	Incidence
$W_1(t)$	Recidivist drug users	Prevalence
$W_2(t)$	No use	Prevalence
$D(t)$	Deaths by any cause	Cumulative Prevalence
$H_1(t)$	Light drug users with HCV	Prevalence
$PAY_1H_1(t)$	Incidence of transition from light drug users to light drug users with HCV	Incidence
$H_2(t)$	Hard drug users with HCV	Prevalence
$PAY_2H_2(t)$	Incidence of transition from hard drug users to hard drug users with HCV	Incidence
$V(t)$	Clients of healthcare services with HCV	Prevalence
$K_1(t)$	Recidivist drug users with HCV	Prevalence
$PAW_1K_1(t)$	Incidence of transition from recidivist drug users to recidivist drug users with HCV	Incidence
$K_2(t)$	No use with HCV	Prevalence
$\rho(t)$	Epidemic/endemic indicator	Function
$\xi(t)$	Measure of expected impact of a secondary prevention intervention	Function
Δ	Efficacy rate of prevention intervention	Constant

Figure 4: Graphical representation of the 'nested epidemics' model

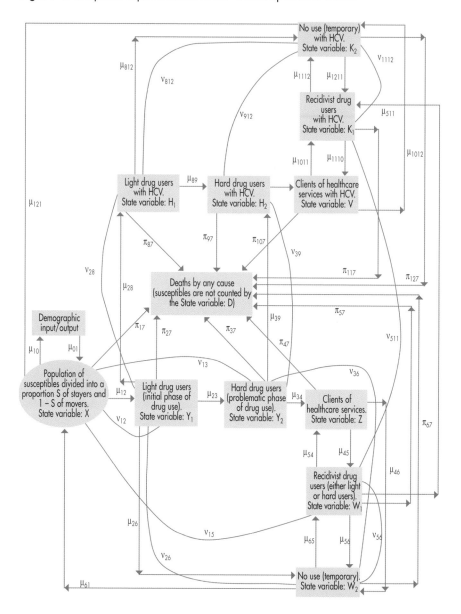

Figure 5: Hierarchy of intervention goals for reducing transmission of HIV

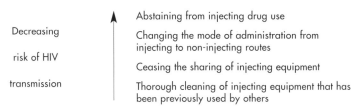

Source: Lintzeris and Spry-Bailey (1988).

than to eliminating drug use or ensuring abstinence. Although the aim is still to reduce drug use in general, the emphasis is placed on the prevention of the potential harmful effects of drug taking behaviour.

With regard to HIV or hepatitis, a harm reduction strategy will first try to reduce the transmission of infections by means of cleaning of injecting equipment that has been previously used by others or by means of the cessation of sharing of injecting equipment, rather than by the means of promoting abstention from drug use (Figure 5). Obtaining some immediate and realistic goals is usually viewed as a first step towards risk-free use. Abstinence may be considered a final aim. With respect to this definition, it follows immediately that a harm reduction intervention aimed at reducing the transmission of infections can be viewed as a secondary intervention with respect to the external epidemic, but it is completely equivalent to a primary prevention intervention with respect to the internal epidemic.

Thus, harm reduction interventions have a considerable impact on the external epidemic (onset incidence of injecting drug use) if the prevalence of IDUs is high, but it is significant in curtailing the spread of the internal epidemic (onset incidence of infectious diseases) only if applied at the very beginning of the injecting drug use epidemic. In conclusion, we can state that the harm reduction interventions aimed at preventing the spread of infectious diseases among IDUs should be applied at as early a stage as possible. The empirical evidence from the various EU countries where these interventions have been implemented confirms this general qualitative result (Owel, 2000).

We can finally observe that the spread of the infectious disease epidemic among IDUs is primarily related to the hidden part of the drug user's career (compartments Y_1 and Y_2 of Figure 2). This calls for interventions aimed at reducing the duration of this period — the so-called latency period. According to

Figure 6: Incidence and prevalence curves of the 'nested epidemics' model

(a) Incidence curve of the transition from light users to light users with HCV

(b) Prevalence curve of light users with HCV

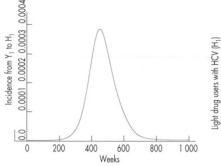
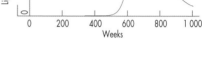

(c) Incidence curve of the transition from hard users to hard users with HCV

(d) Prevalence curve of hard users with HCV

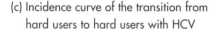
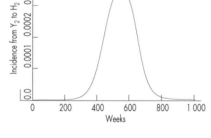
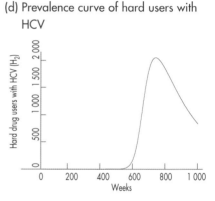

(e) Incidence curve from recidivist drug users to recidivist drug users with HCV

(f) Prevalence curve of recidivist drug users with HCV

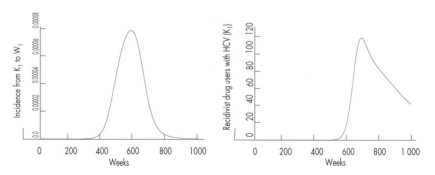

analyses conducted in several EU countries (EMCDDA, 1999a, 2000), the latency period appears to be remarkably similarly distributed over different cities, with a median of between four and six years and an average of between five and seven years. In young drug users, however, this time lapse appears to be much longer. This finding emphasises the need to implement specific interventions targeted at young drug users in order to both reduce their latency period and prevent the spread of infectious diseases. Such interventions are clearly a special kind of harm reduction intervention. In conclusion, harm reduction is a vital and necessary option for both the secondary prevention of injecting drug use and the primary prevention of infectious disease spread among IDUs.

To complete the picture, some preliminary results obtained by simulation are reported in Figure 6. These results confirm the qualitative analysis and the considerations about possible interventions and, in particular, about the harm reduction interventions reported above.

Final remarks

In the present contribution, a compartmental model has been presented to reproduce the epidemic of problematic drug use. Both qualitative and quantitative analyses, which employ simulation methods, have been briefly reported to show the potential of the models for decision-makers. The quantitative analyses ('what if' scenarios) have been developed on the basis of the knowledge of the heroin epidemic in Italy in the last 20 years. On the other hand, the results obtained, both from the qualitative and quantitative analyses, apply to other epidemics of drug use, such as new drugs, from a qualitative point of view. In particular, the qualitative evaluation of the effectiveness of different types of interventions over the course of the epidemic is valid for any epidemic.

The model has been generalised to mirror the diffusion of infectious diseases among IDUs, leading to a suitable operational 'nested epidemics' model. The general qualitative and quantitative considerations about the effectiveness of primary and secondary interventions still apply, as preliminary results obtained by simulation show (Figure 6). The analytical study of the model and further scenario analyses will be dealt with in a future contribution.

References

Behrens, D. A., Caulkins, J. P., Tragler, G., Haunschmied, J. L., Feichtinger, G. (1999), 'A dynamic model of drug initiation: implications for treatment and drug control', *Mathematical Biosciences* 159: 1–20.

Behrens, D. A., Caulkins, J. P., Tragler, G., Feichtinger, G. (2000), 'Optimal control of drug epidemics: prevent and treat — but not at the same time?', *Management Science* 46(3): 333–47.

Billard, L., Dayananda, P. W. A. (1993), 'Drug addiction-pushers generated from addicts', *Biometrical Journal* 35: 227–44.

De Alarcòn, R. (1969), 'The spread of heroin abuse in a community', *Bulletin on Narcotics* 21: 17–22.

Dietz, K. (1988), 'On the transmission dynamics of HIV', *Mathematical Biosciences* 90: 397–414.

European Monitoring Centre for Drugs and Drug Addiction (EMCDDA) (1999a), *Pilot project to estimate time trends and incidence of problem drug use in the European Union*, Final report, EMCDDA, Lisbon.

European Monitoring Centre for Drugs and Drug Addiction (EMCDDA) (1999b), *Coordination of implementation, follow-up and analysis of cohort studies on mortality among drug users in European Union Member States*, Final report, EMCDDA, Lisbon.

European Monitoring Centre for Drugs and Drug Addiction (EMCDDA) (2000), *Study on incidence of problem drug use and latency time to treatment in the European Union*, Final report, EMCDDA, Lisbon.

Hadeler, K. P. (1989), 'Modelling AIDS in structured populations', *Proceedings of I.S.I. 47th Session*, Paris, 83–99.

Hunt, L. G., Chambers, C. D. (1976), *The heroin epidemics*, Spectrum Publications Inc., New York.

Iannelli, M. (1992), 'The mathematical description of epidemics: some basic models and problems', in Da Prato, G. (ed.), *Mathematical aspects of human disease*, Giardini editori e Stampatori, Pisa, Applied Mathematics Monographs, CNR, Vol. 3, 15–25.

Jacquez, J. A., Simon, C. P., Koopman, J., Sattenspiel, L., Perry, T. (1988), 'Modelling and analysing HIV transmission: the effect of contact patterns', *Mathematical Biosciences* 92: 119–99.

Judd, A., Hickman, M., Renton, A., Stimson, G. V. (1999), 'Hepatitis C infection among injecting drug users: has harm reduction worked?', *Addiction Research* 7: 1–6.

Kretzschmar, M., Dietz, K. (1997), 'The effect of pair formation and variable infectivity on the spread of an infection without recovery', *Mathematical Biosciences* 148(1): 83–113.

Lintzeris, N., Spry-Bailey, P. (1998), 'Harm reduction with problem users', in Hamilton, M., Kellehear, A., Rumbold, G. (eds), *Drug use in Australia. A harm minimisation approach*, Oxford University Press, Oxford, 240.

Mackintosh, D. R., Stewart, G. T. (1979), 'A mathematical model of a heroin epidemic: implications for control policies', *Journal of Epidemiology and Community Health* 33: 299–304.

Owel, M. (2000), *Harm reduction within six European national drug policies: a necessary option or a deficiency?*, MA dissertation, Master's degree in European criminology and criminal justice systems, University of Ghent, academic year 1999/2000.

Ravà, L., Rossi, C. (1999), 'Estimating the size of a hidden population involved in the HIV/AIDS epidemic: a method based on back-calculation and dynamical models', in Anderson, J., Katzper, M. (eds), *Simulation in the medical sciences*, Society for Computer Simulation, San Diego, California, 57–62.

Rossi, C. (1991), 'A stochastic Mover–Stayer model for HIV epidemic', *Mathematical Biosciences* 107: 521–45.

Rossi, C. (1999), 'Estimating the prevalence of injecting drug users on the basis of Markov models of the HIV/AIDS epidemic: applications to Italian data', *Health Care Management Science* 2: 173–79.

Rossi, C. (2001), 'A Mover–Stayer type model for epidemics of problematic drug use', *Bulletin on Narcotics* LIII (1/2): 39–64.

Rossi, C. (2003), 'Operational models for epidemic of problematic drug use: the Mover–Stayer approach to heterogeneity', *Socio-Economic Planning Sciences* (in press).

Rossi, C., Schinaia, G. (1998), 'The Mover–Stayer model for the HIV/AIDS epidemic in action', *Interfaces* 28(3): 127–43.

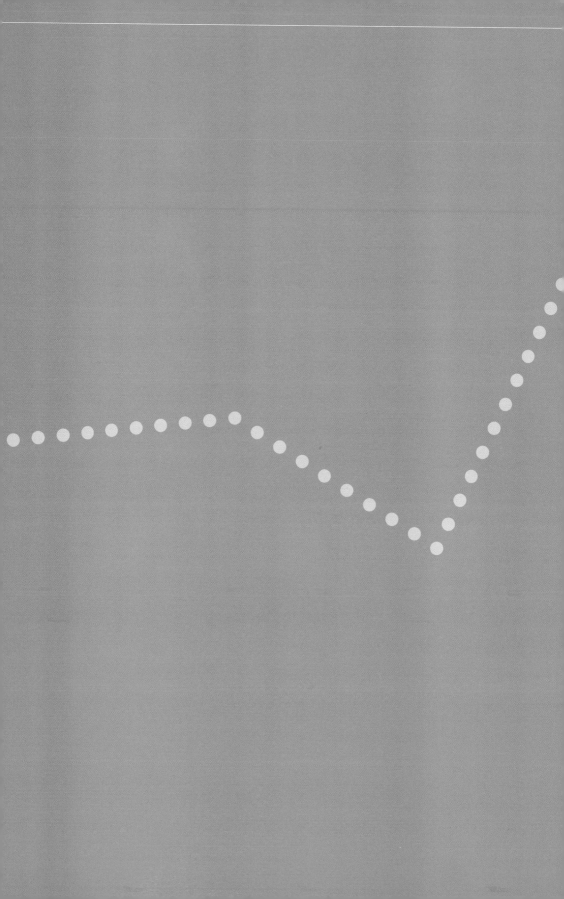

Chapter 7
Modelling policy options to control problem drug use

Gernot Tragler

One of the key questions in drug policy is how to divide scarce resources among competing drug control programmes such as prevention, treatment, and law enforcement. This chapter focuses on this question and provides some answers by making reference to work conducted by a group of operations researchers ([5]) during the last five years.

The focus so far has primarily been on models of the current US cocaine epidemic, because data for this drug problem have proven to be better in terms of availability, quality, and reliability. Even though this does not allow direct conclusions to be drawn for countries within the EU or for other drugs (e.g. heroin), it is still possible to learn some lessons from analyses of the major US drug problem. More importantly, the models and mathematical tools used so far can be applied directly to EU drug problems, as soon as sufficiently reliable data are available.

As this monograph deals primarily with the impact and costs of hepatitis C in IDUs, reference is also made to a model that indicates the optimal spending for MMT and simultaneously accounts for the influence of treatment both on consumption levels and the spread of infectious diseases such as HCV or HIV.

Why apply optimal control theory to drugs?

Illicit drugs impose significant costs on societies ([6]) to the point that, in Stares's (1996) terms, drugs have become a 'global habit'. A variety of control strategies exist including prevention, treatment, and various forms of enforcement, which

---

([5]) Christian Almeder (Department of Business Studies, University of Vienna, Vienna, Austria); Doris A. Behrens (Department of Economics, University of Klagenfurt, Klagenfurt, Austria); Jonathan P. Caulkins (H. John Heinz III School of Public Policy and Management, Carnegie Mellon University, Pittsburgh, Pennsylvania, US); Maria Dworak (Institute for Demography, Austrian Academy of Sciences, Vienna, Austria); Gustav Feichtinger, Josef L. Haunschmied, Gernot Tragler, Vladimir Veliov (Institute for Econometrics, Operations Research and System Theory, Vienna University of Technology, Vienna, Austria); Caius Gavrila (Dipartimento di Matematica, Università degli Studi di Roma Tor Vergata, Rome, Italy).
([6]) For the US, the Office of National Drug Control Policy (1999) estimates that illicit drugs impose costs on society which exceed USD 100 billion annually.

give rise to a fundamental question in drug policy — how should scarce resources be allocated between these programmes? Analysts have sought to inform this decision by estimating the cost-effectiveness of different interventions. The majority of this work has made estimates only for a particular point in time, concluding, for example, that in 1992 domestic enforcement in the US was three times more cost-effective than was border interdiction (Rydell et al., 1996). Until very recently, studies that used 'dynamic' models ([7]) had not focused on cost-effectiveness (e.g. Schlenger, 1973; Levin et al., 1975; Gardiner and Shreckengost, 1987; Homer, 1993). However, drug use and associated problems evolve over time, so it seems plausible that no single, static strategy is best, but rather that the optimal mix of interventions should also vary over time.

This is exactly where optimal control theory, which was developed in the late 1950s as an outgrowth of the centuries old 'calculus of variations', comes into play. The usual definition of optimal control implies the optimisation of dynamic systems described by differential equations and at least one control function. Optimal control theory has been applied to problems in many areas, including aerospace, engineering, and economics.

To come to a better understanding as to why models of drug use seeking for an optimal dynamic mix between drug treatment, prevention, and enforcement fit perfectly into the optimal control framework, we will develop a simple model of illicit drug consumption, representative of other, more complex, models. This model was amongst the first optimal control applications in drug use research (Tragler, 1998; Tragler et al., 2001).

A simple model of illicit drug control: treatment versus enforcement

Verbal description of the model

A key characteristic of drugs such as cocaine is that addiction and tolerance make 'demand' a function of the current level of use. Therefore, it is important to differentiate between users who will consume at a greater or lesser rate depending on the current price and non-users who do not participate in the market at all until they undergo a discrete transition (called 'initiation') and become users. Practically, the number of non-users is so large that it is effectively constant, so we simply track the number of drug users over time.

([7]) 'Dynamic' models take into account temporal variations of the processes under consideration. In mathematical terms, dynamic models typically consist of a set of difference or differential equations.

There are clearly different intensities of use, and people do not become addicted the minute they initiate, so more refined state spaces are possible (see the next section). We restrict ourselves to a single 'state' variable, because we want to include price effects without making the model too complicated ([8]).

Initiation is modelled to be increasing in the current number of users, reflecting the fact that most people start using when a friend or sibling introduces them to the drug. In addition, it is assumed that initiation is modulated by price as described later.

Over time, users quit, many of their own accord, but some with the assistance of treatment. That is, treatment can be seen as augmenting the flow out of the population of users. Unfortunately, not all treated users cease use. Relapse is common. Some types of users are more likely to relapse than others, and the treatment system has some capacity to target interventions at those for whom the prognosis is most favourable. Hence, we follow the lead of Rydell et al. (1996) in assuming that treatment's marginal effectiveness diminishes as its scale increases.

Enforcement is quite different. In the first place, most enforcement efforts are directed at dealers, not users ([9]). In the second place, enforcement against black markets, when they are mature, does not work primarily by removing people from the population. Imprisoned dealers are easily replaced. Rather, enforcement is believed to act more like a tax; it raises risks and, as a result, the costs of distributing drugs, which in turn drives up prices. This 'risks and prices' aspect of enforcement encompasses not only domestic enforcement, but also interdiction and source-country control operations (Reuter and Kleiman, 1986). Finally, whereas diminishing returns mean that treatment becomes inefficient if it is too large relative to the target, 'enforcement swamping' (Kleiman, 1993) implies that enforcement is ineffective if it is too small relative to the size of the market. For any given level of enforcement spending, the larger the market over which that effort is spread, the lower the risk and, hence, the smaller the effect on price.

By focusing on prices, we ignore two other, less important, ways in which enforcement helps to control use. First, retail enforcement can drive up 'search

---

([8]) In an optimal control framework, 'state' variables are those for which differential equations describe their dynamics. The standard solution method for optimal control models, Pontryagin's maximum principle (see, for example, Feichtinger and Hartl, 1986; Leonard and Long, 1992), requires the introduction of one additional differential equation (the so-called co-state equation) for each of the state equations. Consequently, the introduction of just one additional state variable into the model increases the system to be analysed by two differential equations, etc., which, in general, makes the analysis much harder.

([9]) Many users are arrested, but imprisonment — which is the more expensive part of enforcement — is more common for distribution offences; some dealers are also users, but that incapacitative effect is not the dominant aspect of enforcement.

time' by reducing availability (Moore, 1973; Kleiman, 1988). Second, interdiction can occasionally generate temporary conditions of physical scarcity. The former is probably of second-order importance (Caulkins, 1998). The latter has generated some successes ([10]), but suppliers can adapt their routes and methods fairly quickly to restore equilibrium conditions (Caulkins et al., 1993).

Analysts used to reason that, since drugs are addictive, consumption must be relatively unresponsive to price, but four recent empirical studies (reviewed by Caulkins and Reuter, 1998) suggest that the price elasticity of demand for cocaine in the US is about −1. That is, if prices go up by 1 %, consumption will go down by 1 %. Some of the reduction occurs in the short run, as current users reduce their consumption. Some accrues in the longer term, as higher prices suppress initiation and promote cessation.

We formulated the objective as minimising the discounted sum of the costs associated with drug use plus the costs of drug control. 'Quantity consumed' has merits as a general purpose measure of the magnitude of a drug problem (Rydell et al., 1996; Caulkins and Reuter, 1997), so we assume that the societal costs of drug use are proportional to the quantity consumed, where consumption is given by the number of users times the price-modulated consumption rate.

The final part of our model pertains to control spending. We consider both unrestricted control (any non-negative level of treatment and enforcement spending is feasible) and a restricted model in which total spending must be proportional to the number of users ([11]). The latter is a crude way of recognising that budgeting is often reactive, i.e. responding to the current size of the problem. In some cases, the unrestricted model calls for enormous levels of spending when there are relatively few users in order to prevent future initiation. While such a proactive, aggressive approach can be optimal, it might not be possible to convince taxpayers to spend a lot of money on a potential future problem that is currently small. Likewise, we consider a variant of the restricted problem in which not only the level but also the mix of spending is fixed, not optimised dynamically. That is, the decision-maker chooses, once and for all, what fraction of drug control spending goes to enforcement. The more restricted the set of controls, the worse the objective function value, but the easier it would be to implement optimal control.

([10]) The French connection/Turkish opium ban of the early 1970s and the 1989–90 cocaine price spike.
([11]) A more realistic approach would use 'quantity consumed' as a proxy variable for the size of the current drug problem. In particular, consumption is a better measure of harm, and spending would not be reduced when the user population declines, but consumption and related problems are still increasing. However, the analysis of such an approach would be much more difficult.

This concludes the verbal description of the dynamic optimisation model as given by Tragler (1998) and Tragler et al. (2001). The next section presents the equations and mathematical expressions that describe the optimisation problem, to give a better picture of the ingredients and the structure of the model.

Mathematical formulation of the model

Table 1 presents the functions, parameters, and variables that are needed for a complete characterisation of the dynamic model of illicit drug control described above. Like any optimal control model, our optimisation problem consists of the following components (Leonard and Long, 1992).

Table 1: Functions, parameters and variables for the one-state model

	Description	Type
t	Time	Independent variable
$A(t)$	Number of users at time t	State variable
$u(t)$	Treatment spending	Control variable
$v(t)$	Enforcement spending	Control variable
a	Absolute value of the elasticity of initiation with respect to price	Parameter
b	Elasticity of desistance with respect to price	Parameter
c	Treatment efficiency proportionality constant	Parameter
k	Constant governing the rate of initiation	Parameter
r	Time discount rate	Parameter
α	Constant in the initiation term	Parameter
κ	Social cost per unit of consumption	Parameter
μ	Baseline rate at which users quit without treatment	Parameter
ϖ	Absolute value of the short-run price elasticity of demand	Parameter
θ	Per capita rate of consumption at baseline prices	Parameter
$p(A(t), v(t))$	Retail price	Function
$\beta(A(t), u(t))$	Outflow rate due to treatment	Function
$J(A(t), u(t), v(t))$	Discounted weighted sum of the costs of drug use and control	Objective functional

Sources: Tragler (1998); Tragler et al. (2001).

Some variables can be identified that describe the state of the system: they are called 'state variables'. In our case, there is only one state variable, which is the number of users at time t, $A(t)$. The rate of change over time in the value of a state variable may depend on the value of that variable, time itself, or some other variables, which can be controlled at any time by the operator of the system (often referred to as the 'decision-maker', e.g. the government in our case). These other variables are called control variables, which in our case are treatment and enforcement spending, denoted by $u(t)$ and $v(t)$, respectively. The equations describing the rate of change in the state variables are usually differential equations and are called state equations. For each state variable, there is exactly one state equation, so for our model, there is one state equation for the single state $A(t)$, given by

$$A(t) = \underbrace{kp\big(A(t),v(t)\big)^{-a}A(t)^{-\alpha}}_{\text{initiation}} - \underbrace{c\beta\big(A(t),u(t)\big)A(t)}_{\text{outflow due to treatment}} - \underbrace{\mu p\big(A(t),v(t)\big)^{b}A(t)}_{\text{outflow without treatment}}.$$

Once values are chosen for the control variables (at each date), the rates of change in the values of the state variables are thus determined at any time and, given the initial value for the state variables, so are all future values.

The object of controlling a system is usually to contribute to a given objective. As described above, the objective in our case is to minimise the discounted sum of the costs associated with drug use plus the costs of drug control over some fixed time horizon. In mathematical terms,

$$\min_{u(t),v(t)} J\big(A(t),u(t),v(t)\big) = \min_{u(t),v(t)} \int_{0}^{\infty} \underbrace{e^{-rt}}_{\text{discounting}} \left(\underbrace{\kappa\theta A(t)p\big(A(t),v(t)\big)^{-\omega}}_{\substack{\text{consumption}\\\text{costs of drug use}}} + \underbrace{u(t)}_{\substack{\text{treatment}\\\text{spending}}} + \underbrace{v(t)}_{\substack{\text{enforcement}\\\text{spending}}} \right) dt,$$

where $J(A(t), u(t), v(t))$ is called the objective functional [12].

Finally, the control and/or state variables are in general subject to constraints. For instance, as a minimum requirement, we need the control variables to satisfy

$$u(t) \geq 0, v(t) \geq 0.$$

[12] Note that in the given formulation the planning horizon is infinite, which is done for mathematical convenience. A finite planning horizon [0, T] can also easily be dealt with.

In the constrained budget variant, in which total spending must be proportional to the number of users, we have the additional constraint

$$u(t) + v(t) = GA(t),$$

for a positive constant, G. When the mix of interventions is also constrained, we have

$$u(t) = fGA(t), v(t) = (1-f)GA(t),$$

with a constant f between 0 and 1 ([13]).

Summarising, our optimal control problem consists of the minimisation of the objective functional subject to the state equation and constraints on the controls and/or state. Before we get to some policy conclusions, we still need to complete the model description.

Modelling consumption as $\theta Ap^{-\omega}$ is consistent with a constant elasticity model of per capita demand. The state equation describing the dynamics of the number of users has terms for initiation, outflow due to treatment, and the background rate of desistance (Figure 1). The rate of initiation is an increasing function of the current number of users (kA^a) modulated by price. The per capita rate of desistance is assumed to be a constant (μ) modulated by price. High prices suppress initiation and encourage desistance. In the absence of controls, the elasticity of the steady-state number of users with respect to price is $-a-b$. The overall, or long-term, elasticity of demand is the sum of the elasticity of demand per capita and the price

Figure 1: Flow diagram for the one-state model

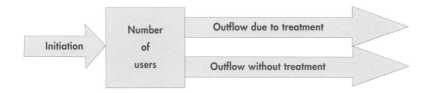

Sources: Tragler (1998); Tragler et al. (2001).

([13]) The value of f multiplied by 100 gives the percentage of the budget that is used for treatment, while the remaining part goes to enforcement.

elasticity of the number of users. Hence, we set $-(a + b + \omega)$ equal to the overall elasticity of demand.

Outflow due to treatment is modelled as being proportional to treatment spending per capita raised to an exponent (z) that reflects diminishing returns, with a small constant in the denominator (δ) that prevents division by zero. In particular,

$$\beta\big(A(t), u(t)\big) = \left(\frac{u(t)}{A(t) + \delta}\right)^{z}.$$

We take our model of enforcement's effect on price from Caulkins et al. (1997):

$$p\big(A(t), v(t)\big) = d + e\,\frac{v(t)}{A(t) + \varepsilon},$$

where ε is an arbitrarily small constant that avoids division by zero. The parameter d captures the fact that prohibition itself forces suppliers to operate in inefficient ways (what Reuter, 1983, calls 'structural consequences of product illegality'). Because of enforcement swamping, the marginal effectiveness of enforcement (e) is multiplied by enforcement effort relative to market size ($v(t)/A(t)$), not total enforcement effort.

Conclusions from the analysis of the model

For reasons of brevity, we restrict ourselves to the most interesting insights that are provided by the analysis of the model, for which parameter values were chosen that describe the actual cocaine epidemic in the US (see Tragler, 1998, for the analysis in full detail).

The basic conclusions of this model are that, if one initiates control early, when there are relatively few users, and the problem is truly an epidemic in the sense that initiation into drug use is driven by contact with current users, then one should apply both enforcement and treatment very aggressively to short circuit the epidemic spread. Otherwise, the optimal policy is not to stop the growth of the epidemic, but rather to moderate it. Initially, this should be done primarily by enforcement, to keep prices high and suppress initiation to a maximum extent. Over time, enforcement spending should increase, but not nearly as fast as treatment spending. Hence, treatment should receive a larger share of control resources when a drug problem is mature than when it is first growing. If initiation rates subsequently drop, for example because the drug develops a negative reputation, and the problem shrinks, then treatment funding should be reduced, but enforcement should be cut even more aggressively.

The model generates a variety of other insights, including: (i) a quick detection of the onset of a drug epidemic is valuable because total costs are much lower if control begins early; (ii) people who perceive drug use to be costly for society should favour greater drug control spending and allocating a greater proportion of that spending to enforcement; and (iii) sharp price declines, such as those observed in the 1980s for cocaine in the US, do not necessarily imply a policy failure; indeed, it can even be optimal to have such declines.

A two-state model for the US cocaine epidemic

The model described above does not present a conclusive treatise on optimal dynamic drug control for at least two reasons. First, it is very simple; for example, it uses just one state variable to reflect drug use. Second, the controls are restricted to treatment and price-raising enforcement. In a parallel effort, Behrens et al. (2000a) compared treatment and prevention in a model that differentiates between light and heavy users (see Figure 2) ([14]). This two-state model is an extension of Everingham and Rydell's (1994) model for the demand of cocaine. A significant limitation of the latter model was that initiation was scripted. Future projections and policy simulation exercises were predicated on a fixed projection of future initiation that is insensitive to the course of the drug epidemic. That is problematic because the current prevalence of use significantly influences initiation rates. In particular, most people who start using drugs do so through contact with a friend or sibling who is already using. Indeed, the metaphor of a drug 'epidemic' is commonly used precisely because of this tendency for current users to 'recruit' new users. If that were the only mechanism by which current use affected initiation, one might expect initiation to increase monotonically. Musto (1987) argued that, in addition, knowledge of the possible adverse effects of drug use acts as a deterrent or brake on initiation. He hypothesised that drug epidemics eventually burn out when a new generation of potential users becomes aware of the dangers of problem drug use and, as a result, does not start to use drugs. Whereas many light users work, uphold family responsibilities, and generally do not manifest obvious adverse effects of drug use, a significant fraction of heavy users are visible reminders of the dangers of using addictive substances. Hence, one might expect large numbers of heavy users to suppress rates of initiation into drug use.

([14]) The distinction between light and heavy users is made so as to reflect data from the national household survey of drug abuse (NIDA, 1991) which measures the prevalence of cocaine use among the US household population. In particular, people who reported using cocaine at least weekly were defined as heavy users, while those who consumed at least once within the last year but used less than weekly were called light users. The average heavy user consumes cocaine at a rate approximately seven times that of an average light user and exhibits substantially greater adverse consequences associated with that drug use.

Figure 2: Flow diagram for the two-state model

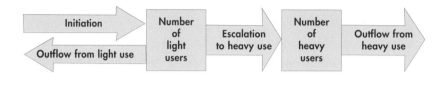

Source: Behrens et al. (1999, 2000a).

To incorporate Musto's (1987) hypothesis into their two-state model, Behrens et al. (1999, 2000a) investigated about 60 functional forms. Eventually they chose one of those five functional forms which gave the best system performance with respect to minimisation of the squared differences between modelled and observed initiation data from 1970 to 1991. As is demonstrated in Figure 3, the fit of the modelled epidemic is not perfect; the historical data reflect a higher, sharper peak in light use. Nevertheless, the similarity is striking given that the actual epidemic was subject to a varying set of drug control interventions over time that could be responsible for deviations from the model's uncontrolled path. Likewise, idiosyncratic historical events, such as Len Bias's death and the sharp increases in

Figure 3: Time paths of the continuously modelled US cocaine epidemic and the smoothed historical data

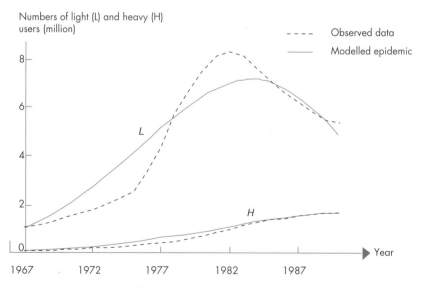

Sources: Behrens et al. (1999, 2000a) for time paths; Everingham and Rydell (1994) for the smoothed historical data.

prices in late 1989, could account for some of the differences between historical and modelled data. Also, of course, we cannot expect a perfect fit for a relatively simple model of a very complicated process such as the current US cocaine epidemic.

For results of the optimally controlled light and heavy users model with prevention and treatment as controls, we refer to Behrens et al. (2000a); extensions of this model including, as a third state, a memory of past heavy users can be found in Behrens et al. (2000b; 2002), and are reviewed in Behrens and Tragler (2001).

More complex optimal control models of illicit drug use

The two models above describe in different detail the current US cocaine epidemic, but they neglect additional characteristics of illicit drug use. Below, we briefly sketch three other dynamic optimisation models, which incorporate drug-related property crimes, the spread of blood-borne diseases in a population of IDUs, or age as a second independent variable (in addition to time *t*).

Price-raising drug enforcement and property crime

The starting point of Caulkins et al.'s (2000) model is the observation that price-raising drug enforcement suppresses drug use, but that it is also expensive and may increase property crime. This has led to contradictory recommendations concerning how drug enforcement should or should not be used. They reconcile these recommendations by incorporating the enforcement's effects on both drug use and on property crime within an optimal-control model that recognises whether convicted, drug-involved, property offenders are merely incarcerated or whether they also receive some form of drug treatment.

This model is a direct adaptation of the one-state model by Tragler et al. (2001) described in detail above. On the one hand, it simplifies the latter model by omitting spending on standard forms of treatment. On the other hand, it extends it to include property crime. In technical terms, the property crime model by Caulkins et al. (2000) uses one state variable (the number of users) and one control variable (price-raising law enforcement). The objective functional in this case determines the optimal trade-off between social costs of drug use, social costs of property crime, arresting and incarceration costs, and the costs of enforcement.

Optimal control of methadone treatment in preventing blood-borne disease

MMT has two major effects on illicit drug users. Firstly, it reduces the consumption of heroin use. Secondly, and increasingly importantly, it can prevent blood-borne diseases. Pollack (2000, 2001a, b) provides an explicit epidemiological model to explore the impact of problem drug use treatment on the incidence and prevalence of HCV and HIV. Studying the cost-effectiveness of methadone treatment, Pollack computes the cost (average and marginal) per infection averted. Although his approach is intertemporal, the number of 'treatment slots', M, may not vary over time in his model. More precisely, he minimises the cost per averted infection by comparing various constant values of M.

The purpose of ongoing research (e.g. Gavrila et al., submitted) is to extend Pollack's analyses to dynamic cost-effectiveness studies in which M acts as a time-dependent control variable. The performance functional contains (at least) two terms, i.e. the social costs created by the incidence or prevalence of HCV/HIV cases, and the costs of MMT.

Age-structured models

Almeder et al. (in press) introduce a model for drug initiation that extends traditional dynamic models by considering explicitly the age distribution of the users. As in the two-state model by Behrens et al. (2000a), it also relies on negative reputational feedback, but it is assumed that older drug users suppress initiation by younger people. This model is simpler than that of Behrens et al. (2000a) in that it considers all drug users to be similar. There is no distinction between light users (who promote initiation) and heavy users (who suppress initiation). This model is more complicated, though, in that it explicitly considers the age structure of users and non-users.

This additional complexity is appealing, given that drug initiation is a social process and age differences are important in social interactions. For example, for a teenager considering whether to initiate drug use, the fact that many other teenagers are using the drug might be a positive inducement. However, if drug use is associated with the teenager's parents' generation, drug use may be less appealing. Conceivably, contrary impulses might mean that drug use by the parents' generation might even suppress initiation by youth.

Figure 4: Initiation rates for cannabis (dark blue curve) and opiates (light blue curve) among Italian regular army troops in 1994 as functions of age

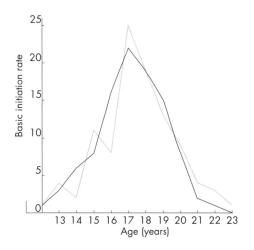

Source: UNDCP (1997).

Another motivation for considering age-structured populations comes from the well-known fact that initiation rates depend crucially on age (see Figure 4). Consequently, an appealing aspect of age-structured models is the possibility of also making the controls age specific. In particular, when it comes to school-based prevention programmes, the policy question arises as to at which age classes these programmes should best be targeted.

From a mathematical point of view, optimal control models taking age into account as an additional independent variable are less appealing, because they are substantially more complicated. In this area of 'distributed parameter control', the equations to be solved are partial differential equations, which are inherently difficult to analyse. Moreover, optimal control models, including the abovementioned interactions between individuals of different age groups, could not be analysed before the development of new solution techniques (e.g. Feichtinger et al., 2003). In other words, these models are always at the edge of tractability.

Conclusions

Optimal control models of illicit drug consumption, such as the ones cited in this chapter, provide a powerful tool for understanding and controlling drug epidemics. In particular, they enable the development of optimal control strategies that typically consist of a dynamic mix of interventions such as prevention, treatment, and law enforcement.

The optimal control framework is very general. It allows modelling of all kinds of aspects that typically arise in the context of illicit drug use. As we saw in the examples above, it is possible, for example, to include the impact of blood-borne diseases such as HCV or HIV in a model of IDUs. Also, there is a free choice of the state variables, the control variables, the constraints, and even the target, which is described by the objective functional ([15]).

However, there are, of course, limitations. Firstly, it is necessary to stress the fact that basically all the optimal control models investigated so far are complex enough for their analysis to serve as a Ph.D. topic in mathematics, even if they are of such a seemingly simple structure as the one-state model described above. In other words, the analysis is hard and demands lots of time. Beyond that, we may expect that future models will be of even higher complexity, making the analysis typically harder rather than easier ([16]).

Secondly, whereas there are basically no limitations in setting up a model of arbitrarily high complexity, there is no guarantee that such a model can be analysed at all. In fact, it needs a lot of experience to create models that are within the bounds of tractability and yet interesting for public policy.

Thirdly, and probably most importantly, data limitations set the strongest restriction on what can be done. As noted at the beginning of this chapter, the lack of appropriate data for EU drug problems so far has been the main reason for the operations researchers' focus on the current US cocaine epidemic, for which sufficiently reliable data are available. Hence, one of the major issues in EU drug policy should be the collection and processing of appropriate data ([17]), which would allow the direct application of tools that have already been applied successfully elsewhere.

([15]) Most of the existing models minimise the sum of social costs and control costs. Another specification is provided by Kaya (2004), who solves the problem of finding a time optimal control to get from some initial state to a target state.
([16]) The parallel development of new solution techniques, as well as computer hard- and software, enable us to deal with more complex models without losing tractability.
([17]) A minimum data set required to apply these models in a serious way includes: time series of incidence, numbers of users, quitting, and amounts consumed; budget data over several years such as prevention, treatment, and enforcement spending; time series of price data; and social cost estimates. Ideally, the numbers of users would be split into groups with different levels of use (e.g. occasional versus heavy use). Of course, any additional information makes the models and the according policy conclusions more realistic (e.g. proportions of users receiving treatment, effects of treatment on quitting).

Acknowledgements

This research was partly financed by the Austrian Science Foundation (FWF) under grant No P14060-OEK ('Dynamics and control of illicit drug consumption'). The helpful and inspiring comments of three anonymous referees are gratefully acknowledged.

References

Almeder, C., Caulkins, J. P., Feichtinger, G., Tragler, G. (in press), 'An age-structured single-state drug initiation model — cycles of drug epidemics and optimal prevention programs', *Socio-Economic Planning Sciences* 38: 91–109.

Behrens, D. A., Tragler, G. (2001), 'The dynamic process of dynamic modelling: the cocaine epidemic in the United States', *Bulletin on Narcotics* LIII: 65–78.

Behrens, D. A., Caulkins, J. P., Tragler, G., Feichtinger, G., Haunschmied, J. L. (1999), 'A dynamic model of drug initiation: implications for treatment and drug control', *Mathematical Biosciences* 159: 1–20.

Behrens, D. A., Caulkins, J. P., Tragler, G., Feichtinger, G. (2000a), 'Optimal control of drug epidemics: prevent and treat — but not at the same time?', *Management Science* 46(3): 333–47.

Behrens, D. A., Caulkins, J. P., Tragler, G., Feichtinger, G. (2000b), *Memory, contagion, and capture rates: characterising the types of addictive behaviour that are prone to repeated epidemics*, Research Report 251, Institute for Econometrics, Operations Research and Systems Theory, Vienna University of Technology, Vienna.

Behrens, D. A., Caulkins, J. P., Tragler, G., Feichtinger, G. (2002), 'Why present-oriented societies undergo cycles of drug epidemics', *Journal of Economic Dynamics and Control* 26: 919–36.

Caulkins, J. P. (1998), 'The cost-effectiveness of civil remedies: the case of drug control interventions', in Green Mazerolle, L., Roehl, J. (eds), *Crime Prevention Studies* 9: 219–37.

Caulkins, J. P., Reuter, P. (1997), 'Setting goals for drug policy: harm reduction or use reduction', *Addiction* 92: 1143–50.

Caulkins, J. P., Reuter, P. (1998), 'What price data tell us about drug markets', *Journal of Drug Issues* 28, 593–612.

Caulkins, J. P., Crawford, G., Reuter, P. (1993), 'Simulation of adaptive response: a model of drug interdiction', *Mathematical and Computer Modelling* 17: 37–52.

Caulkins, J. P., Rydell, C. P., Schwabe, W. L., Chiesa, J. (1997), *Mandatory minimum drug sentences: throwing away the key or the taxpayers' money?*, RAND, Santa Monica, CA.

Caulkins, J. P., Dworak, M., Feichtinger, G., Tragler, G. (2000), 'Price-raising drug enforcement and property crime: a dynamic model', *Journal of Economics* 71: 227–53.

Everingham, S. S., Rydell, C. P. (1994), *Modelling the demand for cocaine*, RAND, Santa Monica, CA.

Feichtinger, G., Hartl, R. F. (1986), *Optimale Kontrolle ökonomischer Prozesse — anwendungen des Maximumprinzips in den Wirtschaftswissenschaften*, DeGruyter, Berlin.

Feichtinger, G., Tragler, G., Veliov, V. (2003), 'Optimal conditions for age-structured control systems; *Journal of Mathematic Analysis and Applications* 288: 47–68.

Gardiner, L. K., Shreckengost, R. C. (1987), 'A system dynamics model for estimating heroin imports into the United States', *System Dynamics Review* 3: 8–27.

Gavrila, C., Pollack, H. A., Caulkins, J. P., Kort, P. M., Feichtinger, G., Tragler, G. (submitted), 'Optimal control of harm reduction in preventing blood-borne diseases among drug users'.

Homer, J. B. (1993), 'A system dynamics model for cocaine prevalence estimation and trend projection', *Journal of Drug Issues* 23: 251–79.

Kaya, C. Y. (2004), 'Time-optimal switching control for the US cocaine epidemic', *Socio-Economic Planning Sciences* 38: 57–72.

Kleiman, M. A. R. (1988), 'Crackdowns: the effects of intensive enforcement on retail heroin dealing', in Chaiken, M. R. (ed.), *Street-level drug enforcement: examining the issues*, National Institute of Justice, Washington, DC.

Kleiman, M. A. R. (1993), 'Enforcement swamping: a positive-feedback mechanism in rates of illicit activity', *Mathematical and Computer Modelling* 17: 65–75.

Leonard, D., Long, N. V. (1992), *Optimal control theory and static optimisation in economics*, Cambridge University Press, Cambridge, MA.

Levin, G., Roberts, E. B., Hirsch, G. B. (1975), *The persistent poppy: a computer-aided search for heroin policy*, Ballinger Publishing Company, Cambridge, MA.

Moore, M. H. (1973), 'Achieving discrimination on the effective price of heroin', *American Economic Review* 63: 270–7.

Musto, D. F. (1987), *The American disease: origins of narcotic control*, Oxford University Press, New York.

National Institute on Drug Abuse (NIDA) (1991), *Overview of the 1991 household survey of drug abuse*, press release, December.

Office of National Drug Control Policy (1999), *1999 national drug control strategy*, The White House, Washington, DC.

Pollack, H. (2000), 'The cost-effectiveness of methadone in preventing blood-borne disease: a comparison of HIV and hepatitis C', working paper.

Pollack, H. (2001a), 'Controlling infectious diseases among injection drug users: learning (the right) lessons from HIV', working paper.

Pollack, H. (2001b), Cost-effectiveness of harm reduction in preventing hepatitis C among injection drug users', *Medical Decision Making*, September–October, 357–67.

Reuter, P. (1983), *Disorganised crime: the economics of the visible hand*, MIT Press, Cambridge, MA.

Reuter, P., Kleiman, M. A. R. (1986), 'Risks and prices: an economic analysis of drug enforcement', in Morris, N., Tonry, M. (eds), *Crime and justice: a review of research*, University of Chicago Press, Chicago, IL.

Rydell, C. P., Caulkins, J. P., Everingham, S. S. (1996), 'Enforcement or treatment? Modelling the relative efficacy of alternatives for controlling cocaine', *Operations Research* 44: 687–95.

Schlenger, W. E. (1973), 'A systems approach to drug user services', *Behavioural Science* 18: 137–47.

Stares, P. B. (1996), *Global habit: the drug problem in a borderless world*, Brookings Institute, Washington, DC.

Tragler, G. (1998), 'Optimal control of illicit drug consumption: treatment versus enforcement', Ph.D. thesis, Institute for Econometrics, Operations Research and System Theory, Vienna University of Technology, Vienna.

Tragler, G., Caulkins, J. P., Feichtinger, G. (2001), 'Optimal dynamic allocation of treatment and enforcement in illicit drug control', *Operations Research* 49: 352–62.

United Nations Drug Control Programme (UNDCP) (1997), *World drug report*, Oxford University Press, Oxford.

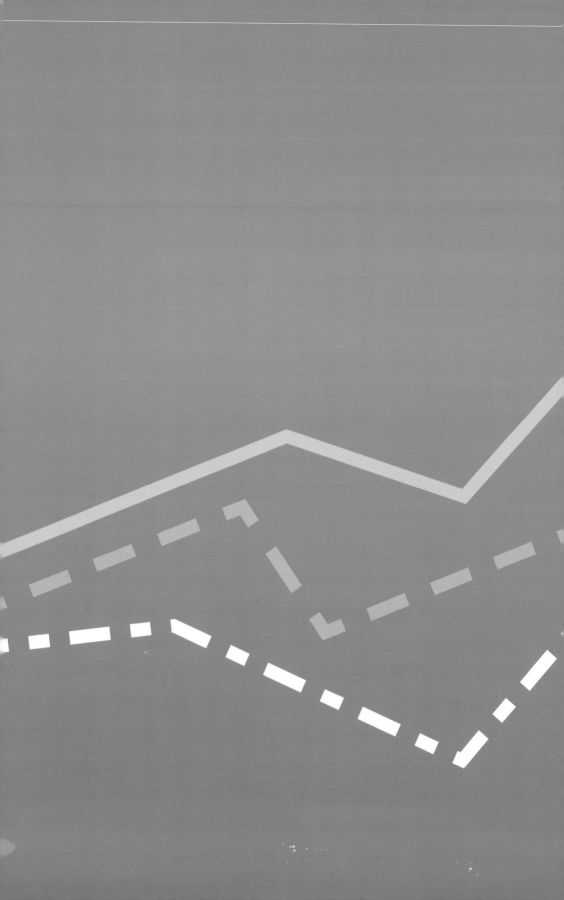

Healthcare costs of drug-related hepatitis C infection

PART III

Introduction

Part III of this monograph deals with the direct healthcare costs of drug-related HCV infection. However, contributions to this part do have a broader reach than this description suggests. Postma et al. present estimates of drug-related costs due to HCV infection in conjunction with such estimates for two other important drug use transmissible infections: HBV and HIV. Wong et al. present a full pharmaco-economic evaluation for antiretroviral combination therapy for HCV. Both contributions have in common that the focus is on direct healthcare costs, in contrast to Part IV in which wider cost categories are considered.

In pharmaco-economics, several classifications are used for expressing the consequences of disease on resource utilisation: direct (for example, hospital care) versus indirect costs of production losses, medical (healthcare) versus non-medical costs (for example, those related to care by family and friends) and patient-related versus general programme costs. These classifications have been widely used to address the economic impact of the HIV/AIDS epidemic (Postma, 1998). Direct healthcare costs considered in this part are all patient related; i.e. the patient is the cost driver. General programme costs (such as those of detoxification facilities), indirect costs of production losses, and non-medical costs are considered in Part IV.

Furthermore, pharmaco-economics deploys various methods for economic evaluation. Three major areas distinguished are: cost-of-illness studies, cost-effectiveness analyses and cost-utility analyses (Postma, in press). The contribution by Postma et al. is a cost-of-illness assessment, whereas that by Wong et al. integrates the approaches of cost-effectiveness and cost–utility analyses. The former contribution therefore touches on two crucial discussions in cost-of-illness assessments — the usefulness of these types of studies in general, and the development of guidelines for appropriate costing. The latter study considers central issues in cost-effectiveness and cost–utility — such as discounting of health gains in terms of life years and quality of life gained.

Cost of illness in IDUs has been investigated for HIV in several instances, for example in the framework of the EU concerted action on multinational AIDS scenarios (Postma, 1998). To enhance the relevance of cost-of-illness assessments, several projects have been undertaken to develop guidelines for a generic approach. Again, some of this work has been centred around the topic of HIV economics, for example in the framework of an EU project (Tolley and Gyldmark, 1993). The current estimate by Postma et al. in this part reflects an update of a previous attempt (Postma et al., 2001) and amounts to approximately EUR 1.4 billion for drug-related HCV costs in France, Germany, Italy, Portugal, Spain and the UK (1999 price level). Extrapolated to the whole of the EU, and taken together with the costs of drug-related HBV and HIV, these costs reflect approximately 0.5 % of total EU healthcare expenditures.

Cost-of-illness studies have encountered criticism in the scientific literature (Drummond, 1992). It has been argued that: (i) its usefulness for decision-making is limited; (ii) exact costing may be done using various methods; and (iii) it may be arbitrary where to draw the line with respect to the inclusion and exclusion of various cost sectors. (i) Plain assessment of cost figures may be of limited importance, in particular if the investigator neglects to put these figures into the appropriate perspective. However, putting figures into perspective (for example, by expressing them as a percentage of total healthcare expenditures) helps decision-makers to understand the relative impacts of different problems. Furthermore, we note that cost-of-illness studies are often a prerequisite for further analyses using the cost-effectiveness or cost-utility designs. (ii) Development of guidelines on how to measure and value costs may be helpful to enhance the comparability and validity of applied studies and designs. Guidelines are developed for both cost-of-illness and cost-effectiveness studies (Tolley and Gyldmark, 1993; Single et al., 1996; Hjelmgren et al., 2001). (iii) Especially with respect to cost assessments in drug users, the cost-of-illness design has been criticised regarding the choice of which cost categories to include and which to exclude (Uhl, 1998). Indeed, such a choice may sometimes seem arbitrary to the outsider and may merely reflect a consensus of those debating on the design of such studies. For example, one category that often raises debate refers to the direct medical costs in life years gained. Similarly, the total costs of drug use may be greatly inflated by the costs of police enforcement or imprisonment, which follow from arbitrary societal decisions regarding drug policy.

Wong et al. combine the cost-of-illness design with cost-effectiveness and cost–utility analyses of antiviral combination therapy. The specific combination therapy considered consists of interferon alpha 2b and ribavirin, a combination that has recently proved to double the beneficial effects of classical interferon treatment in randomised clinical trials. They deploy a previously published and validated Markov model to estimate the lifetime direct medical costs of HCV infection (Wong et al., 1998). The model was adapted to include combination therapy and allow for relapse into drug use and reinfection with HCV.

The analysis by Wong et al. allows the expression of the cost-effectiveness of combination therapy as a variety of outcomes: US dollars per life year gained, per quality-adjusted life year (QALY) gained and per discounted quality-adjusted life year (DQALY) gained. The authors focus on the outcome per DQALY gained, to enable valid comparison with other medical interventions in the US. This comparison renders that combination therapy has a favourable pharmaco-economic profile at USD 5 600 per DQALY gained in the baseline. This favourable profile is robust in sensitivity analysis.

With respect to their design, we note that Wong et al. exclude direct medical costs in life years gained. This is in line with some but opposes other country-specific pharmaco-economic guidelines. Also, these guidelines recommend discounting costs, benefits and health. The procedure of discounting covers time preference: we attach a higher value to current money and health than to future money and health. We note that Wong et al. focus on discounted results, whereas undiscounted amounts are also reported. This appreciates the recent discussions on the appropriateness of discounting health gains at similar percentages as monetary amounts, although guidelines do generally favour discounting of money and health gains at similar percentages (Hjelmgren et al., 2001).

Maarten Postma

References

Drummond, M. (1992), 'Cost-of-illness studies: a major headache?', *Pharmacoeconomics* 2: 1–4.

Hjelmgren, J., Berggren, F., Andersson, F. (2001), 'Health economic guidelines — similarities, differences and some implications', *Value in Health* 4: 225–50.

Postma, M. J. (1998), 'Assessment of the economic impact of AIDS at national and multi-national level', Thesis at the University of Maastricht (the Netherlands).

Postma, M. J. (in press), 'Pharmaco-economic research', *Pharmacy, World and Science*.

Postma, M. J., Wiessing, L. G., Jager, J. C. (2001), 'Pharmaco-economics of drug addiction: estimating the costs of hepatitis C virus, hepatitis B virus and human immunodeficiency virus infection among injecting drug users in Member States of the European Union', *UN Bulletin on Narcotics* 53 (1/2): 79–89.

Single, E., Collins, D., Easton, B., Harwood, H., Lapsey, H., Maynard, A. (1996), *International guidelines for estimating the costs of substance abuse*, Canadian Centre on Substance Abuse, Ottawa.

Tolley, K., Gyldmark, M. (1993), 'The treatment and care costs of people with HIV infection and AIDS; development of a standardised framework for Europe', *Health Policy* 24: 55–70.

Uhl, A. (1998), 'Evaluation of primary prevention in the field of illicit drugs: definitions — concepts — problems', in Springer, A., Uhl, A. (eds), *Evaluation research in regard to primary prevention of drug abuse*, European Commission Social Sciences, Brussels.

Wong, J. B., Bennett, W. G., Koff, R. S., Pauker, S. G. (1998), 'Pre-treatment evaluation of chronic hepatitis C: risks, benefits and costs', *JAMA* 280: 2088–93.

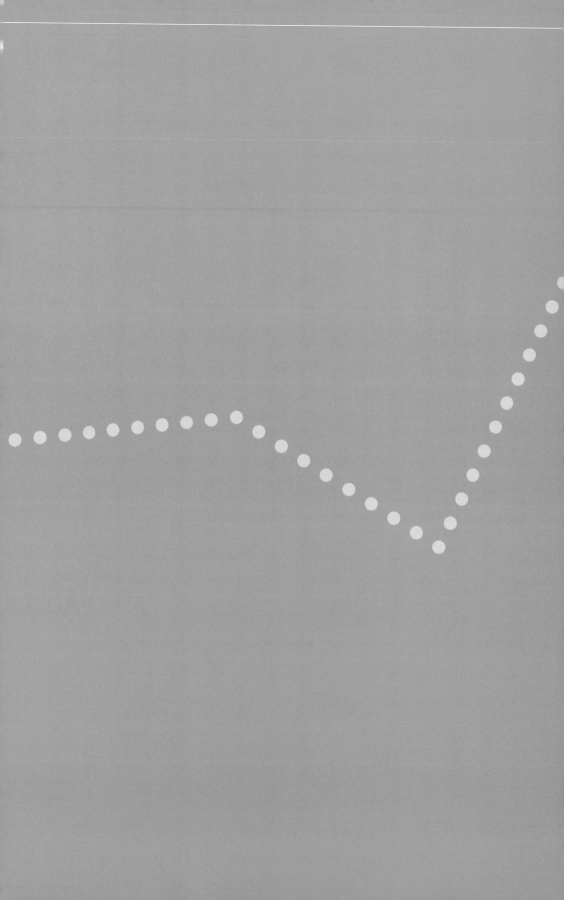

Chapter 8
Updated healthcare cost estimates for drug-related hepatitis C infections in the European Union

Maarten Postma, Lucas Wiessing and Johannes Jager

Drug addiction presents yet another area for application of pharmaco-economics. Whereas, traditionally, pharmaco-economics is primarily applied to evaluations of drug therapies, aspects of drug addiction may equally well be approached using pharmaco-economic concepts. In particular, healthcare resource utilisation may be such an aspect where pharmaco-economics may be applied without much controversy. Controversies have arisen with respect to other types of social costs, in particular for those types where opportunity costing may be less appropriate (Postma et al., 2001). This chapter aims to develop a generic approach to estimate drug-related healthcare costs for some major drug use transmitted viruses.

Previously, we reported on the pharmaco-economics of drug addiction by presenting a preliminary estimate of healthcare costs due to HCV, HBV and human immunodeficiency virus (HIV) in the EU (Postma et al., 2001). The background of our study was the growing interest in pharmaco-economic evaluation in the fight against infectious diseases through interventions such as vaccination, screening, enhanced safety of blood transfusion and NSPs. Increasingly, decision-making bodies in EU countries demand evidence of favourable pharmaco-economic profiles — such as cost-effectiveness ratios — before interventions are implemented (Hjelmgren et al., 2001). In this respect, pharmaco-economic profiles are assessed using randomised studies, observational designs and model simulations. Preventive interventions offer no exemption from this trend; cost-effectiveness estimates of interventions to prevent infectious diseases among drug users are increasingly required. As a prerequisite to cost-effectiveness assessments, cost-of-illness studies have to be performed. Such studies provide insight into the direct healthcare costs that may be averted by preventive intervention.

Our previous analysis presented the cost of illness in 10 selected EU countries for HCV, HBV and HIV related to injecting drug use, with the purpose of providing the basic information for cost-effectiveness analyses. In the baseline estimate, costs of drug-related HCV, HBV and HIV infection amount to EUR 1.89 billion per year for selected EU Member States (1995 price level). This corresponds to 0.4 % of the expenditure of EU Member States on healthcare. HCV accounted for 39 % of these costs with EUR 750 million (HIV: 59 % and HBV: 2 %). Figure 1 shows the country-specific results (Postma et al., 2001). Our current analysis investigates updated cost analyses for injecting-drug-use-related HCV for the six major impact countries: France, Germany, Italy, Portugal, Spain and the UK, comprising 96 % of drug-related HCV costs in those 10 EU countries studied previously (Figure 2).

In this chapter, we aim to further improve the cost-of-illness assessment, in particular with respect to HCV costing. Whereas accurate data for the costs of HIV were available and reliable estimates could be made, for HCV, scarce data availability allowed only rough assessments. Furthermore, pharmacotherapy for HCV has changed drastically recently with the introduction of combination therapy of recombinant interferon alpha and ribavirin, changing the spectrum of HCV costs. Ribavirin is now registered and officially priced in many EU countries. Here, we adapt a French model for the progression of disease for HCV infection through the various stages of complications, incorporating the costs and effects of combination therapy (Loubière et al., 2001). This model was developed within the framework of transfusion safety, with respect to the introduction of nucleic acid testing for HCV for blood donors. We adapted this model to fit French drug users

Figure 1: Costs of HCV, HBV and HIV (million EUR; 1995 price level) for 10 EU countries prior to HCV combination therapy

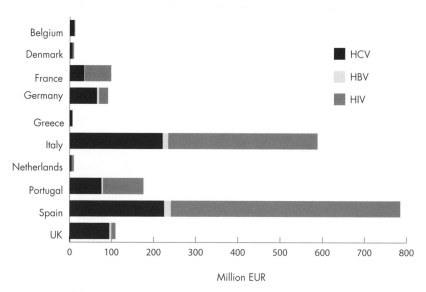

Source: Postma et al. (2001).

Figure 2: Percentage distribution of drug-related HCV costs for 10 EU countries prior to HCV combination therapy

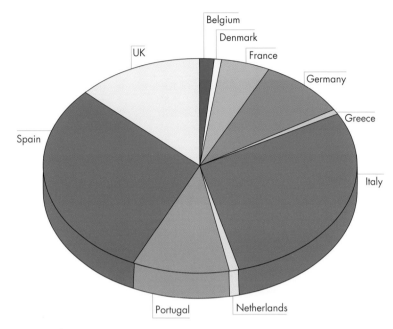

Source: Postma et al. (2001).

instead of transfusion recipients. Next, we extrapolated the model to other countries.

Methods

Markov model for HCV in drug users

To estimate lifetime costs of HCV in drug users, a published Markov model was adapted that describes HCV disease progression in infected blood donors through several compartments (on pharmacotherapy, active HCV infection, cirrhosis, decompensated cirrhosis, HC, transplantation and death) (Loubière et al., 2001). The model distinguishes two phases (Figure 3): during the first 1.5 years, patients are merely distributed over the two stages of 'recovery' and 'active HCV', with some intermediate stages during the process (chronic hepatitis, on combination therapy). Only after these first 1.5 years do the typical Markovian annual transition rates become operational to describe the risks for going from one stage (for example, HC) to another (for example, death). Figure 3 summarises this

Figure 3: Progression of disease for HCV infection in (ex-)drug users during (a) the first 1.5 years after HCV infection, and (b) annual rates of progression after 1.5 years after HCV infection (adapted from Loubière et al., 2001)

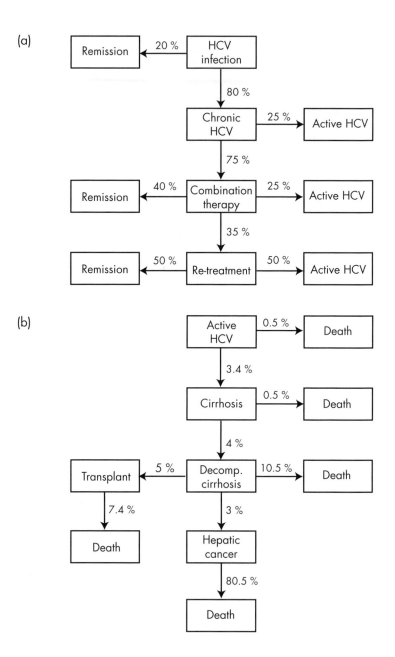

progression of disease for HCV-infected drug users (for the current purpose, at high aggregation level, no differences are made with respect to progression of disease varying over age, vital loads, genotypes, alcohol consumption, etc.).

As shown, the model includes combination (re-)treatment with interferon and ribavirin, with 40 and 50 % success in treatment and re-treatment, respectively (25 % are assumed to have contraindications for interferon treatment). Additionally, it was assumed that almost 60 % of those initially failing on combination treatment were eligible for retreatment (Loubière et al., 2001). The major adaptation of the originally published model referred to the annual risk of developing cirrhosis: 3.4 % in the current model versus 5.9 % in the published model (Kim et al., 1997). This adaptation was based on calibrating the cirrhosis risk to arrive at a 20-year likelihood of developing cirrhosis of 48 % (Wong et al., Chapter 9). Also, limited data suggest that patients with transfusion-acquired HCV may have an accelerated rate of liver progression compared with patients with injecting-drug-use-acquired HCV (Wong et al., Chapter 9). As recent data have suggested that progression may be even slower, we included lower progression rates in sensitivity analysis at 20-year progression rates of 25 and 8 % (Seeff, 1999; Freeman et al., 2001). Furthermore, on top of the distributions and transition rates for HCV progression, in the staged Markov model, mortality related to (past) drug use was inserted at 0.5 % per year for (ex-)drug users (UNDCP, 1997). This percentage may reflect a conservative assumption, and for active IDUs figures of up to 1 to 2 % have been found (EMCDDA, 2002). Ideally, a weighted average should be calculated with the weights reflecting the respective proportions of active and ex-drug users. However, data to estimate these weights were not available.

The Markov model was applied to an (ex-)drug user diagnosed with HCV at the age of 25 years. Given this relatively young age, non-drug-related mortality (mortality due to other causes) was neglected in the analysis. Given rapidly changing pharmacotherapy and treatment patterns for HCV complications, the time horizon of the Markov model was limited to 25 years. Other models evaluating cost of illness and/or cost-effectiveness of interventions in hepatitis have often chosen longer time frames, up to 50 to 70 years. Given the procedure of discounting (see below) the impact of an extended time horizon can only be limited.

Stage-specific HCV costing

Cost estimates for the different stages of HCV infection were readily available for France (Table 1). For the figures on interferon alpha and ribavirin, 3 million IU tiw

Table 1: **Annual treatment costs per patient for different stages of HCV progression in France (EUR; 1999 price level)**

	EUR
Cirrhosis	1 400
Decompensated cirrhosis	11 400
Hepatocellular carcinoma	10 400
Transplantation (first year)	91 500
Transplantation (follow-up)	7 900
Interferon	3 660
Ribavirin	8 350

and 1 000 mg/day orally, respectively, were assumed (standard treatment doses in many countries). Lifetime cost estimates of HCV infection result from combining the Markov model for progression of disease (Figure 1) and excess mortality for (ex-)drug use (Table 1).

Extrapolation to other countries

Lifetime cost estimates were corrected for time preference applying a discount rate of 4 %, recommended for several EU countries such as the Netherlands or being in between recommendations for some other countries (CVZ, 1996; Gold et al., 1996; see also www.nice.org.uk). Discounting is the cumulative application of a negative annual weighting factor to future costs to reflect a time preference for delaying costs in general (vice versa, we generally prefer to enjoy benefits as early as possible). Discounting is different from inflation correction and should be applied on top of inflation correction if appropriate.

For major impact countries other than France, only the costs of interferon and ribavirin could be generically estimated (Table 2). This was done by assuming that interferon/ribavirin costs constitute the same proportion of total HCV costs as for France. Per country, a correction was applied for the relative prices of pharmaceuticals and medical care in different countries. For this correction, we applied the ratio of purchasing power parities (PPPs) in pre-euro national currencies per US dollars for pharmaceuticals and medical care (source: OECD health database, 2000; pre-euro national currencies were used, depending on the availability of information). The purchasing power parity may be conceived as an alternative to exchange rates, relating the prices of a similar bundle of healthcare goods in two countries to each other. For Germany, Italy, Portugal, Spain and the UK, this ratio was normalised on the French ratio of 1:24 (Table 2). A ratio of

Table 2: Annual treatment costs per patient for interferon alpha and ribavirin and normalised PPP ratio (see text) for six selected countries (EUR; 1999 price level)

	Interferon alpha (EUR)	Ribavirin (EUR)	Normalised PPP ratio (%)
France	3 660	8 350	100
Germany	6 900	14 250	61
Italy	11 100	11 000	102
Portugal	4 800	9 050 ([1])	85
Spain	3 500	9 050	84
UK	4 160	9 940	48

([1]) In the absence of an official Portuguese price for ribavirin, the Spanish price, in euro, was assumed.

1:24 implies that — with the US situation as baseline — pharmaceuticals are relatively expensive compared with other medical care. Lifetime HCV costs are then straightforward. For example, if French lifetime costs for HCV were equally divided over pharmaceuticals (interferon alpha and ribavirin) and medical care, the UK's medical-care lifetime costs are estimated by taking 48 % of the costs for interferon alpha and ribavirin. All in all, our method does take some crucial differences between healthcare systems into account as far as expressed in purchasing power parities.

Linking of epidemiology and costing

Two approaches for linking epidemiology and costing are generally distinguished. The prevalence-based approach links costs to prevalence estimates and is more appropriate if current budget impacts are the primary interest. If the full future pharmaco-economic impact is what is being referred to in a decision context — i.e. the avoidable costs — the incidence-based approach is the more appropriate for linking epidemiology and healthcare costs (Postma et al., 2001). This is the case if the decision context refers to investments and allocating budgets in the prevention of drug-addiction-related problems (Pollack, 2001). Therefore, this chapter reports results using the incidence-based approach.

Incidence estimates were taken from the previous publication (Table 3) and were conceived to apply also to the current and near future situation given the relatively stable prevalence of HCV in injecting drug users (Postma et al., 2001; see also Wiessing et al., Chapter 4). In the absence of hard national data, our HCV

Table 3: Estimated annual incidence of HCV in EU countries, mid- to end-1990s	
Belgium	1 360
Denmark	850
France	2 558
Germany	8 271
Greece	544
Italy	19 222
Netherlands	611
Portugal	9 176
Spain	27 162
UK	14 949

incidence estimates can only be very crude and should be interpreted with caution. As indicated (Postma et al., 2001), they were indirectly derived from existing incidence estimates for HIV that were calculated using the back-calculation approach (Downs et al., 2000). Specifically, the ratio of HCV and HIV prevalence as derived from multiple sources per country (EMCDDA, 2002; Wiessing et al., Chapter 4) was used to extrapolate the back-calculated HIV incidence into an estimate of HCV incidence (both in absolute numbers of annual incident cases). To our knowledge, resulting incidence estimates are currently the only national estimates available for drug users in western Europe.

Results

Estimated lifetime discounted costs per HCV infection in French drug users was estimated at EUR 14 140 (undiscounted: EUR 18 800). Of this figure, 60 % relates to interferon and ribavirin. Based on other countries' costs for interferon and ribavirin and normalised PPP ratios, discounted lifetime costs in those countries were estimated at EUR 13 100 to EUR 26 200 (Figure 4).

The incidence-based estimate of drug-related HCV costs amounts to EUR 1.43 billion for the six countries considered (1999 price level). For all 10 countries previously considered (including Belgium, Denmark, Greece and the Netherlands), the total costs may be approximately 5 % higher (Postma et al., 2001).

Figure 4: Estimated lifetime costs per hepatitis C infection after introduction of HCV combination therapy (EUR; 1999 price level)

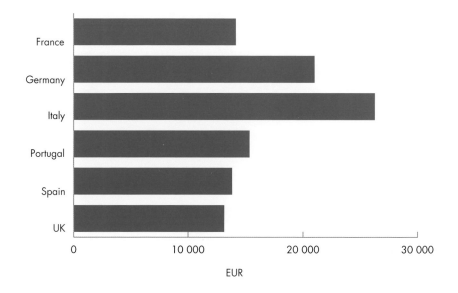

Figure 5: Costs of HCV in the previous (million 1995 EUR; Postma et al., 2001) and current updated estimates (million 1999 EUR)

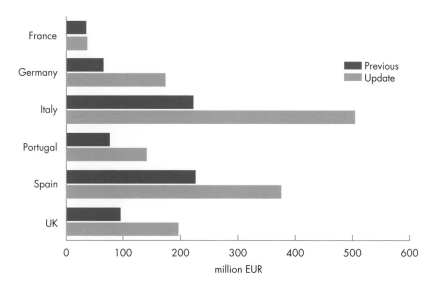

Figure 6: Sensitivity analysis on the progression to cirrhosis (48 % in 20 years in the baseline): impact on aggregate costs of HCV (EUR 1.43 billion in the baseline; 1999 price level)

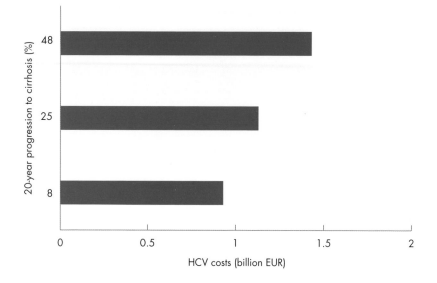

Figure 5 displays costs per country, per year of infection, both for the current estimate (in million euro; 1999 price level) and for the previous assessment (in million euro; 1995 price level; Postma et al., 2001).

Finally, Figure 6 shows the sensitivity analysis on lowering the progression to cirrhosis. Given the large share of combination treatment costs in aggregate costing, the impact of varying progression to cirrhosis is proportionally less than the lowering of the progression itself.

Discussion

Our updated estimate of incidence-based HCV costs in 10 EU countries for 1999 reflects approximately a doubling compared with our previous estimate for 1995 (EUR 750 million) (Postma et al., 2001). Our previous estimate was done in the absence of costing data, while, currently, scarce data are available. Updated higher costs primarily relate to the inclusion of relatively costly combination therapy.

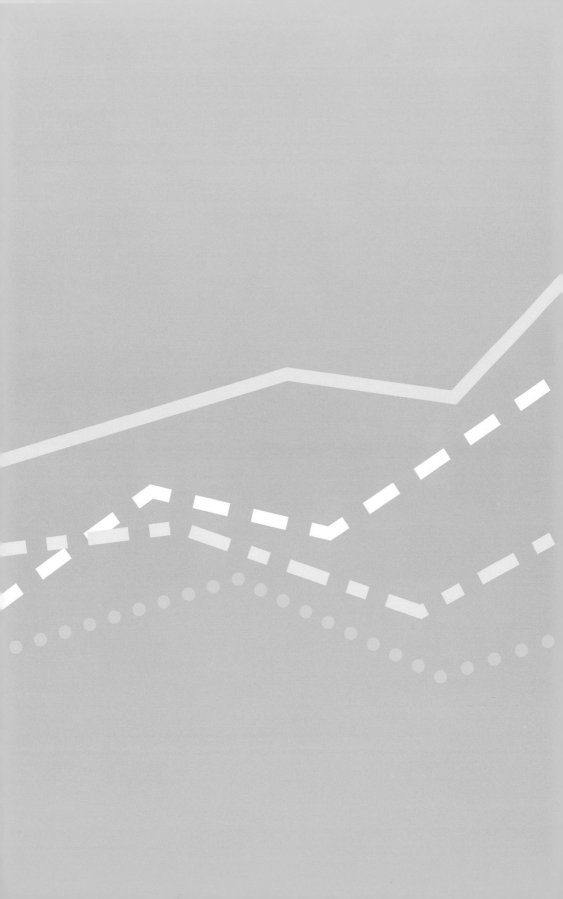

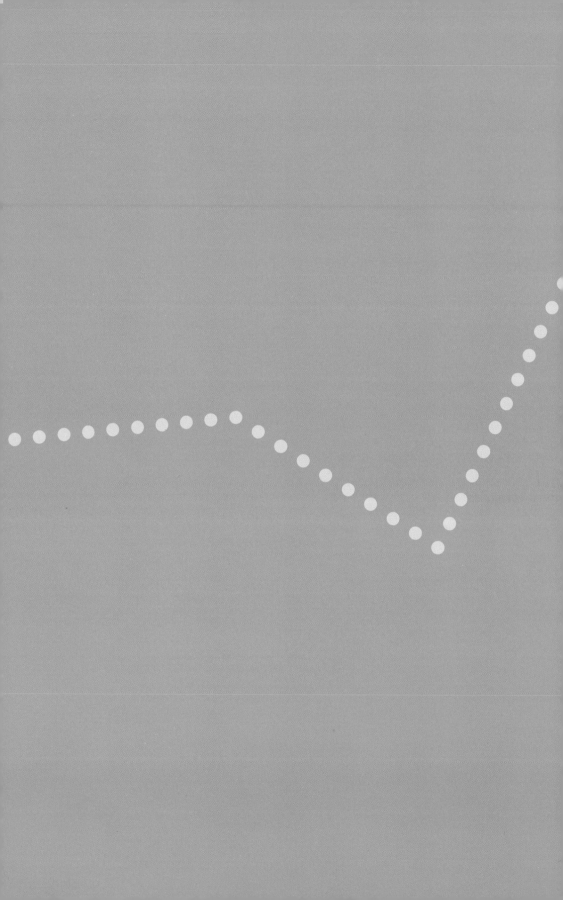

Chapter 9
Cost-effectiveness of treatment of hepatitis C in injecting drug users

John Wong, Diana Sylvestre and Uwe Siebert

Introduction

Chronic hepatitis C affects an estimated 170 million people worldwide and
5 million people in western Europe (Anonymous, 1997c; Alter et al., 1999). Now
that the blood supply is routinely screened for hepatitis C, injecting drug use is the
most important and most common route of acquisition. Most studies suggest that
50 to 96 % of IDUs have evidence of HCV infection (Bell et al., 1990; Girardi et
al., 1990; Huemer et al., 1990; Van den Hoek et al., 1990; Donahue et al.,
1991; Eyster et al., 1991; Zeldis et al., 1992; Fingerhood et al., 1993; Verbaan
et al., 1993; Tennant, 1994; Galeazzi et al., 1995; Thomas et al., 1995; Crofts
and Aitken, 1997; Selvey et al., 1997; MacDonald et al., 2000; Thorpe et al.,
2000; Hagan et al., 2001; Hope et al., 2001; Lorvick et al., 2001; McCarthy and
Flynn, 2001). In selected populations of young IDUs or NSPs, the prevalence of
hepatitis C antibody was between 27 and 45 % (Selvey et al., 1996; Garfein et
al., 1998; Thorpe et al., 2000; Hahn et al., 2001; Hope et al., 2001; Lorvick et
al., 2001). The likelihood of hepatitis C infection increases with longer duration of
drug use, higher frequency of drug use and the sharing of needles (Bell et al.,
1990; Van den Hoek et al., 1990; Donahue et al., 1991; Zeldis et al., 1992;
Thomas et al., 1995; Thorpe et al., 2000; Diaz et al., 2001). The acquisition of
hepatitis C infection in IDUs occurs rapidly, with 50 to 80 % of individuals
becoming positive for hepatitis C antibody within 6 to 12 months after initiation of
injecting drug use (Garfein et al., 1996). Thus, the US Centers for Disease Control
and Prevention recommend that individuals who have ever injected illicit drugs,
even once, be screened for hepatitis C (Anonymous, 1998b).

An insidiously progressive liver disease, chronic hepatitis C results in cirrhosis in
more than 20 % of patients after 20 years of persistent infection (Hoofnagle,
1997). In a meta-analysis of 13 studies involving 987 patients, Pagliaro et al.
(1999) found a 28 % median progression from chronic hepatitis to cirrhosis after
8 to 12 years. Although not all infected individuals develop advanced liver
disease, chronic hepatitis C is the leading cause of chronic liver disease and the

leading indication for liver transplantation in adults because of its high prevalence (Anonymous, 1997; Alter et al., 1999). Individuals developing decompensated cirrhosis or HCC from hepatitis C have a shortened life expectancy, poor quality of life, and incur substantial costs. Once advanced liver disease occurs, liver transplantation is the only treatment that could substantially improve prognosis, but it is quite expensive and the supply of donor liver organs is inadequate to meet demand. Numerous studies suggest that, despite the decrease in acute cases of hepatitis C, the morbidity, mortality and costs of treating individuals developing liver complications from hepatitis C will continue to rise over the next 10 to 20 years (Deuffic et al., 1999; Armstrong et al., 2000; Wong et al., 2000a; Davis et al., 2002). Data showing a rising incidence of hepatocellular carcinoma support the notion of rising rates of complications from hepatitis C (El-Serag and Mason, 1999).

Recent international and US randomised clinical trials (McHutchison et al., 1998; Poynard et al., 1998a), however, have shown that the combination of interferon alpha 2b and ribavirin can result in a sustained loss of detectable HCV, improved liver histology and normalisation of liver enzymes in patients with chronic hepatitis or compensated cirrhosis. Although no randomised clinical trial has sufficient follow-up to examine these outcomes, studies suggest that viral eradication improves liver histology, decreases the risk of HCC or cirrhosis and decompensation and perhaps improves survival (Anonymous, 1998a; Nishiguchi et al., 1995; Mazzella et al., 1996; Bonis et al., 1997; Camma et al., 1997; Kuwana et al., 1997; Marcellin et al., 1997; Schalm et al., 1997; Teramura et al., 1997; Benvegnu et al., 1998; Ikeda et al., 1998; Imai et al., 1998; Kasahara et al., 1998; Lau et al., 1998; Niederau et al., 1998; Poynard et al., 1998b; Serfaty et al., 1998; Reichard et al., 1999; Shindo et al., 1999; Sobesky et al., 1999). In those with chronic hepatitis C, treatment-induced viral eradication also restored impaired quality of life measures (Foster et al., 1998; Bonkovsky and Woolley, 1999; Ware et al., 1999).

Because complications from HCV may not occur for 20 to 30 years and such a randomised clinical trial might be prohibitively expensive and perhaps unethical (Bennett et al., 1996), decision analytical computer models have been developed to simulate the likely outcomes resulting from viral eradication (Bennett et al., 1997; Kim et al., 1997, 1999; Wong et al., 1998, 2000b; Inadomi and Sonnenberg, 1999; Younossi et al., 1999; Loubière et al., 2001). These analyses attempt to integrate the likelihood of antiviral therapy response, the likelihood of progressive liver disease, general population and hepatitis-C-related mortality, disease-related morbidity that affects quality of life, and the costs of antiviral treatment and of monitoring and treating the liver disease. To avoid potentially overly optimistic results in favour of antiviral treatment, some of these analyses introduce assumptions that bias their results against antiviral therapy by considering the possibility of spontaneous viral negativity without antiviral treatment, and by including the possibility for progressive liver disease despite becoming virally negative from treatment (Bennett et al., 1997; Wong et al., 1998, 2000b). By tracking each computer cohort member for each treatment strategy over time until all have died, the computer simulation credits the cohort for the proportion alive each year and for their annual medical-care expenditure, thereby estimating the average life expectancy and expected lifetime expenditures for each strategy.

Most physicians would probably encourage treatment for patients with moderate hepatitis and nearly certainly for those with bridging fibrosis or compensated cirrhosis (Wong and Koff, 2000). For IDUs, treatment remains controversial (Davis and Rodrigue, 2001; Edlin et al., 2001). Three consensus conferences suggest treatment only in individuals who have stopped drug use (Anonymous, 1997, 1999b; Sherman, 1997) although the most recent conference suggests evaluation on a case-by-case basis (Anonymous, 2002; Edlin, 2002). Reasons to withhold treatment include considerations of potential poor compliance with treatment and follow-up, treatment side effects and expense, risk of reinfection and the relatively slowly progressive natural history of hepatitis C (Edlin et al., 2001). Nonetheless, antiviral treatment for hepatitis C has been undertaken successfully in IDUs (Backmund et al., 2001; Jowett et al., 2001). In this chapter, we modify and apply a previously published and validated Markov model examining the cost-effectiveness of hepatitis C treatment to apply specifically to individuals with infection acquired through injecting drug use. The model has been modified to account for the increased risk of mortality unrelated to liver disease that occurs among former IDUs (Joe et al., 1982) and to permit reacquisition of hepatitis C infection through resumed injecting drug use (Proust et al., 2000; Hser et al., 2001).

Methods

Patient selection

We recognise that not all patients are treatment candidates and that, even if a candidate, the patient may not consent to or desire hepatitis C treatment. In a UK experience, antiviral therapy was indicated in 100 of 237 IDUs with hepatitis C, but only 50 of the 100 actually initiated treatment (Jowett et al., 2001). For the purposes of this analysis, we assume that a careful selection process in a multidisciplinary setting with expertise in managing injecting drug use and hepatitis C antiviral treatment patients has occurred (Davis and Rodrigue, 2001; Edlin et al., 2001). We assume that, as part of the evaluation process for consideration for treatment, patients have elevated serum aminotransaminases, confirmed hepatitis C antigen, known genotype, known liver biopsy and no prior antiviral treatment.

We compared the risks and benefits of immediate antiviral treatment with natural history with no antiviral treatment. Treatment consisted of combination therapy for 24 weeks for those with genotype 2 or 3 and a non-cirrhotic liver biopsy and 48 weeks for all others. As is recommended, combination treatment was discontinued for 24-week non-responders (McHutchison et al., 1998; Poynard et al., 1998a, 2000; Wong et al., 2000b). Because treatment for patients with mild hepatitis is controversial, for the purposes of this analysis, only patients with moderate hepatitis or compensated cirrhosis were considered in the base-case analysis. The demographic and hepatitis C characteristics are based on two published treatment studies in European patients with a history of injecting drug use (Backmund et al., 2001; Jowett et al., 2001).

Decision analytical model

A previously described and validated Markov simulation model was used to estimate the subsequent long-term prognosis of identical hypothetical cohorts of IDUs with chronic hepatitis C (Bennett et al., 1997; Wong et al., 1998; Wong, 2000). In a Markov model, the natural history of a disease is represented by prespecified states of health, so for hepatitis C, cohort members were tracked as they moved through states of health determined by clinical and histological descriptors associated with hepatitis C and liver disease. During a year, patients may: (i) remain in the same histological or clinical state; (ii) progress to another histological or clinical state; (iii) die from liver disease; or (iv) die from other causes based on attained age and gender. The simulations and tracking continued until all patients died.

Although this model was based on prior publications, it differs in the following aspects: (i) there is a higher risk of mortality from non-liver disease as has been found in former IDU populations (Joe et al., 1982); and (ii) patients may relapse into drug use and reacquire hepatitis C infection (Proust et al., 2000; Hser et al., 2001). We assume patients have been abstinent for six months but our results would have been similar for those still actively injecting drugs because of data suggesting similar rates for drug relapse for active IDUs and for those abstinent for less than five years (Hser et al., 2001). As a bias against antiviral therapy, we assumed that relapse would result in HCV reinfection. Lastly, despite some limited data suggesting that patients with transfusion-acquired HCV may have a poorer prognosis than those with injecting-drug-use-acquired disease (Gordon et al., 1993), IDUs may have an accelerated rate of liver disease progression from the relatively high prevalence of comorbid alcoholism. Therefore, in sensitivity analysis, we examined the effect of more rapid histologic progression (Poynard et al., 1997; Schiff, 1997).

Survival, data and costs

Estimates used within the decision model were based on natural history studies of hepatitis C. The likelihood of progression from mild to moderate hepatitis and then to cirrhosis (Knodell fibrosis score 4) was based on three studies (Mattsson et al., 1988; Tremolada et al., 1992; Takahashi et al., 1993), but is supported by recent studies linking histologic inflammation to liver disease progression (Pagliaro et al., 1999; Ryder, 1999). The likelihood of developing decompensated cirrhosis was based on a published natural history study of hepatitis C patients with cirrhosis (Fattovich et al., 1997), but more recent data suggest an even higher rate of progression (Niederau et al., 1998; Serfaty et al., 1998). The presenting mode of decompensation affected long-term prognosis (Christensen et al., 1989; Salerno et al., 1993; Anonymous, 1994). Survival following liver transplantation or development of an HCC was based on studies involving a large number of patients (Okuda et al., 1985; Kilpe et al., 1993; Ascher et al., 1994; Detre et al., 1996). Projections using the decision model have been validated in comparison with other published studies (Bennett et al., 1997). Because observed response rates in IDUs have been similar to those observed in two large randomised, placebo-controlled clinical trials comparing interferon and a placebo with the combination of ribavirin and interferon (McHutchison et al., 1998; Poynard et al., 1998a), we estimated the probability of sustained viral negative response using a published multivariate logistic regression model for the combined US and international trials (Wong and Koff, 2000). Table 1 lists these estimates (Yousuf et al., 1992).

To reflect the morbidity associated with complications from hepatitis C, we also adjusted life expectancy for quality of life on a scale from zero (dead) to one (perfect health). An expert panel of senior hepatologists (Wong et al., 1998) familiar with treatment and with liver disease assessed their own utilities for each of the health states using the standard reference gamble (balancing a near-term risk of dying against living with improved quality of life) and the time–trade-off technique (balancing longer survival with a poorer quality of life against shorter survival with a higher quality of life). In these analyses, patients who were alive but with symptoms related to liver disease were not given full credit for each year

Table 1: Baseline data

Variable		Value	Reference
Mean age (years)		32	(Backmund et al., 2001; Jowett et al., 2001)
Probability (%) of:			
Female gender		30.7	(Backmund et al., 2001; Jowett et al., 2001)
Genotype 2 or 3		42.5	(Backmund et al., 2001; Jowett et al., 2001)
Moderate hepatitis		66.7	(Jowett et al., 2001)
Cirrhosis		33.3	(Jowett et al., 2001)
Sustained viral negative response (32-year-old) [1]			
Women			
Genotype 2 or 3			
No cirrhosis		73.7	(Wong and Koff, 2000)
Cirrhosis		52.5	(Wong and Koff, 2000)
Not genotype 2 or 3			
No cirrhosis		39.2	(Wong and Koff, 2000)
Cirrhosis		20.3	(Wong and Koff, 2000)
Men			
Genotype 2 or 3			
No cirrhosis		64.9	(Wong and Koff, 2000)
Cirrhosis		42.2	(Wong and Koff, 2000)
Not genotype 2 or 3			
No cirrhosis		29.9	(Wong and Koff, 2000)
Cirrhosis		14.4	(Wong and Koff, 2000)
Initial health state	Annual risk (%) of:		
Mild hepatitis	Remission	0.2	(Yousuf et al., 1992)
	Moderate hepatitis	4.1	(Mattsson et al., 1988; Takahashi et al., 1993; Tremolada et al., 1992)
Moderate hepatitis	Cirrhosis	7.3	(Mattsson et al., 1988; Takahashi et al., 1993; Tremolada et al., 1992)
Cirrhosis	Ascites	2.5	(Fattovich et al., 1997)
	Variceal haemorrhage	1.1	(Fattovich et al., 1997)
	Hepatic encephalopathy	0.4	(Fattovich et al., 1997)
	Hepatocelluar carcinoma	1.5	(Fattovich et al., 1997)
Decompensated cirrhosis	Liver transplantation	3.1	(Bennett et al., 1997)

Table 1 (continued)

Variable		Value	Reference
Initial health state	Annual risk (%) of:		
Ascites	Refractory ascites	6.7	(Salerno et al., 1993)
	Death	11	(Salerno et al., 1993)
Refractory ascites	Death	33	(Salerno et al., 1993)
Variceal haemorrhage	Death (first year)	40	(Anonymous, 1994)
	Death (subsequent years)	13	(Anonymous, 1994)
Hepatic encephalopathy	Death (first year)	68	(Christensen et al., 1989)
	Death (subsequent years)	40	(Christensen et al., 1989)
Hepatocellular carcinoma	Death	86	(Okuda et al., 1985)
Liver transplantation	Death (first year)	21	(Ascher et al., 1994; Detre et al., 1996; Kilpe et al., 1993)
	Death (subsequent years)	5.7	(Ascher et al., 1994; Detre et al., 1996; Kilpe et al., 1993)
Annual probability of injecting drug relapse (%)			
0–5 years after discontinuation		15.3	(Price et al., 2001)
> 5 years after discontinuation		2.7	(Price et al., 2001)
Injecting drug use mortality (annual relative or multiplicative risk compared with general population) (%)			
Age < 21 years		14	(Joe et al., 1982)
Age 21–30 years		10	(Joe et al., 1982)
Age > 30 years		4	(Joe et al., 1982)
Health-related quality of life			
Long-term health state			
Mild chronic hepatitis		0.98	(Wong et al., 1998)
Moderate chronic hepatitis		0.92	(Wong et al., 1998)
Compensated cirrhosis		0.82	(Wong et al., 1998)
Ascites			
Diuretic sensitive		0.75	(Wong et al., 1998)
Diuretic refractory		0.52	(Wong et al., 1998)
Variceal haemorrhage		0.55	(Wong et al., 1998)
Hepatic encephalopathy		0.53	(Wong et al., 1998)
Hepatocellular carcinoma		0.55	(Wong et al., 1998)
Liver transplantation		0.86	(Wong et al., 1998)
Viral positive		0.95	(Wong et al., 1998)
Short-term health state (days deducted)			
Combination therapy (days deducted)		− 7	(Wong et al., 1998)

Table 1 (continued)

Variable	Value	Reference
Cost (USD)		
Combination therapy for 24 weeks for		
genotype 2 or 3 and no cirrhosis	9 011	(Wong et al., 2000b)
48 weeks for all others:		
24 weeks viral negative	16 098	(Wong et al., 2000b)
24 weeks viral positive	7 921	(Wong et al., 2000b)
Annual cost of care for:		
Mild hepatitis	107	(Bennett et al., 1997)
Moderate hepatitis	111	(Bennett et al., 1997)
Compensated cirrhosis	794	(Bennett et al., 1997)
Decompensated cirrhosis:		
Ascites		
Diuretic sensitive	1 792	(Bennett et al., 1997)
Diuretic refractory	18 094	(Bennett et al., 1997)
Hepatic encephalopathy		
First year	11 861	(Bennett et al., 1997)
Subsequent years	2 748	(Bennett et al., 1997)
Variceal haemorrhage		
First year	18 479	(Bennett et al., 1997)
Subsequent years	3 616	(Bennett et al., 1997)

(¹) Based on a logistic regression analysis of the combination therapy treatment arms of the international and US trials considering age, gender, cirrhosis, genotype and 48-week treatment duration for all patients except those who have genotype 2 or 3 without cirrhosis.

lived, but instead received only partial credit (e.g. 0.7 years for a year of life with cirrhosis). Similarly, to account for side effects and inconvenience from antiviral therapy, we assumed that antiviral treatment would impair quality of life during therapy.

As regards costs, we considered direct medical-care costs including antiviral-treatment-associated clinic visits, laboratory testing (electrolytes, blood counts, liver and thyroid tests), adverse events, pregnancy tests, contraception and abortion costs associated with ribavirin because of its teratogenicity in animal studies (Wasserman, 1995). Antiviral drug costs were based on average US wholesale costs of USD 6.20 for 200 mg of ribavirin and USD 11.64 per MU for interferon (Anonymous, 1999a). As would occur in practice, dose reduction for side effects and drug discontinuation in patients who were viral positive after 24 weeks of therapy reduced the costs of antiviral therapy (Wong and Koff, 2000).

Previously published actual variable treatment costs, wholesale drug costs and charges adjusted with cost to charge ratios for actual patients with hepatitis C were used to estimate post-treatment costs (Bennett et al., 1997; Wong et al., 1998). Variable costs refer to the cost of giving one additional treatment with a particular disorder and are typically one half of total costs that in turn are lower than charges which include an arbitrary profit margin. These estimates used a bottom-up accounting practice, combining estimated health resource utilisation frequencies with unit costs for hospitalisation, outpatient visits, laboratory tests, medications and therapeutic interventions such as endoscopy. All costs were in 1998 US dollars. The analysis took the societal perspective, assuming that quality of life adjustments considered time or indirect costs (Gold et al., 1996). As recommended, an annual 3 % discount rate was applied to survival and costs, and a sensitivity analysis with a 5 % rate was performed to permit comparison with previously published studies (Gold et al., 1996). Because most well-accepted medical interventions have incremental cost-effectiveness ratios falling below USD 50 000 per year of life saved (Bennett et al., 1997), we considered any ratios below this threshold to be 'cost-effective'.

The computer simulations tracked annual costs and survival with a DecisionMaker 7.0 programme (Pratt Medical Group, Boston, Massachusetts) to yield the expected average lifetime costs, life expectancy and quality-adjusted life expectancy associated with each strategy. We performed additional sensitivity analyses for different estimates of disease progression, for alternative compliance assumptions, and for clinical subgroups, to examine the effect of these alternatives on the results.

Results

Base-case analysis

Incidence of cirrhosis, life expectancy and quality of life

For comparison, if all patients had mild hepatitis, the 20-year risks of compensated cirrhosis and liver-related mortality were 26 and 5 %, respectively. Table 2 presents the detailed base-case results for IDUs with advanced histology, one third with cirrhosis and the remainder with moderate hepatitis (Jowett et al., 2001). These results suggest that antiviral treatment would decrease the absolute 20-year risk of compensated cirrhosis by 13 % and of liver-related mortality by 7 %.

Table 2: Base-case analysis: likelihood of cirrhosis and liver-related mortality, life expectancy, quality-adjusted life expectancy, lifetime costs and cost-effectiveness analysis

	Natural history (no antiviral treatment)	Combination therapy now
20-year likelihood		
Cirrhosis (%)	48.2	35.7
Liver-related mortality (%)	32.5	25.7
Life expectancy (years)	20.4	22.1
Quality-adjusted life expectancy (QALY)	16.4	18.3
Lifetime costs (USD)	34 095	37 648
Discounted lifetime costs (USD)	20 983	26 713
Discounted quality-adjusted life expectancy (DQALY)	11.5	12.6
Incremental cost-effectiveness		
(USD per discounted QALY)		5 600

Abbreviations: DQALY = discounted quality-adjusted life years; QALY = quality-adjusted life years.

In the long term, the reduced risk of cirrhosis associated with immediate therapy translated into a 1.7-year gain in life expectancy compared with no antiviral therapy. When considering quality of life, the benefit of immediate therapy increased to 1.9 QALY versus no antiviral therapy. Although quality adjustment reduced the calculated length of life with each strategy, the calculated benefit with antiviral treatment increased. This was because treatment decreased the likelihood of advanced liver disease-related complications and reduced time spent in less desirable states of health such as decompensated cirrhosis or HCC.

Costs

Table 2 shows the effect of each strategy on lifetime costs. More than two thirds of the USD 11 483 average antiviral treatment costs were offset by savings from the prevention of liver disease-related complications. When compared with non-IDUs, the savings from the prevention of future disease are lower because of the risk of recurrent injecting drug use and reacquisition of hepatitis C infection.

Discounting

The concept of discounting considers money spent now to have a higher value than money spent in the future. Because immediate therapy has higher current costs and its benefits occur in the future, discounting reduced the benefit of combination therapy and increased its relative costs compared with no antiviral treatment. In Table 2, antiviral therapy increased lifetime discounted costs by USD 5 729 and life expectancy by 1.03 DQALY, yielding an incremental cost-effectiveness ratio of USD 5 600 per DQALY gained compared with no antiviral therapy. When discounting at 5 %, this ratio rose to USD 9 000 per DQALY gained.

Sensitivity analyses

Because of data suggesting higher rates of progression in individuals drinking alcohol (Poynard et al., 1997; Schiff, 1997) and some data in IDUs (Tong and el-Farra, 1996), in the sensitivity analysis, we doubled the annual likelihood of histological progression and found that combination therapy had an incremental cost-effectiveness ratio of USD 2 700 per DQALY gained compared with no antiviral treatment. Results were also similar for alternative estimates of injecting-drug-related mortality (van Haastrecht et al., 1996) with an incremental cost-effectiveness of USD 6 100 per DQALY gained. Table 3 presents results for various clinical subgroups for immediate antiviral treatment versus no antiviral therapy.

Psychological morbidity and suicidal ideation in IDUs potentially complicate anti-HCV therapy (Grassi et al., 2001). In a sensitivity analysis of suicide-related mortality, even if the mortality rate increased to 1 per 100 (100 times that observed among over 25 000 individuals treated with antiviral therapy (Maddrey, 1999)), antiviral therapy would still increase life expectancy by 1.7 QALY at an incremental cost-effectiveness of USD 6 100 per DQALY gained.

Adherence with treatment and follow-up remain areas of concern (Ho et al., 2001). Even if costs for antiviral treatment remained unchanged and non-adherence reduced the sustained response rate to 50 % of that expected, then antiviral therapy would still increase life expectancy by 0.9 QALY at an incremental cost-effectiveness of USD 14 400 per DQALY gained. Finally, the costs of administering antiviral therapy to IDUs may be higher than those for non-IDUs. Even if the costs of drugs, office visits and laboratory tests were doubled, antiviral therapy would have an incremental cost-effectiveness of USD 12 300 per DQALY gained.

Table 3: **One-way sensitivity analysis: combination therapy versus natural history (no antiviral treatment)**

	Gain in years of life (years)	Gain in quality-adjusted life years (QALY)	Incremental cost-effectiveness (USD per DQALY gained)
Age 40	1.0	1.2	8 600
Age 50	0.4	0.6	17 300
Age 60	0.2	0.3	38 800
Male	1.4	1.6	6 500
Female	2.4	2.6	3 800
Not genotype 2 or 3	1.1	1.2	10 700
Genotype 2 or 3	2.4	2.7	2 400
Moderate hepatitis	1.9	2.3	5 100
Compensated cirrhosis	1.2	1.1	7 500
Never relapsed into injecting drug use	2.9	3.4	1 500
Abstinent from injecting drug use for > 5 years at time of antiviral treatment	2.3	2.6	3 100

Abbreviations: DQALY = discounted quality-adjusted life years; QALY = quality-adjusted life years.

Discussion

Hepatitis C appears to progress insidiously and not all patients develop cirrhosis. However, although antiviral treatment entails risks of side effects and is expensive, nearly all physicians would agree that HCV-infected patients with cirrhosis or bridging fibrosis should be treated because of their high likelihood of progressing to liver decompensation. Following such progression, the shortage of donor organs limits the availability of liver transplantation, so antiviral treatment is an attempt to prevent progression in this high-risk group. Similarly, many physicians would treat patients with moderate hepatitis, in particular those who are young and healthy and whose future length of life makes it likely that they may eventually develop liver complications.

A history of prior or current injecting drug use, however, complicates these hepatitis C treatment decisions because of concerns regarding adherence, treatment tolerability, and risk of reinfection. Among active or previous IDUs, Backmund and Jowett have demonstrated successful antiviral-therapy-induced eradication of hepatitis C despite these concerns (Backmund et al., 2001; Jowett et al., 2001). Regarding reinfection, chimpanzee studies, repeatedly transfused individuals and two IDUs have been found to have reinfection (Farci et al., 1992; Lai et al., 1994; Payen et al., 1998; Proust et al., 2000). The one report in English (Proust et al., 2000) described an IDU who, after resolving the initial HCV infection spontaneously with normalisation of liver enzymes and clearance of viraemia by PCR testing, became reinfected, developed elevated ALT levels and was again PCR positive with a different HCV genotype. In the Backmund study, however, none of the patients developed reinfection following anti-HCV therapy, but follow-up was admittedly limited (Backmund et al., 2001). More recently in a study of IDUs, Mehta et al. (2002) found a lower incidence of HCV viraemia among those who had previously spontaneously cleared HCV viraemia compared with those who had never been infected, suggesting the presence of protective HCV immunity. If this is also true for patients who clear infection from treatment, then reinfection could be 'less of a concern' for IDUs (Mehta et al., 2002). In contrast to spontaneous viral clearance, 1 of 27 patients with successful therapy-induced HCV viral clearance who were followed up for five years became reinfected (Dalgard et al., 2002).

Our analysis attempts to capture the uncertainty regarding the likelihood of histologic progression, the likelihood of a sustained response, the higher mortality associated with a history of injecting drug use and the risk of drug use relapse and reinfection. Other Markov models for the natural history of hepatitis C have been published (Kim et al., 1997, 1999; Inadomi and Sonnenberg, 1999; Younossi et al., 1999; Loubière et al., 2001) but differ in the number of health states for chronic hepatitis and decompensated cirrhosis and in specific probability estimates. The Markov model used for this injecting drug use analysis has been shown to yield projected likelihoods of progressive liver disease similar to those found in mortality studies (Fattovich et al., 1997; Seeff et al., 1992) and to five prospective studies of transfusion-associated non-A, non-B hepatitis (Seeff, 1997). Despite the concerns about adherence, reinfection and tolerability, our analysis suggests that antiviral therapy for IDUs should reduce the risk of developing liver complications, should extend life and improve quality of life, particularly in our study population with only moderate hepatitis or compensated cirrhosis patients.

From an economic standpoint, our analysis also suggests that immediate antiviral therapy for IDUs should be cost-effective when compared with other medical interventions. For example, some recently published incremental cost-effectiveness studies have found ratios of USD 60 000 per DQALY saved for chronic haemodialysis (Weinstein, 1999), USD 135 000 for herceptin for breast cancer (Elkin et al., 2000), and USD 1 million for interferon beta for multiple sclerosis (Forbes et al., 1999). Although there are methodological concerns about using a league table approach to compare resources allocation (Drummond et al., 1997), as an example to illustrate the application of league tables, a policy-maker with USD 1 million in funding would add 17 years of healthy life to the overall population if that money were spent entirely on haemodialysis, whereas spending it on treating hepatitis C in IDUs would add 128 years of healthy life. From a public health viewpoint, the economic costs of hepatitis C are substantial with a recent study suggesting annual direct and indirect costs of USD 5.5 billion in the US in 1997 (Leigh et al., 2001). Brown and Crofts (1998) estimate USD 14 million in healthcare spending for every 1 000 newly HCV-infected IDUs.

Our analysis is limited by the absence of definitive criteria or guidelines to help select individuals likely to comply with antiviral treatment and to remain abstinent from drugs throughout their life. For example, the necessary duration of drug abstinence prior to beginning antiviral treatment is unclear. Although most guidelines have recommended that illicit drug use be discontinued for at least six months (Anonymous, 1997, 1999b), Backmund et al. (2001) in Germany began treatment two weeks prior to discharge from a detoxification unit. Price et al. (2001) found that abstinence for at least five years markedly decreased the likelihood of subsequent injecting drug use over the next 11 years. Depression is present in 16 to 30 % of IDUs (Edlin et al., 2001), and treatment with interferon may lead to suicide, so again patient selection is crucial as is the presence of a multidisciplinary team familiar with treating addiction, psychiatric disorders and hepatitis C.

This analysis does not consider the most recent combination treatment with PEG interferon and ribavirin, although recently published cost-effectiveness analyses suggest that this combination should also be 'cost-effective' (Manns et al., 2001; Buti et al., 2003; Siebert et al., 2003). Finally, our study also does not consider the costs of screening and potential benefits associated with preventing the spread of hepatitis C to others following antiviral-treatment-induced eradication, nor does it consider the medical-care costs of relapse into injecting drug use or decreased risk of reacquisition of hepatitis C through education about the risks of needle sharing that occurs during antiviral treatment (Alter and Moyer, 1998; Hahn et al., 2001; Hope et al., 2001; Pollack, 2001). A previously published study, however, does suggest that screening IDUs should be cost-effective (Leal et al., 1999).

Although not all IDUs are treatment candidates, individualised decisions with physician and patient discussing the risks and benefits of antiviral treatment have formed the fundamental ethical basis for all clinical interactions (Des Jarlais and Schuchat, 2001; Edlin et al., 2001). Despite the potential difficulties, drug users have medical needs and can become motivated to address them with the help of a compassionate, tolerant and non-judgmental healthcare team. The societal principle of equity would promote the right of IDUs to have access to medical care. Beyond the equity argument, our analysis demonstrated that even a pure utilitarian and preference-based approach would lead to the choice of antiviral therapy for IDUs, because of the expected health benefits. Despite the expense and risk of reinfection or potential problems with adherence, our results would support the clinical benefit and cost-effectiveness of hepatitis C treatment for appropriately selected IDUs.

References

Alter, M. J., Moyer, L. A. (1998), 'The importance of preventing hepatitis C virus infection among injection drug users in the United States', *Journal of Acquired Immune Deficiency Syndromes and Human Retrovirology* 18 (Suppl. 1): S6–10.

Alter, M. J., Kruszon-Moran, D., Nainan, O. V., McQuillan, G. M., Gao, F., Moyer, L. A., Kaslow, R. A., Margolis, H. S. (1999), 'The prevalence of hepatitis C virus infection in the United States 1988 through 1994', *New England Journal of Medicine* 341: 556–62.

Anonymous (1994), 'Sclerotherapy for male alcoholic cirrhotic patients who have bled from esophageal varices: results of a randomised, multicentre clinical trial. The Veterans Affairs Cooperative Variceal Sclerotherapy Group', *Hepatology* 20: 618–25.

Anonymous (1997), 'National Institutes of Health Consensus Development Conference Panel Statement: Management of hepatitis C', *Hepatology* 26 (Suppl. 1): 2S–10S.

Anonymous (1998a), 'Effect of interferon-alpha on progression of cirrhosis to hepatocellular carcinoma: a retrospective cohort study. International Interferon-alpha Hepatocellular Carcinoma Study Group', *The Lancet* 351: 1535–9.

Anonymous (1998b), 'Recommendations for prevention and control of hepatitis C virus (HCV) infection and HCV-related chronic disease', *MMWR* 47 (RR-19): 1–39.

Anonymous (1999a), *1999 Drug topics red book*, Medical Economics, Montvale, NJ.

Anonymous (1999b), 'EASL International Consensus Conference on Hepatitis C', *Journal of Hepatology* 30: 956–61.

Anonymous (1999c), 'EASL International Consensus Conference on Hepatitis C, Paris, 26 and 27 February 1999. Consensus statement', *Journal of Hepatology* 31 (Suppl. 1): 3–8.

Anonymous (2002), 'National Institutes of Health Consensus Development Conference Statement: Management of hepatitis C: 10 to 12 June 2002', *Hepatology* 36 (Suppl. 1): S3–S20.

Armstrong, G. L., Alter, M. J., McQuillan, G. M., Margolis, H. S. (2000), 'The past incidence of hepatitis C virus infection: implications for the future burden of chronic liver disease in the United States', *Hepatology* 31: 777–82.

Ascher, N. L., Lake, J. R., Emond, J., Roberts, J. (1994), 'Liver transplantation for hepatitis C virus-related cirrhosis', *Hepatology* 20 (1 Pt 2): 24S–27S.

Backmund, M., Meyer, K., Von Zielonka, M., Eichenlaub, D. (2001), 'Treatment of hepatitis C infection in injection drug users', *Hepatology* 34: 188–93.

Bell, J., Batey, R. G., Farrell, G. C., Crewe, E. B., Cunningham, A. L., Byth, K. (1990), 'Hepatitis C virus in intravenous drug users', *Medical Journal of Australia* 153: 274–6.

Bennett, W. G., Inoue, Y., Beck, J. R., Wong, J. B., Pauker, S. G., Davis, G. L. (1997), 'Estimates of the cost-effectiveness of a single course of interferon-alpha 2b in patients with histologically mild chronic hepatitis C', *Annals of Internal Medicine* 127: 855–65.

Bennett, W. G., Pauker, S. G., Davis, G. L., Wong, J. B. (1996), 'Modelling therapeutic benefit in the midst of uncertainty: therapy for hepatitis C', *Digestive Diseases and Sciences* 41 (12 Suppl.): 56S–62S.

Benvegnu, L., Chemello, L., Noventa, F., Fattovich, G., Pontisso, P., Alberti, A. (1998), 'Retrospective analysis of the effect of interferon therapy on the clinical outcome of patients with viral cirrhosis', *Cancer* 83: 901–9.

Bonis, P. A., Ioannidis, J. P., Cappelleri, J. C., Kaplan, M. M., Lau, J. (1997), 'Correlation of biochemical response to interferon alfa with histological improvement in hepatitis C: a meta-analysis of diagnostic test characteristics', *Hepatology* 26: 1035–44.

Bonkovsky, H. L., Woolley, J. M. (1999), 'Reduction of health-related quality of life in chronic hepatitis C and improvement with interferon therapy. The Consensus Interferon Study Group', *Hepatology* 29: 264–70.

Brown, K., Crofts, N. (1998), 'Health care costs of a continuing epidemic of hepatitis C virus infection among injecting drug users', *Australian and New Zealand Journal of Public Health* 22 (3 Suppl.): 384–8.

Buti, M., Medina, M., Casado, M. A., Wong, J. B., Fosbrook, L., Esteban, R. (2003), 'A cost-effectiveness analysis of peginterferon alfa-2b plus ribavirin for the treatment of naive patients with chronic hepatitis C', *Alimentary Pharmacology and Therapeutics* 17: 687–94.

Camma, C., Giunta, M., Linea, C., Pagliaro, L. (1997), 'The effect of interferon on the liver in chronic hepatitis C: a quantitative evaluation of histology by meta-analysis', *Journal of Hepatology* 26: 1187–99.

Christensen, E., Krintel, J., Hansen, S., Johansen, J., Juhl, E. (1989), 'Prognosis after the first episode of gastrointestinal bleeding or coma in cirrhosis. Survival and prognostic factors', *Scandinavian Journal of Gastroenterology* 24: 999–1006.

Crofts, N., Aitken, C. K. (1997), 'Incidence of bloodborne virus infection and risk behaviours in a cohort of injecting drug users in Victoria, 1990–1995', *Medical Journal of Australia* 167: 17–20.

Dalgard, O., Bjoro, K., Hellum, K., Myrvang, B., Skaug, K., Gutigard, B., Bell, H., the Construct Group (2002), 'Treatment of chronic hepatitis C in injecting drug users: 5 years' follow-up', *European Addiction Research* 8: 45–9.

Davis, G. L., Rodrigue, J. R. (2001), 'Treatment of chronic hepatitis C in active drug users'. *New England Journal of Medicine* 345: 215–7.

Davis, G. L., Albright, J. E., Cook, S., Rosenberg, D. (2003), 'Projecting future complications of chronic hepatitis C in the United States', *Liver Transplantation* 9: 331–8.

Des Jarlais, D. C., Schuchat, A. (2001), 'Hepatitis C among drug users: Deja vu all over again?', *American Journal of Public Health* 91: 21–2.

Detre, K. M., Belle, S. H., Lombarddero, M. (1996), 'Liver transplantation for chronic viral hepatitis', *Viral Hepatitis Review* 2: 219–28.

Deuffic, D., Buffat, L., Poynard, T., Valleron, A. J. (1999), 'Modelling the hepatitis C virus epidemic in France', *Hepatology* 29: 1596–1601.

Diaz, T., Des Jarlais, D. C., Vlahov, D., Perlis, T. E., Edwards, V., Friedman, S. R., Rockwell, R., Hoover, D., Williams, I. T., Monterroso, E. R. (2001), 'Factors associated with prevalent hepatitis C: differences among young adult injection drug users in lower and upper Manhattan, New York City', *American Journal of Public Health* 91: 23–30.

Donahue, J. G., Nelson, K. E., Munoz, A., Vlahov, D., Rennie, L. L., Taylor, E. L., Saah, A. J., Cohn, S., Odaka, N. J., Farzadegan, H. (1991), 'Antibody to hepatitis C virus among cardiac surgery patients, homosexual men, and intravenous drug users in Baltimore, Maryland', *American Journal of Epidemiology* 134: 1206–11.

Drummond, M. F., O'Brien, B., Stoddart, G. L., Torrance, G. W. (1997), *Methods for the economic evaluation of health care programmes*, Oxford University Press, Oxford.

Edlin, B. R. (2002), 'Prevention and treatment of hepatitis C in injection drug users?', *Hepatology* 36 (Suppl. 1): S210–19.

Edlin, B. R., Seal, K. H., Lorvick, J., Kral, A. H., Ciccarone, D. H., Moore, L. D., Lo, B. (2001), 'Is it justifiable to withhold treatment for hepatitis C from illicit-drug users?', *New England Journal of Medicine* 345: 211–5.

Elkin, E. B., Weinstein, M. C., Winer, E. P., Kuntz, K. M., Weeks, J. C. (2000), 'The cost-effectiveness of herceptin for metastatic breast cancer [Abstract]', *Medical Decision Making* 20: 485.

El-Serag, H. B., Mason, A. C. (1999), 'Rising incidence of hepatocellular carcinoma', *New England Journal of Medicine* 340: 745–50.

Eyster, M. E., Alter, H. J., Aledort, L. M., Quan, S., Hatzakis, A., Goedert, J. J. (1991), 'Heterosexual co-transmission of hepatitis C virus (HCV) and human immunodeficiency virus (HIV)', *Annals of Internal Medicine* 115: 764–8.

Farci, P., Alter, H. J., Govindarajan, S., Wong, D. C., Engle, R., Lesniewski, R. R., Mushahwar, I. K., Desai, S. M., Miller, R. H., Ogata, N. (1992), 'Lack of protective immunity against reinfection with hepatitis C virus', *Science* 258: 135–40.

Fattovich, G., Giustina, G., Degos, F., Tremolada, F., Diodati, G., Almasio, P., Nevens, F., Solinas, A., Mura, D., Brouwer, J. T., Thomas, H., Njapoum, C., Casarin, C., Bonetti, P., Fuschi, P., Basho, J., Tocco, A., Bhalla, A., Galassini, R., Noventa, F., Schalm, S. W., Realdi, G. (1997), 'Morbidity and mortality in compensated cirrhosis type C: a retrospective follow-up study of 384 patients', *Gastroenterology* 112: 463–72.

Fingerhood, M. I., Jasinski, D. R., Sullivan, J. T. (1993), 'Prevalence of hepatitis C in a chemically dependent population', *Archives of Internal Medicine* 153: 2025–30.

Forbes, R. B., Lees, A., Waugh, N., Swingler, R. J. (1999), 'Population based cost utility study of interferon beta-1b in secondary progressive multiple sclerosis', *British Medical Journal* 319: 1529–33.

Foster, G., Goldin, R., Thomas, H. (1998), 'Chronic hepatitis C virus infection causes a significant reduction in quality of life in the absence of cirrhosis', *Hepatology* 27: 209–12.

Galeazzi, B., Tufano, A., Barbierato, E., Bortolotti, F. (1995), 'Hepatitis C virus infection in Italian intravenous drug users: epidemiological and clinical aspects', *Liver* 15: 209–12.

Garfein, R. S., Doherty, M. C., Monterroso, E. R., Thomas, D. L., Nelson, K. E., Vlahov, D. (1998), 'Prevalence and incidence of hepatitis C virus infection among young adult injection drug users', *Journal of Acquired Immune Deficiency Syndromes and Human Retrovirology* 18 (Suppl. 1): S11–9.

Garfein, R. S., Vlahov, D., Galai, N., Doherty, M. C., Nelson, K. E. (1996), 'Viral infections in short-term injection drug users: the prevalence of the hepatitis C, hepatitis B, human immunodeficiency, and human T-lymphotropic viruses', *American Journal of Public Health* 86: 655–61.

Girardi, E., Zaccarelli, M., Tossini, G., Puro, V., Narciso, P., Visco, G. (1990), 'Hepatitis C virus infection in intravenous drug users: prevalence and risk factors', *Scandinavian Journal of Infectious Diseases* 22: 751–2.

Gold, M. R., Siegel, J. E., Russell, L. B., Weinstein, M. C. (1996), *Cost-effectiveness in health and medicine*, Oxford University Press, New York.

Gordon, S. C., Elloway, R. S., Long, J. C., Dmuchowski, C. F. (1993), 'The pathology of hepatitis C as a function of mode of transmission: blood transfusion vs intravenous drug use', *Hepatology* 18: 1338–43.

Grassi, L., Mondardini, D., Pavanati, M., Sighinolfi, L., Serra, A., Ghinelli, F. (2001), 'Suicide probability and psychological morbidity secondary to HIV infection: a control study of HIV-seropositive, hepatitis C virus (HCV)-seropositive and HIV/HCV-seronegative injecting drug users', *Journal of Affective Disorders* 64: 195–202.

Hagan, H., Thiede, H., Weiss, N. S., Hopkins, S. G., Durchin, J. S., Russell, A. E. (2001), 'Sharing of drug preparation equipment as a risk factor for hepatitis C', *American Journal of Public Health* 91: 42–6.

Hahn, J. A., Page-Shafer, K., Lum, P. J., Ochoa, K., Moss, A. R. (2001), 'Hepatitis C virus infection and needle exchange use among young injection drug users in San Francisco', *Hepatology* 34: 180–7.

Ho, S. B., Nguyen, H., Tetrick, L. L., Opitz, G. A., Basara, M. L., Dieperink, E. (2001), 'Influence of psychiatric diagnoses on interferon-alpha treatment for chronic hepatitis C in a veteran population', *American Journal of Gastroenterology* 96: 157–64.

Hoofnagle, J. H. (1997), 'Hepatitis C: the clinical spectrum of disease', *Hepatology* 26 (3 Suppl. 1): 15S–20S.

Hope, V. D., Judd, A., Hickman, M., Lamagni, T., Hunter, G., Stimson, G. V., Jones, S., Donovan, L., Parry, J. V., Gill, O. N. (2001), 'Prevalence of hepatitis C among injection drug users in England and Wales: is harm reduction working?', *American Journal of Public Health* 91: 38–42.

Hser, Y. I., Hoffman, V., Grella, C. E., Anglin, M. D. (2001), 'A 33-year follow-up of narcotics addicts', *Archives of General Psychiatry* 58: 503–8.

Huemer, H. P., Prodinger, W. M., Larcher, C., Most, L., Dierich, M. P. (1990), 'Correlation of hepatitis C virus antibodies with HIV-1 seropositivity in intravenous drug addicts', *Infection* 18: 122–3.

Ikeda, K., Saitoh, S., Suzuki, Y., Kobayashi, M., Tsubota, A., Koida, I., Arase, Y., Fukuda, M., Chayama, K., Murashima, N., Kumada, H. (1998), 'Disease progression and hepatocellular carcinogenesis in patients with chronic viral hepatitis: a prospective observation of 2 215 patients', *Journal of Hepatology* 28: 930–8.

Imai, Y., Kawata, S., Tamura, S., Yabuuchi, I., Noda, S., Inada, M., Maeda, Y., Shirai, Y., Fukuzaki, T., Kaji, I., Ishikawa, H., Matsuda, Y., Nishikawa, M., Seki, K., Matsuzawa, Y. (1998), 'Relation of interferon therapy and hepatocellular carcinoma in patients with chronic hepatitis C. Osaka Hepatocellular Carcinoma Prevention Study Group', *Annals of Internal Medicine* 129: 94–9.

Inadomi, J. M., Sonnenberg, A. (1999), 'Cost-effectiveness of initial combination therapy versus monotherapy followed by combination therapy in hepatitis C', *Gastroenterology* 116 (4 Pt 2): A316.

Joe, G., Lehman, W., Simpson, D. D. (1982), 'Addict death rates during a four-year post-treatment follow-up', *American Journal of Public Health* 72: 703–9.

Jowett, S. L., Agarwal, K., Smith, B. C., Craig, W., Hewett, M., Bassendine, D. R., Gilvarry, E., Burt, A. D., Bassendine, M. F. (2001), 'Managing chronic hepatitis C acquired through intravenous drug use', Quebec *Journal of Medicine* 94: 153–8.

Kasahara, A., Hayashi, N., Mochizuki, K., Takayanagi, M., Yoshioka, K., Kakumu, S., Iijima, A., Urushihara, A., Kiyosawa, K., Okuda, M., Hino, K., Okita, K. (1998), 'Risk factors for hepatocellular carcinoma and its incidence after interferon treatment in patients with chronic hepatitis C. Osaka Liver Disease Study Group', *Hepatology* 27: 1394–402.

Kilpe, V. E., Krakauer, H., Wren, R. E. (1993), 'An analysis of liver transplant experience from 37 transplant centres as reported to Medicare', *Transplantation* 56: 554–61.

Kim, W. R., Poterucha, J. J., Hermans, J. E., Therneau, T. M., Dickson, E. R., Evans, R. W, Gross, J. B., Jr (1997), 'Cost-effectiveness of 6 and 12 months of interferon-alpha therapy for chronic hepatitis C', *Annals of Internal Medicine* 127: 866–74.

Kim, W. R., Poterucha, J. J., Dickson, E. R., Gross, J. B., Jr (1999), 'Optimal treatment strategy for chronic hepatitis C in 1999', *Gastroenterology* 116 (4 Pt 2): A399.

Kuwana, K., Ichida, T., Kamimura, T., Ohkoshi, S., Ogata, N., Harada, T., Endoh, K., Asakura, H. (1997), 'Risk factors and the effect of interferon therapy in the development of hepatocellular carcinoma: a multivariate analysis in 343 patients', *Journal of Gastroenterology and Hepatology* 12: 149–55.

Lai, M. E., Mazzoleni, A. P., Argiolu, F., De Virgilis, S., Balestrieri, A., Purcell, R. H., Cao, A, Farci, P. (1994), 'Hepatitis C virus in multiple episodes of acute hepatitis in polytransfused thalassaemic children', *The Lancet* 343: 388–90.

Lau, D. T., Kleiner, D. E., Ghany, M. G., Park, Y., Schmid, P., Hoofnagle, J. H. (1998), '10-year follow-up after interferon-alfa therapy for chronic hepatitis C', *Hepatology* 28: 1121–7.

Leal, P., Stein, K., Rosenberg, W. (1999), 'What is the cost utility of screening for hepatitis C virus (HCV) in intravenous drug users?', *Journal of Medical Screening* 6: 124–31.

Leigh, J. P., Bowlus, C. L., Leistikow, B. N., Schenker, M. (2001), 'Costs of hepatitis C', *Archives of Internal Medicine* 161: 2231–7.

Lorvick, J., Kral, A. H., Seal, K., Gee, L., Edlin, B. R. (2001), 'Prevalence and duration of hepatitis C among injection drug users in San Francisco, California', *American Journal of Public Health* 91: 46–7.

Loubière, S., Rotily, M., Durand-Zaleski, I., Costagliola, D. (2001), 'Including polymerase chain reaction in screening for hepatitis C virus RNA in blood donations is not cost-effective', *Vox Sanguinis* 80: 199–204.

MacDonald, M. A., Wodak, A. D., Dolan, K. A., van Beek, I., Cunningham, P. H., Kaldor, J. M. (2000), 'Hepatitis C antibody prevalence among injecting drug users at selected needle and syringe programs in Australia, 1995–1997', *Medical Journal of Australia* 172: 57–61.

Maddrey, W. C. (1999), 'Safety of combination interferon alfa-2b/ribavirin therapy in chronic hepatitis C-relapsed and treatment-naive patients', *Seminars in Liver Disease* 19: 67–75.

Manns, M. P., McHutchison, J. G., Gordon, S. C., Rustgi, V. K., Shiffman, M., Reindollar, R., Goodman, S. D., Koury, K., Ling, M. H., Albrecht, J. K. and the International Hepatitis Interventional Therapy Group (2001), 'Peginterferon alfa-2b plus ribavirin compared with interferon alfa-2b plus ribavirin for initial treatment of chronic hepatitis C: a randomised trial', *The Lancet* 258: 958–65.

Marcellin, P., Boyer, N., Gervais, A., Martinot, M., Pouteau, M., Castelnau, C., Kilani, A., Areias, J., Auperin, A., Benhamou, J., Degott, C., Erlinger, S. (1997), 'Long-term histologic improvement and loss of detectable intrahepatic HCV RNA in patients with chronic hepatitis C and sustained response to interferon-alpha therapy', *Annals of Internal Medicine* 127: 875–81.

Mattsson, L., Weiland, O., Glaumann, H. (1988), 'Long-term follow-up of chronic post-transfusion non-A, non-B hepatitis: clinical and histological outcome', *Liver* 8: 184–8.

Mazzella, G., Accogli, E., Sottili, S., Festi, D., Orsini, M., Salzetta, A., Novelli, V., Cipolla, A., Fabbri, C., Pezzoli, A., Roda, E. (1996), 'Alpha interferon treatment may prevent hepatocellular carcinoma in HCV-related liver cirrhosis', *Journal of Hepatology* 24: 141–7.

McCarthy, J. J., Flynn, N. (2001), 'Hepatitis C in methadone maintenance patients: prevalence and public policy implications', *Journal of Addictive Diseases* 20: 19–31.

McHutchison, J. G., Gordon, S. C., Schiff, E. R., Shiffman, M. L., Lee, W. M., Rustgi, V. K., Goodman, Z. D., Ling, M. H., Cort, S., Albrecht, J. K. (1998), 'Interferon alfa-2b alone or in combination with ribavirin as initial treatment for chronic hepatitis C. Hepatitis Interventional Therapy Group', *New England Journal of Medicine* 339: 1485–92.

Mehta, S. H., Cox, A., Hoover, D. R., Wang, X. H., Mao, Q., Ray, S., Strathdee, S. A., Vlahov, D., Thomas, D. L. (2002), 'Protection against persistence of hepatitis C', *The Lancet* 359: 1478–83.

Niederau, C., Lange, S., Heintges, T., Erhardt, A., Buschkamp, M., Hurter, D., Nawrocki, M., Kruska, L., Hensel, F., Petry, W., Haussinger, D. (1998), 'Prognosis of chronic hepatitis C: results of a large, prospective cohort study', *Hepatology* 28: 1687–95.

Nishiguchi, S., Kuroki, T., Nakatani, S., Morimoto, H., Takeda, T., Nakajima, S., Shiomi, S., Seki, S., Kobayashi, K., Otani, S. (1995), 'Randomised trial of effects of interferon-alpha on incidence of hepatocellular carcinoma in chronic active hepatitis C with cirrhosis', *The Lancet* 346: 1051–5.

Okuda, K., Ohtsuki, T., Obata, H., Tomimatsu, M., Okazaki, N., Hasegawa, H., Nakajima, Y., Ohnishi, K. (1985), 'Natural history of hepatocellular carcinoma and prognosis in relation to treatment. Study of 850 patients', *Cancer* 56: 918–28.

Pagliaro, L., Peri, V., Linea, C., Camma, C., Giunta, M., Magrin, S. (1999), 'Natural history of chronic hepatitis C', *Italian Journal of Gastroenterology and Hepatology* 31: 28–44.

Payen, J. L., Izopet, J., Barange, K., Puel, J., Selves, J., Pascal, J. P. (1998), 'Hepatitis C virus reinfection after an intravenous drug injection', *Gastroenterologie Clinique et Biologique* 22: 469–70.

Pollack, H. A. (2001), 'Cost-effectiveness of harm reduction in preventing hepatitis C among injection drug users', *Medical Decision Making* 21: 357–67.

Poynard, T., Bedossa, P., Opolon, P. (1997), 'Natural history of liver fibrosis progression in patients with chronic hepatitis C. The Obsvirc, Metavir, Clinivir, and Dosvirc groups', *The Lancet* 349: 825–32.

Poynard, T., Marcellin, P., Lee, S. S., Niederau, C., Minuk, G. S., Ideo, G., Bain, V., Heathcote, J., Zeuzem, S., Trepo, C., Albrecht, J. (1998a), 'Randomised trial of interferon alpha 2b plus ribavirin for 48 weeks or for 24 weeks versus interferon alpha 2b plus placebo for 48 weeks for treatment of chronic infection with hepatitis C. International Hepatitis Interventional Therapy Group', *The Lancet* 352: 1426–32.

Poynard, T., Moussalli, V., Ratziu, V., Thevenot, T., Regimbeau, C., Opolon, P., Horsman, Y. R. B., Closon, M., Fevery, J., Hautekeete, M. (1998b), 'Is antiviral treatment (IFN alpha and/or ribavirin) justified in cirrhosis related to hepatitis C virus? Societe Royale Belge de Gastroenterologie', *Acta Gastroenterologica Belgica* 59: 431–7.

Poynard, T., McHutchison, J. G., Goodman, Z., Ling, M. H., Albrecht, J. (2000), 'Is an "a la carte" combination interferon alfa-2b plus ribavirin regimen possible for the first line treatment in patients with chronic hepatitis C? The Algovirc Project Group', *Hepatology* 31: 211–8.

Price, R. K., Risk, N. K., Spitznagel, E. L. (2001), 'Remission from drug abuse over a 25-year period: patterns of remission and treatment use', *American Journal of Public Health* 91: 1107–13.

Proust, B., Dubois, F., Bacq, Y., Le Pogam, S., Rogez, S., Levillain, R., Goudeau, A. (2000), 'Two successive hepatitis C virus infections in an intravenous drug user', *Journal of Clinical Microbiology* 38(8): 3125–7.

Reichard, O., Glaumann, H., Fryden, A., Norkrans, G., Wejstal, R., Weiland, O. (1999), 'Long-term follow-up of chronic hepatitis C patients with sustained virological response to alpha-interferon', *Journal of Hepatology* 30: 783–7.

Ryder, S. D. (1999), 'Progression of liver fibrosis in mild hepatitis C: a prospective study paired with a liver biopsy study [Abstract]', *Hepatology* 30 (4 Pt 2): 316A.

Salerno, F., Borroni, G., Moser, P., Badalamenti, S., Cassara, L., Maggi, A., Fusini, M., Cesana, B. (1993), 'Survival and prognostic factors of cirrhotic patients with ascites: a study of 134 outpatients', *American Journal of Gastroenterology* 88: 514–9.

Schalm, S. W., Fattovich, G., Brouwer, J. T. (1997), 'Therapy of hepatitis C: patients with cirrhosis', *Hepatology* 26 (3 Suppl. 1): 128S–32S.

Schiff, E. R. (1997), 'Hepatitis C and alcohol', *Hepatology* 26 (3 Suppl. 1): 39S–42S.

Seeff, L. B. (1997), 'Natural history of hepatitis C', *Hepatology* 26 (3 Suppl. 1): 21S–28S.

Seeff, L. B., Buskell-Bales, Z., Wright, E. C., Durako, S. J., Alter, H. J., Iber, F. L., Hollinger, F. B., Gitnick, G., Knodell, R. G., Perrillo, R. P. et al. (1992), 'Long-term mortality after transfusion-associated non-A, non-B hepatitis. The National Heart, Lung, and Blood Institute Study Group', *New England Journal of Medicine* 327: 1906–11.

Selvey, L. A., Wignall, J., Buzolic, A., Sullivan, P. (1996), 'Reported prevalence of hepatitis C among clients of needle exchanges in south-east Queensland', *Australian and New Zealand Journal of Public Health* 20: 61–4.

Selvey, L. A., Denton, M., Plant, A. J. (1997), 'Incidence and prevalence of hepatitis C among clients of a Brisbane methadone clinic: factors influencing hepatitis C serostatus', *Australian and New Zealand Journal of Public Health* 21: 102–4.

Serfaty, L., Aumaitre, H., Chazouilleres, O., Bonnand, A. M., Rosmorduc, O., Poupon, R. E., Poupon, R. (1998), 'Determinants of outcome of compensated hepatitis C virus-related cirrhosis', *Hepatology* 27: 1435–40.

Sherman, M. (1997), 'Management of viral hepatitis: clinical and public health perspectives — a consensus statement. CASL Hepatitis Consensus Group. Canadian Association for Study of the Liver', *Canadian Journal of Gastroenterology* 11: 407–16.

Shindo, M., Ken, A., Okuno, T. (1999), 'Varying incidence of cirrhosis and hepatocellular carcinoma in patients with chronic hepatitis C responding differently to interferon therapy', *Cancer* 85: 1943–50.

Siebert, U., Sroczynski, G., Rossol, S., Wasem, J., Ravens-Sieberer, U., Kurth, B. M., Manns, M. P., McHutchison, J. G., Wong, J. B., German Hepatitis C Model (GEHMO) Group, International Hepatitis Interventional Therapy Group (2003), 'Cost-effectiveness of peginterferon alfa-2b plus ribavirin versus interferon alfa-2b plus ribavirin for initial treatment of chronic hepatitis C', *Gut* 52: 425–32.

Sobesky, R., Mathurin, P., Charlotte, F., Moussalli, J., Olivi, M., Vidaud, M., Ratziu, V., Opolon, P., Poynard, T. (1999), 'Modelling the impact of interferon alfa treatment on liver fibrosis progression in chronic hepatitis C: a dynamic view. The Multivirc Group', *Gastroenterology* 116: 378–86.

Takahashi, M., Yamada, G., Miyamoto, R., Doi, T., Endo, H., Tsuji, T. (1993), 'Natural course of chronic hepatitis C', *American Journal of Gastroenterology* 88: 240–3.

Tennant, F. (1994), 'Hepatitis C in intravenous drug addicts', *Archives of Internal Medicine* 154: 1163–4.

Teramura, K., Fukuda, A., Kobayashi, H., Yoshimoto, S., Kawashima, H., Ohsawa, N. (1997), 'Virus elimination and histologic improvement in patients with chronic hepatitis C treated with interferon alpha', *Journal of Clinical Gastroenterology* 25: 346–51.

Thomas, D. L., Vlahov, D., Solomon, L., Cohn, S., Taylor, E., Garfein, R., Nelson, K. E. (1995), 'Correlates of hepatitis C virus infections among injection drug users', *Medicine* 74: 212–20.

Thorpe, L. E., Ouellet, L. J., Levy, J. R., Williams, I. T., Monterroso, E. R. (2000), 'Hepatitis C virus infection: prevalence, risk factors, and prevention opportunities among young injection drug users in Chicago, 1997–1999', *Journal of Infectious Diseases* 182: 1588–94.

Tong, M. J., el-Farra, N. S. (1996), 'Clinical sequelae of hepatitis C acquired from injection drug use', *Western Journal of Medicine* 164: 399–404.

Tremolada, F., Casarin, C., Alberti, A., Drago, C., Tagger, A., Ribero, M. L., Realdi, G. (1992), 'Long-term follow-up of non-A, non-B (type C) post-transfusion hepatitis', *Journal of Hepatology* 16: 273–81.

van den Hoek, J. A., van Haastrecht, H., Goudsmit, J., de Wolf, F., Coutinho, R. A. (1990), 'Prevalence, incidence, and risk factors of hepatitis C virus infection among drug users in Amsterdam', *Journal of Infectious Diseases* 162: 823–6.

van Haastrecht, H. J., van Ameijden, E. J., van den Hoek, J. A., Mientjes, G. H., Bax, J. S., Coutinho, R. A. (1996), 'Predictors of mortality in the Amsterdam cohort of human immunodeficiency virus (HIV)-positive and HIV-negative drug users', *American Journal of Epidemiology* 143: 380–91.

Verbaan, H., Andersson, K., Eriksson, S. (1993), 'Intravenous drug abuse — the major route of hepatitis C virus transmission among alcohol-dependent individuals?', *Scandinavian Journal of Gastroenterology* 28: 714–8.

Ware, J. E., Jr, Bayliss, M. S., Mannocchia, M., Davis, G. L. (1999), 'Health-related quality of life in chronic hepatitis C: impact of disease and treatment response. The International Hepatitis Interventional Therapy Group', *Hepatology* 30: 550–5.

Wasserman, Y. (1995), *Physicians' fee reference 1995*, Medical Publishers, West Allis.

Weinstein, M. C. (1999), 'High-priced technology can be good value for money', *Annals of Internal Medicine* 130: 857–8.

Wong, J. B. (2000), 'Understanding the natural history of chronic hepatitis C: can decision analysis help? [Abstract]', *Hepatology* 32 (Pt 2): 426A.

Wong, J. B., Koff, R. S. (2000), 'Watchful waiting with periodic liver biopsy versus immediate empirical therapy for histologically mild chronic hepatitis C. A cost-effectiveness analysis', *Annals of Internal Medicine* 133: 665–75.

Wong, J. B., Bennett, W. G., Koff, R. S., Pauker, S. G. (1998), 'Pre-treatment evaluation of chronic hepatitis C: risks, benefits and costs', *JAMA* 280: 2088–93.

Wong, J. B., McQuillan, G. M., McHutchison, J. G., Poynard, T. (2000a), 'Estimating future hepatitis C morbidity, mortality, and costs in the United States', *American Journal of Public Health* 90: 1562–9.

Wong, J. B., Poynard, T., Ling, M. H., Albrecht, J. K., Pauker, S. G. (2000b), 'Cost-effectiveness of 24 or 48 weeks of interferon alfa-2b alone or with ribavirin as initial treatment of chronic hepatitis C. International Hepatitis Interventional Therapy Group', *American Journal of Gastroenterology* 95: 1524–30.

Younossi, Z. M., Singer, M. E., McHutchison, J. G., Shermock, K. M. (1999), 'Cost-effectiveness of interferon alpha 2b combined with ribavirin for the treatment of chronic hepatitis C', *Hepatology* 30: 1318–24.

Yousuf, M., Nakano, Y., Tanaka, E., Sodeyama, T., Kiyosawa, K. (1992), 'Persistence of viraemia in patients with type-C chronic hepatitis during long-term follow-up', *Scandinavian Journal of Gastroenterology* 27: 812–16.

Zeldis, J. B., Jain, S., Kuramoto, I. K., Richards, C., Sazama, K., Samuels, S., Holland, P. V., Flynn, N. (1992), 'Seroepidemiology of viral infections among intravenous drug users in northern California', *Western Journal of Medicine* 156: 30–5.

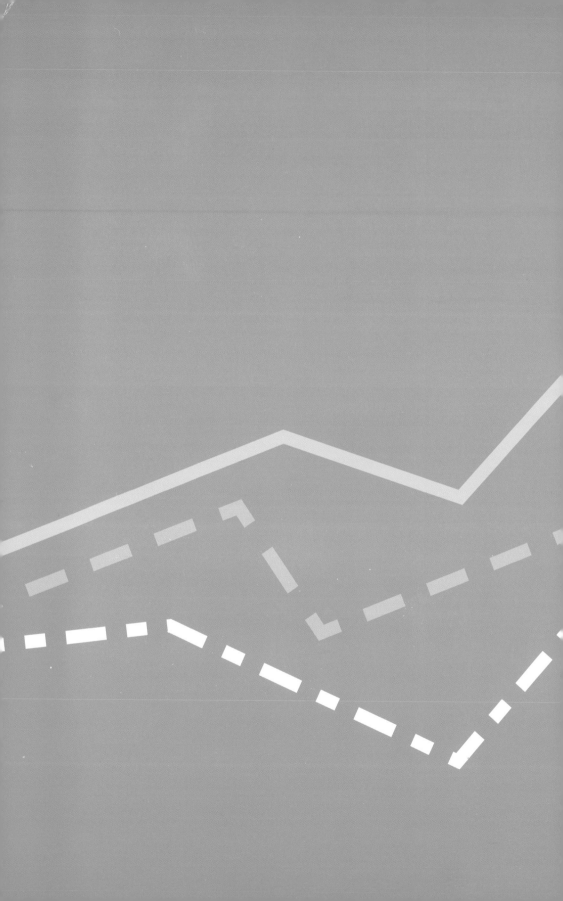

Wider costs of drug use

PART **IV**

Introduction

Part IV extends the previous part in terms of the cost categories considered in the analysis. Whereas Part III was confined to patient-related direct healthcare costs related to drug use, the current one also addresses the indirect costs of production losses, general programme costs (for example, the costs of prevention and law enforcement) and impact on families (for example, unpaid household work). In particular, Welte et al. focus on the indirect costs of production losses as measured from various perspectives and using various methods. In an application in the Netherlands and Germany, the 'classic' human capital, the friction cost and the willingness-to-pay approaches are utilised.

Welte et al. (Chapter 10) distinguish perspectives for measuring the indirect costs of production losses as those of the drug user, the family, the employer, social insurance and, finally, society as a whole. With respect to Welte et al. and their application to the Netherlands, it is interesting to note that recently issued Dutch guidelines for pharmaco-economic research favour the societal perspective (Hjelmgren et al., 2001). Welte et al. summarise: 'All costs, i.e. indirect costs in the paid and unpaid work sectors, should be considered from a societal perspective. However, transfer costs (e.g. welfare money) should not be included as they only represent a redistribution of resources and not a loss of resources.'

As do Kopp and Blanchard (see below), Welte et al. prefer the human capital approach for assessing the indirect part of societal costs. They note that, as general agreement on this specific valuation is lacking, reporting according to various approaches is still recommended.

Antoñanzas et al. (Chapter 11) reviewed internationally published studies on the social costs of drugs. Initially, they reconsider the crucial difference between social costs and private costs. Social costs are closely linked to the economic concept of 'externalities'. They note that, in general, the empirical studies on drug use costs tend to consider only the social costs, ignoring social benefits (reduced healthcare costs due to premature death) and private costs and benefits.

In the review, Antoñanzas et al. go back to the classical study by Rice et al. (1991) in Public Health Reports, which notably remains one of the most comprehensive published studies. Antoñanzas et al. also include one Spanish study that only allows very limited comparison with the Spanish estimate of direct healthcare costs as estimated in Chapter 8, due to differences in the methodology for derivation (in particular, incidence versus prevalence-based costing assessments). Furthermore, a close link to the recently issued guidelines for social costing in drug use is provided (Single et al., 1998). Antoñanzas et al. finalise by stating that, in addition to further economic research, epidemiological data gathering is urgently needed, as was noted at the end of Chapter 8.

Jeanrenaud (Chapter 12) continues Part IV with a further review of Swiss national studies on the social costs of drugs and by suggesting a synthesis of the human capital and willingness-to-pay approaches. In particular, in the combination of human capital and willingness-to-pay approaches, the social costs of illicit drugs are conceived as the sum of production losses — valued using human capital — and the loss in quality of life — valued by willingness to pay. The studies reviewed were not considered by Antoñanzas et al. as they were published in the French or German language or disseminated in local Swiss media only.

Estimates of the social costs provided vary between 0.2 and 1 % of the Swiss gross national product and appear to be very sensitive to the inclusion/exclusion of intangible costs. Special attention is given to a study by Gutzwiller and Steffen (2000), presenting a cost–benefit analysis of a programme for medical prescription of heroin in Switzerland. It is noted that prescribing heroin may have cost-saving potential and may thus be an intervention with a favourable pharmaco-economic profile achieving cost–benefit ratios that range from two to five.

Kopp and Blanchard (Chapter 13) extend the analysis by including other aspects of social costs, with an application for France. In particular, they aggregate lost incomes, lost taxes, lost added values and the costs of the fight against drugs at various political levels (costs of justice, police, etc., and contributions to the EU). Furthermore, they include estimated healthcare costs in their total social cost estimate of 0.16 % of the French gross national product.

With respect to some aspects, Kopp and Blanchard may even have overestimated social costs. For example, healthcare costs could only be estimated for HIV/AIDS and substitution treatment with Subutex® (buprenorphine). Postma et al. (Chapter 8) estimated healthcare costs for drug-related hepatitis at approximately EUR 50 million in France. Nonetheless, Kopp and Blanchard indicate that each French citizen has to bear, on average, almost EUR 35 per year as a consequence of drug use.

In summary, this part of the monograph should provide the reader with knowledge of different approaches for measuring various aspects of the social costs of drug *use. This insight will prove useful in appreciating the various studies on social costs that were reviewed in Part IV.*

Maarten Postma

References

Gutzwiller, F., Steffen, T. (2000), *Cost–benefit analysis of heroin maintenance treatment*, Karger, Basle.

Hjelmgren, J., Berggren, F., Andersson, F. (2001), 'Health economic guidelines — similarities, differences and some implications', *Value in Health* 4: 225–50.

Rice, D., Kelman, S., Miller, L. (1991), 'Estimates of economic costs of alcohol and drug abuse and mental illness, 1985–1988', *Public Health Reports* 106: 280–92.

Single, E., Robson, L., Xie, X., Rehm, J. (1998), 'Estimates of economic costs of alcohol, tobacco and illicit drugs in Canada', *Addiction* 93: 991–1006.

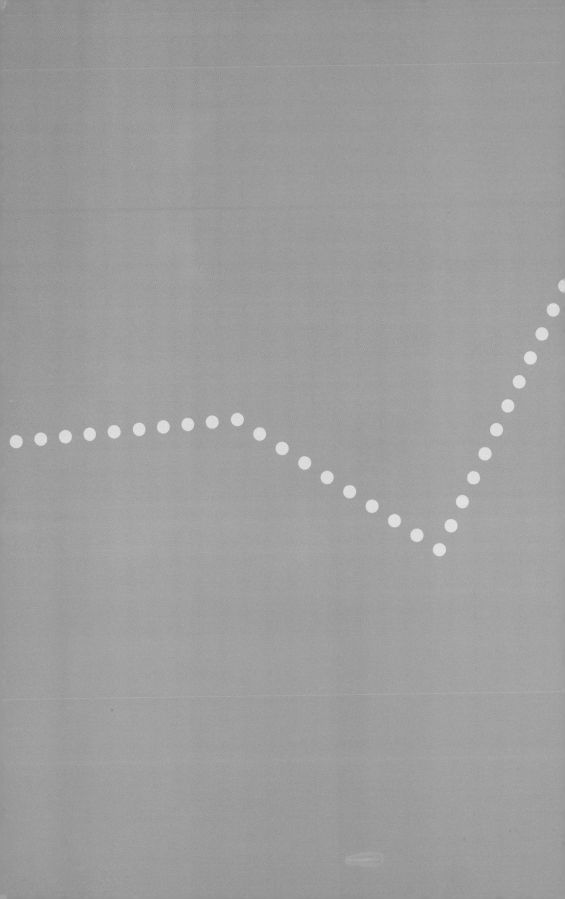

Chapter 10
Assessment of the indirect costs of injecting drug use: which methods should be employed?

Robert Welte, Hans-Helmut König, Johannes Jager and Reiner Leidl

Introduction

Injecting drug use leads to substantial intangible and tangible (direct and indirect) costs. Intangible costs are mainly caused by death, pain, suffering and bereavement (Single et al., 1996a). The direct costs of injecting drug use are the valued resource consumption of tangible goods and services actually delivered to address the consequences of injecting drug use. Examples of direct costs are healthcare, prevention, research and law enforcement costs. The indirect costs (also called productivity costs) are the value of productive services not performed due to the consequences of injecting drug use. Thus, the indirect costs are caused by lost or impaired ability to work due to injecting-drug-use-attributable morbidity (e.g. sick leave), mortality, or crimes (e.g. staying in a detention centre). Indirect costs occur in both the paid and unpaid work sectors. The paid work sector can be defined as all work activities that contribute to the gross domestic product. On the other hand, unpaid work is not recognised in the classical system of national accounts (Goldschmidt-Clermont and Pagnossin-Aligisakis, 1995). It mainly consists of household work, caring for family and non-family members (informal care), maintenance of transport, consumer items and homes, and engagement for society (work in an honorary position and voluntary work).

Extensive studies on the costs of unhealthy lifestyles for Australia, Canada, Switzerland and the US (Institut suisse de prophylaxie de l'alcoolisme, 1990; Collins and Lapsely, 1991, 1996; Rice et al., 1991; Single et al., 1996b; Harwood et al., 1998) demonstrate that the costs of illicit drug use are considerable, but less than the costs of tobacco smoking or excessive alcohol drinking. Indirect costs cause the major part of illicit drug use costs for society, for example 60 % in Canada (Single et al., 1996b). The data do not specify to what extent these costs are attributable to injecting drug use. However, sharing needles and other injecting paraphernalia is a major risk factor for infection with HIV, HBV and HCV. These three blood-borne viruses caused about 55 % of the deaths attributable to drug abuse in the US in 1992 (Harwood et al., 1998). In Canada, the major causes of drug-related deaths are suicide (42 %) and overdose (23 %) which are also both strongly associated with injecting drug use (Single, 1999).

In 2001, the second edition of the *International guidelines for estimating the costs of substance abuse* was released (Single et al., 2001). However, as in the first edition published in 1996 (Single et al., 1996a), the friction cost method was not considered, nor were different perspectives investigated in detail. Furthermore, it lacked any recommendation for the estimation of the loss of productivity in the unpaid work sector. Only the substitution approach was briefly mentioned for valuing this productivity loss, while the opportunity and minimal opportunity cost approaches were neglected.

With this chapter, we try to fill these gaps. We first look at the relevant perspectives for estimating the indirect costs of injecting drug use. Then we present approaches for measuring indirect costs. Finally, we show unit cost estimates for paid and unpaid work loss in Germany and the Netherlands.

Methods

The influence of perspective in the measurement of production loss in the paid and unpaid work sectors due to injecting drug use is explored. For this, the perspectives of the IDU, his family, the employer of the IDU, social insurance, and society are considered. Furthermore, the human capital approach, the friction cost method, and the willingness-to-pay approach are compared and their suitability for estimating the indirect costs of injecting drug use is assessed. By using the module for standardised indirect cost estimation (MICE), the net value of one day of production as well as the present value of the future net product in the paid and unpaid work sectors are computed for Germany and the Netherlands, from a societal perspective and in 1999 prices. Future costs are discounted at 3 % (Gold et al., 1996). MICE consists of a Microsoft Excel spreadsheet, a handbook, and documentation specifying the sources for the data input (Welte et al., 2001). It computes the age- and sex-specific unit costs (net product) per day or year of lost work and the present value of the future net product. The loss of unpaid work is valued according to the opportunity cost approach, the minimal opportunity cost approach and the substitution cost approach.

It should be noted that we always compare the productivity of an IDU with the hypothetical productivity of the same type of individual without injecting drug use. We do not distinguish between internal and external costs or private and social costs as: (a) we consider injecting drug use as an addictive behaviour, i.e. the IDU cannot freely decide about the consumption of injecting drugs; and (b) it is highly unlikely that the IDU was fully informed about the costs that injecting drug use might impose upon him and his dependants and made a rational decision to become an IDU (Single et al., 1996a; Single et al., 2001).

Results

Perspective

The indirect costs of injecting drug use strongly depend on the chosen perspective. Table 1 shows which indirect cost categories are of interest, given different perspectives.

IDU

Paid work sector: Depending on his employment status, an IDU might be concerned about the loss of paid work due to his injecting drug use. By definition, the sickness of an unemployed person results in no loss of paid work. For the employed and self-employed individual, one should distinguish between loss of paid work due to reduced productivity, sick leave, work disability and death. Productivity issues and days of sick leave are in general of less interest to the employed than to the self-employed individual. Only if there are incentives to improve work performance and reduce sick leave, for example work-performance-related bonuses or partial payment for sick leave days, will decreased work productivity or sick leave result in costs to the employed individual. On the other hand, self-employed individuals will almost always suffer financially from reduced work performance or sick leave days. Work disability will usually affect both employed and self-employed persons as disability insurance generally covers only a portion of income.

Unpaid work sector: An IDU is likely to consider the loss of household work, maintenance work, and of the care of family members. In each situation, either another family member has to replace him (causing no costs to him) or the work has to be externalised and bought in the market (causing costs to him). Not providing care to non-family members as well as not being able to engage for society are likely to be less of a consideration to an IDU, as the substitution costs will usually not be borne by him.

Family of the IDU

Paid work sector: The perspective of an IDU's family (i.e. partner plus dependent children) is basically the same as that of the IDU as any decrease in his income will also result in a decrease in the family's budget.

Table 1: The perspective determines which indirect cost categories should be considered

Cost category	IDU* — status prior to injecting drug use			Perspective			
	Unemployed	Employed	Self-employed	Family of the IDU	Employer of the IDU	Social insurance	Society
Paid work sector							
Reduced performance	n.a.	No to fully†	Fully	See IDU	Fully	No to fully†	Fully
Sickness leave	n.a.	No to fully†	Partly to fully‡	See IDU	Partly to fully§	No to partly§	Fully
Work disability + early retirement	n.a.	Partly to fully‡	Partly to fully‡	Partly to fully‡	Partly‖	Partly	Fully
Death	n.a.	Partly to fully‡	Partly to fully‡	Partly to fully‡	Partly‖	Partly	Fully
Unpaid work sector							
Household work	No to fully	No to fully	No to fully	Fully	No	No to fully¶	Fully
Maintenance and building of transport means, consumer items, houses	No to fully	No to fully	No to fully	Fully	No	No	Fully
Care of family members	No to fully	No to fully	No to fully	Fully	No	No to fully¶	Fully
Care of non-family members	No	No	No	No	No	No to fully¶	Fully
Engagement for society	No	No	No	No	No	No	Fully

*   Injecting drug user.
†   Depending on the work contract.
‡   Depending on insurance.
§   Depending on the duration of sickness leave (e.g. in Germany, the social insurance pays the salary after the first six weeks of sickness leave).
‖   Only the costs for hiring and training a replacement worker + the costs for the decreased production during the training phase of the replacement worker.
¶   Depending on whether additional (professional) help is used and paid for by social insurance.

Unpaid work sector: Again, the perspective of the family is similar to that of the IDU — with one exception. The loss of work within the household/family will always be fully borne by the family.

Employer of the IDU

Paid work sector: An employer only considers the total costs of decreased performance and sick leave. By that he should distinguish between indirect costs due to sick leave, early retirement (inability to work or incapacity to follow one's profession) and mortality. For short periods of sick leave, each sick day should be valued. For long periods of sick leave, only the costs for the loss of production until another employee has fully replaced the IDU, plus the costs for hiring and training a replacement worker, are of interest. If the employer pays the salary of a sick person only for a specific time interval (e.g. in Germany during the first six weeks), this time interval will limit the maximum time that production loss should be counted. Indirect costs due to early retirement and mortality are restricted to the costs for finding and training a new worker and the decreased production during the training phase of the new worker.

Unpaid work sector: The loss of unpaid work is of no interest to the employer.

Social insurance

Paid work sector: If reduced performance leads to a decreased wage, the premiums for social insurance might also decrease. In the case of long-term sick leave, the social insurance of some countries pays a proportion of the wage after a specified time of sick leave (e.g. in Germany after the first six weeks). Early retirement has two effects: first, social insurance loses contributions, and, second, it has to pay pensions for the early retirees or their surviving dependants. Depending on the age of the IDU, his death may lead either to a positive or a negative net transfer by social insurance.

Unpaid work sector: Costs are applicable only if additional help (e.g. by employing a professional help service) is purchased and paid by the social insurance.

Society

All indirect costs in the paid and unpaid work sectors should be considered from a societal perspective regardless of who causes or pays the costs. However, transfer costs (e.g. welfare money) should not be included as they represent only a redistribution of resources and not a loss of resources to society. The societal perspective corresponds to a public health view where all the consequences of an unhealthy lifestyle, or a disease for all individuals, are considered. Many international guidelines for economic evaluations of healthcare technologies recommend the societal perspective, for example the Australian Commonwealth Department of Health and Ageing (2002), the Canadian (CCOHTA, 1997) and the Dutch guidelines (CVZ, 1999).

Table 2: Approaches to estimating indirect costs

Approach	Work sector	Valuation
Human capital	Paid	Net product for perspective of society
		Net earnings for perspective of IDU (¹) or his or her family
	Unpaid	Opportunity costs
		Minimal opportunity costs
		Substitution costs
Friction costs	Paid	Friction costs
	Unpaid	Friction costs
Willingness-to-pay	Paid	Individual willingness to pay
	Unpaid	Individual willingness to pay

(¹) Injecting drug user.

Approaches for measuring productivity costs

In general, there are three main approaches for measuring indirect costs: the human capital approach, the friction cost method and the willingness-to-pay approach (Table 2).

Human capital approach

The human capital approach (Rice, 1967; Rice and Cooper, 1967) is the standard approach for estimating indirect costs. It is suitable for all perspectives, with the exception of that of the employer and social insurance, and can be used for assessing the indirect costs due to paid and unpaid work loss. It estimates the maximum or potential loss of production as a consequence of disease or death. The full extent of output that a person cannot produce due to a disease is assessed. For long-term work absence, the present value of the future net product has to be calculated with discounting. The loss of paid as well as unpaid work can be considered.

When measuring the loss of unpaid work, bed-disability days are ideally used. The US National Center for Health Statistics defines a bed-disability day as 'a day when a person stayed in bed more than half a day because of illness or injury' (National Center for Health Statistics, 2000).

The average time spent daily on unpaid work can be derived from time-use studies. Such studies have been conducted all over the world, i.e. in Africa (e.g.

Morocco, Nigeria, South Africa), North and South America (e.g. Canada, the Dominican Republic, Ecuador, Guatemala, Mexico, the US), Asia (e.g. India, Japan, Republic of Korea), Australia (Australia, New Zealand) and especially in Europe: there are time-use studies for Austria, Bulgaria, Denmark, Finland, France, Germany, Italy, the Netherlands and the UK (Goldschmidt-Clermont and Pagnossin-Aligisakis, 1995; United Nations Statistics Division, 2002). In some countries, such as the Netherlands, time-use studies are regularly conducted (SCP, 2002). In order to make the results of time-use studies more comparable, attempts are being made to standardise time-use survey methodology worldwide (Bittman, 2000). Methodological guidelines on harmonised European time-use surveys were issued in April 2000. At that time, 10 of the 15 EU Member States had already conducted, or were planning to conduct, time-use studies in the near future based on this harmonised methodology. These countries were: Belgium, Finland, France, Germany, Italy, Norway, Portugal, Spain, Sweden, and the UK (Osterberg, 2000). Other countries were still considering the application of the standardised methodology.

Once one has derived lost time in the paid and unpaid work sectors it has to be valued in monetary terms. For the valuation of paid work, the perspective determines which valuation option should be chosen.

Societal perspective: The average net product offers the best option, as it represents the added net value for society. If it is known that the IDU was employed before he started to use injecting drugs, the average net product per employee should be used. Otherwise, the average net product per capita is first choice. In both cases, the average net product should be stratified by age and sex. Average labour costs corrected by survival probabilities and the risk of unemployment can be used for approximation of the average net product.

Perspective of the IDU or his family: The net earnings by age and sex are the best valuation concept as the IDU or his family will most likely value their work time as the amount of money that they directly receive. If it is known that the IDU was employed before he began to use injecting drugs, the net earnings of employees should be used, otherwise the net earnings per capita are best. In both cases, the net earnings should be corrected for survival probabilities and the risk of unemployment.

For the valuation of unpaid work, the perspective is also important. For the societal perspective and the perspective of the IDU or his family, the following approaches can be used.

Opportunity cost approach: The basic idea is that instead of doing unpaid work, a person could perform paid work. From a societal perspective, the opportunity costs are estimated by using the average net product by age and sex. From the perspective of an IDU or his family, only the net earnings are relevant and thus the average net earnings by age and sex should be applied.

Minimal opportunity cost approach: The net earnings of an employed housekeeper can be used to estimate the minimal opportunity costs for all three perspectives. The underlying idea is that a person would at least receive the net earnings of an employed housekeeper if he did typical unpaid work (household work) for someone else.

Substitution cost approach: The average labour costs of professionals doing the same type of work can be used to approximate the substitution costs for all perspectives. Hence, the productivity loss is valued by asking how much it would cost to buy the lost services in the market, i.e. in the paid work sector.

Friction cost method

The friction cost method has been developed in the Netherlands (Koopmanschap et al., 1995; Koopmanschap and Rutten, 1996) and is required by the Dutch guidelines for pharmaco-economic evaluations (CVZ, 1999). Its application is restricted to the perspective of society and the employer. It estimates only the actual loss of paid work for society or a company. The main assumption is that the paid work of any long-term absent person can be undertaken by an unemployed person. The timespan needed to find and train a replacement worker, i.e. to restore the initial production level, is called the friction time. For any work absence that takes longer than the friction time, only the friction time is considered for the calculation of the production loss. The friction time has been estimated for the Netherlands at three (CVZ, 1999), four (CVZ, 2000), or six months (Jacobs-van der Bruggen et al., 2002) and for Germany (Magvas, 1999) at 71 (old *Länder*) and 70 days (new *Länder*), respectively. It is assumed that during a work absence, about 80 % of the production of a person will be lost (elasticity for annual labour time versus labour productivity = 0.8) as the other 20 % will be taken over by work colleagues or made up for by the sick person after recovery — in other words, by using internal free capacities. The value of lost production plus the costs for finding and training a replacement worker plus the costs of negative medium-term macroeconomic consequences of absence and disability reveal the friction costs, i.e. the indirect costs based on the friction cost method (Koopmanschap et al., 1995; Koopmanschap and Rutten, 1996).

For the valuation of lost production in the paid work sector, the average net product by age and sex per capita or per employee (again depending on whether or not the pre-injecting drug use employment status is known) should be used for the societal perspective. For the employer's perspective, the labour costs represent the best valuation option.

For the valuation of unpaid work, we do not recommend any method, as the friction cost method has only been developed and used for the paid work sector and the concept of friction costs does not fit the majority of unpaid work, that is household work and informal care. If the housekeeping family member falls sick, the work will usually be taken over by other family members. As a result no production losses emerge but the replacing family member has less free time, which is not valued in the friction cost method. If a professional worker (e.g. housekeeper, nurse) has to be hired, there will be no production loss either as it is assumed that he or she is otherwise unemployed. However, there will be costs for finding and training of the replacement worker. The same costs can be assumed for societal engagement of a sick person. Forgone maintenance of the home, means of transport or consumer items due to sickness will most likely be made up after recovery. In addition to the costs for finding and training a replacement worker, there are possible costs due to medium-term macroeconomic consequences: if the demand for employed housekeepers increases, the price for them might also increase.

Willingness-to-pay approach

The willingness-to-pay approach measures the amount an individual would pay in order to obtain a risk reduction, for example to avoid falling sick or to prevent somebody else from falling sick (Mitchell and Carson, 1990; Klose, 1999). It can be used for any perspective except the perspective of social insurance and it considers both paid and unpaid work. The main problem with this method is that it is very difficult to measure the indirect costs only without measuring the intangible or some of the direct costs at the same time. Additionally, the discrimination between indirect costs in the paid and unpaid work sectors is causing problems. As a consequence, the willingness-to-pay approach is not suitable for the measurement of indirect costs only (i.e. without measuring intangible costs as well).

Furthermore, while the other approaches mostly rely on data that can easily be derived from national statistics, the willingness-to-pay approach is much more demanding. Basically, it requires that a new study be conducted with patient or population questioning.

Unit costs for valuing the productivity loss

By using the human capital approach, we calculated the unit costs for valuing the productivity loss of IDUs in Germany and the Netherlands, from a societal perspective. Table 3 shows the unit costs ʿ ʾʰe loss of one actual workday in the paid work sector. Except for the very young ages, the unit costs are rather similar in the two countries considered. For valuing the loss of unpaid work, we used the

Table 3: Unit costs for the loss of one actual workday in the paid work sector from a societal perspective (EUR, 1999 prices) ([1])

| Age (years) | Unit costs per capita | | | |
| | Germany | | Netherlands | |
	Males	Females	Males	Females
15–19	48	29	7	4
20–24	115	85	57	43
25–29	151	108	130	86
30–34	189	110	168	78
35–39	206	107	187	65
40–44	212	111	201	66
45–49	217	110	204	65
50–54	214	98	207	50
55–59	165	66	154	31
60–64	72	18	45	6
65–69	11	2	4	1

| Age (years) | Unit costs per employee | | | |
| | Germany | | Netherlands | |
	Males	Females	Males	Females
15–19	144	112	29	19
20–24	165	135	85	70
25–29	189	156	144	113
30–34	214	158	181	118
35–39	230	152	203	111
40–44	240	153	219	111
45–49	248	153	229	113
50–54	259	155	238	113
55–59	255	146	237	110
60–64	263	153	212	94
65–69	250	146	102	69

([1]) Valuation with the average net product per capita or per employee.

Table 4: Unit costs for the loss of one day in the unpaid work sector from a societal perspective (EUR, 1999 prices)

Age (years)	Opportunity costs			
	Germany		Netherlands	
	Males	Females	Males	Females
12–14	—	—	—	—
15–19	20	23	2	3
20–24	38	66	22	36
25–29	43	75	36	59
30–34	66	112	46	61
35–39	71	108	65	69
40–44	70	104	70	69
45–49	73	105	73	71
50–54	87	109	75	67
55–59	86	103	75	66
60–64	118	110	67	56
65–69	112	105	39	50
70–74	—	—	—	—
75–79	—	—	—	—
80–84	—	—	—	—
85–89	—	—	—	—

Age (years)	Minimal opportunity costs			
	Germany		Netherlands	
	Males	Females	Males	Females
12–14	7	10	4	6
15–19	7	10	4	6
20–24	12	24	11	23
25–29	12	24	11	23
30–34	16	36	11	23
35–39	16	36	14	27
40–44	15	34	14	27
45–49	15	34	14	27
50–54	17	36	14	26
55–59	17	36	14	26
60–64	23	37	14	26
65–69	23	37	17	31
70–74	20	28	15	28
75–79	18	25	13	25
80–84	16	22	12	22
85–89	13	19	10	19

Age (years)	Substitution costs			
	Germany		Netherlands	
	Males	Females	Males	Females
12–14	15	22	7	12
15–19	15	22	7	12
20–24	25	52	22	45
25–29	25	52	22	45
30–34	34	77	22	45
35–39	34	77	28	54
40–44	32	74	28	54
45–49	32	74	28	54
50–54	36	76	28	52
55–59	36	76	28	52
60–64	48	78	28	52
65–69	48	78	33	63
70–74	43	60	30	56
75–79	38	54	27	50
80–84	34	47	23	44
85–89	29	40	20	38

Table 4 (continued)

opportunity cost approach, the minimal opportunity cost approach and the substitution cost approach. The results are presented in Table 4. The big differences between the different valuation concepts are striking and show how important is the selection of the valuation concept. In general, the opportunity cost approach renders costs significantly higher than the substitution cost approach. In some age and sex strata, the costs are even double. On the other hand, the substitution cost approach leads to approximately double the costs of the minimal opportunity cost method. Due to their retirement, there are no earning or labour costs available for persons aged 70 years or older. Thus, the opportunity cost approach is not suitable for valuing unpaid work of older individuals. Finally, Table 5 shows the present value of the future net product for paid work and Table 6 for unpaid work (3 % discounting). The results are similar to those shown in Tables 3 and 4 — again, in general, the opportunity cost approach renders the highest costs, followed by the substitution cost approach and the minimal opportunity cost approach.

Table 5: **Present value of the future net product in the paid work sector from a societal perspective (EUR, 1999 prices, 3 % discounting)**

| Age (years) | Unit costs per capita | | | |
| | Germany | | Netherlands | |
	Males	Females	Males	Females
0–4	546 700	316 710	460 090	192 240
5–9	634 370	367 430	534 230	223 020
10–14	735 990	426 190	619 430	258 670
15–19	828 290	478 580	715 090	297 890
20–24	871 330	491 190	794 690	318 830
25–29	861 690	459 180	816 450	295 230
30–34	808 310	407 100	776 050	246 470
35–39	716 020	348 240	695 420	202 190
40–44	598 400	281 020	583 750	158 380
45–49	459 740	202 800	445 540	108 070
50–54	301 370	120 840	283 230	59 290
55–59	146 960	49 910	122 420	22 010
60–64	43 610	10 900	26 580	3 890
65–69	5 520	1 240	2 210	550

| Age (years) | Unit costs per employee | | | |
| | Germany | | Netherlands | |
	Males	Females	Males	Females
0–4	778 800	559 080	586 800	352 000
5–9	903 710	648 620	681 350	408 340
10–14	1 048 470	752 340	790 020	473 630
15–19	1 137 690	810 680	900 800	538 690
20–24	1 146 040	798 910	981 410	574 010
25–29	1 130 400	760 010	1 008 400	560 040
30–34	1 084 460	701 950	983 460	514 790
35–39	1 010 500	638 040	920 000	464 070
40–44	914 430	569 370	826 130	411 020
45–49	799 030	491 910	704 730	348 880
50–54	662 670	404 360	556 330	276 660
55–59	508 140	308 830	382 550	195 090
60–64	333 350	201 400	195 670	110 890
65–69	124 140	73 430	51 350	35 710

Table 6: Present value of the future net product in the unpaid work sector from a societal perspective (EUR, 1999 prices, 3 % discounting)

Age (years)	Opportunity costs			
	Germany		Netherlands	
	Males	Females	Males	Females
0–4	383 660	560 120	288 210	333 710
5–9	445 180	649 820	334 640	387 120
10–14	516 500	753 740	388 020	449 010
15–19	580 480	852 560	448 250	518 420
20–24	618 460	903 010	497 940	564 070
25–29	639 860	908 330	521 730	561 060
30–34	636 790	869 690	525 120	531 990
35–39	605 490	792 050	501 440	488 700
40–44	567 180	711 340	450 730	431 690
45–49	524 500	622 930	385 130	364 900
50–54	462 890	517 320	305 720	290 180
55–59	382 450	397 040	213 650	209 010
60–64	264 070	257 860	115 000	125 600
65–69	96 400	92 460	33 410	43 730
70–74	–	–	–	–
75–79	–	–	–	–
80–84	–	–	–	–
85–89	–	–	–	–

Age (years)	Minimal opportunity costs			
	Germany		Netherlands	
	Males	Females	Males	Females
0–4	101 600	211 130	81 870	165 060
5–9	117 900	244 950	95 060	191 480
10–14	135 440	282 160	109 560	220 920
15–19	143 050	306 650	120 170	243 910
20–24	147 980	321 700	125 410	254 850
25–29	149 290	324 690	123 770	250 720
30–34	146 840	317 370	121 870	246 030
35–39	139 940	297 510	116 990	236 420
40–44	133 270	276 410	108 680	221 140
45–49	127 190	254 180	99 470	203 990
50–54	119 200	228 190	89 540	186 160

Table 6 (continued)

Age (years)	Minimal opportunity costs			
	Germany		Netherlands	
	Males	Females	Males	Females
55–59	109 260	197 750	79 110	167 650
60–64	94 500	163 010	68 270	147 510
65–69	73 350	122 710	54 900	120 730
70–74	53 800	87 090	39 810	89 410
75–79	37 130	59 560	27 220	61 150
80–84	22 970	35 740	16 780	36 620
85–89	9 280	13 240	6 990	14 040

Age (years)	Substitution costs			
	Germany		Netherlands	
	Males	Females	Males	Females
0–4	217 100	451 140	163 470	329 570
5–9	251 920	523 400	189 810	382 320
10–14	289 400	602 910	218 760	441 100
15–19	305 650	655 220	239 940	487 000
20–24	316 210	687 390	250 410	508 860
25–29	318 990	693 770	247 130	500 600
30–34	313 770	678 130	243 330	491 240
35–39	299 030	635 710	233 590	472 060
40–44	284 760	590 620	217 010	441 540
45–49	271 770	543 130	198 600	407 300
50–54	254 710	487 590	178 790	371 700
55–59	233 460	422 550	157 950	334 750
60–64	201 930	348 310	136 300	294 520
65–69	157 910	264 190	109 620	241 060
70–74	115 820	187 510	79 480	178 530
75–79	79 930	128 240	54 340	122 090
80–84	49 460	76 950	33 500	73 110
85–89	19 980	28 500	13 950	28 040

Discussion and conclusions

Our results, as well as the recent findings by Godfrey et al. (2002), underline the great importance of the perspective on the level and relevance of different cost categories. Some cost categories are of no interest from one perspective (e.g. unpaid work from the employer's perspective), while they may represent the bulk of costs from other perspectives (e.g. unpaid work from the perspective of an unemployed person). This information might be helpful for decision-makers when deciding how to create prevention programmes against injecting drug use, as well as whether the government, social insurance, the IDUs or the employer should finance such a measure. In order to gain comparable study results for all EU Member States, we recommend that the societal perspective be chosen whenever possible as a reference perspective. Depending on the focus of the study, additional perspectives should be applied. For this, Table 1 might prove helpful.

For all perspectives except the perspective of the employer and social insurance, the human capital approach seems to be first choice as an estimation tool as it mainly requires routinely collected data and enables the valuation of work loss in the unpaid work sector in a feasible way. This approach has only one disadvantage. From a societal perspective, it is only able to calculate the maximum indirect costs, as unemployment cannot be taken fully into account. While it is possible to adjust the labour costs per capita (by multiplying the labour costs with the employed labour force participation rate) as well as the labour costs per employee (by applying the probabilities that a person would stay employed in the follow-up years) for unemployment (Welte et al., 2000), it is not possible to adjust for the probability that an otherwise unemployed person replaces the sick, early retired or dead person.

This problem led to the development of the friction cost method, which is supposed to estimate the actual indirect costs in the paid work sector. However, this method is limited to the societal and employer's perspective and brings some other problems. Liljas (1998) has pointed out that the assumption that the elasticity for annual labour time versus labour productivity does not equal one violates one of the fundamental axioms of the theory of the firm — the value of the marginal product of a factor should equal its marginal costs, i.e. firms only employ labour until the marginal value produced by the worker equals the worker's labour costs.

When using the friction cost method in connection with the societal perspective, two other problems emerge. Firstly, the assumption that the vacancies are always filled by previously unemployed persons. If an employed person fills the vacancy, a new vacancy emerges that needs to be filled again, resulting in at least two friction periods (Liljas, 1998). Secondly, the assumption that any person can be replaced by someone who is unemployed and would have otherwise remained unemployed seems rather unrealistic, especially for jobs that require highly skilled persons. Furthermore, the friction cost method has the disadvantage that it is not suitable for the estimation of production losses in the unpaid work sector. Due to these problems, this approach seems less suitable for the estimation of indirect costs from a societal perspective than the human capital approach. However, the friction cost method can be used for the assessment of the minimum indirect costs from a limited societal perspective, especially because production losses in the unpaid work sector are excluded. In addition, this method seems the best available approach when conducting a study from an employer's perspective.

Although the willingness-to-pay approach is a valuable method for estimating the total (i.e. direct, indirect and intangible) costs of injecting drug use, it is not really able to discriminate between the different types of cost. Because of this, it seems unsuitable for the estimation of indirect costs only.

While the indirect costs for the loss of work in the unpaid work sector are below those in the paid work sector in most age and sex strata (Tables 3 and 4), they are still high. Furthermore, exclusion of these costs would be unacceptable ethically, as this would neglect the value of important tasks such as taking care of the family. Hence, they should definitely be taken into account in cost of injecting drug use studies. Because they rely heavily on data from time-use studies, the issue of European guidelines for time-use studies is a milestone for the carrying out and comparison of such studies within the EU. This development will also promote the comparability of cost-effectiveness studies in different Member States of the EU, as indirect costs in the unpaid work sector are increasingly recognised and included in economic evaluations. Hopefully, data from harmonised time-use surveys will soon be available for all EU Member States.

Our results demonstrate that the selection of the valuation method for the loss of unpaid work has a great impact on the unit costs for unpaid work. So far, there is no agreement in the scientific community as to which valuation method should be preferred. This problem is not limited to the estimation of indirect costs for illicit drug use but for all types of disease studies. Until such standardisation is achieved, the best option seems to be to report the results gained by each of the approaches and to present the methods used in a transparent and detailed way.

References

Bittman, M. (2000), *Issues in the design of time-use surveys for collecting data on paid and unpaid work*, University of New South Wales, Sydney.

Canadian Coordinating Office for Health Technology Assessment (CCOHTA) (November 1997), *Guidelines for economic evaluation of pharmaceuticals*, CCOHTA, Ottawa.

College voor Zorgverzekeringen (CVZ) (1999), *Richtlijnen voor farmaco-economisch onderzoek*, CVZ, Amstelveen.

College voor Zorgverzekeringen (CVZ) (2000), *Handleiding voor kostenonderzoek*, CVZ, Amstelveen.

Collins, D., Lapsley, H. M. (1991), *Estimating the economic costs of drug abuse in Australia. National Campaign against Drug Abuse*, Monograph Series No 15, Australian Government Publishing Service, Canberra.

Collins, D. J., Lapsley, H. M. (1996), *The social costs of drug abuse in Australia in 1988 and 1992*, Monograph No 30, Commonwealth Department of Human Services and Health, Australian Government Publishing Service, Canberra.

Commonwealth Department of Health and Ageing (September 2002), *Guidelines for the pharmaceutical industry on preparation of submissions to the Pharmaceutical Benefits Advisory Committee: including major submission involving economic analyses*, Commonwealth Department of Health and Ageing, Canberra.

Godfrey, C., Eaton, G., McDougall, C., Culyer, A. (2002), *The economics and social costs of Class A drug use in England and Wales, 2000*, Home Office Research Study 249, Home Office Research, Development and Statistics Directorate, London.

Gold, M. R., Siegel, J. A., Russel, L. B., Weinstein, M. C. (1996), *Cost-effectiveness in health and medicine*, Oxford University Press, New York.

Goldschmidt-Clermont, L., Pagnossin-Aligisakis, E. (1995), *Measures of unrecorded economic activities in fourteen countries*, United Nations Development Programme (UNDP), New York.

Harwood, H., Fountain, D., Livermore, G. (1998), *The economic costs of alcohol and drug abuse in the United States, 1992*, National Institute of Health, Bethesda.

Institut suisse de prophylaxie de l'alcoolisme (1990), *Le probleme de la drogue — en particulier en Suisse — considere sous son aspect social et preventif*, Office federal de la sante publique, Lausanne.

Jacobs-van der Bruggen, M. U. M., Welte, R., Koopmanschap, M. A., Jager, J. C. (2002), *Aan roken toe te schrijven productiviteitskosten voor Nederlandse werkgevers in 1999*, National Institute of Public Health and the Environment, Bilthoven.

Klose, T. (1999), 'The contingent valuation method in health care', *Health Policy* 47: 97–123.

Koopmanschap, M. A., Rutten, F. F. H. (1996), 'A practical guide for calculating indirect costs of disease', *Pharmacoeconomics* 10: 460–6.

Koopmanschap, M. A., Rutten, F. F. H., van Ineveld, B. M., van Roijen, L. (1995), 'The friction cost method for measuring indirect costs of disease', *Journal of Health Economics* 14: 171–89.

Liljas, B. (1998), 'How to calculate indirect costs in economic evaluations', *Pharmacoeconomics* 13 (1, Pt 1): 1–7.

Magvas, E. (1999), *Wie lange dauert es, eine Stelle zu besetzen? Wer wird eingestellt?*, Institut für Arbeitsmarkt- und Berufsforschung, Nuremberg.

Mitchell, R. C., Carson, R. T. (1990), *Using surveys to value public goods: the contingent valuation method*, Resources for the future, Washington, DC.

National Center for Health Statistics (February 2000), *Health outcomes among Hispanic subgroups: data from the national health interview survey, 1992–95. Advance data number 310*, National Center for Health Statistics, Hyattsville.

Osterberg, C. (2000), *Methodological guidelines on harmonised European time use surveys*, United Nations Secretariat, Statistics Division, New York.

Rice, D. P. (1967), 'Estimating the cost of illness', *American Journal of Public Health 57*: 424–40.

Rice, D. P., Cooper, B. S. (1967), 'The economic value of human life', *American Journal of Public Health 57*: 1954–66.

Rice, D. P., Kelman, S., Miller, L. S. (1991), 'Estimates of economic costs of alcohol and drug abuse and mental illness, 1985 and 1988', *Public Health Reports 106*: 280–92.

Single, E. (1999), *The economic implications of injection drug use*, Canadian Centre on Substance Abuse (CCSA), Ottawa.

Single, E., Collins, D., Easton, B., Harwood, H., Lapsely, H., Maynard, A. (1996a), *International guidelines for estimating the costs of substance abuse*, First edition, Canadian Centre on Substance Abuse (CCSA), Ottawa.

Single, E., Robson, L., Xie, X., Rehm, J. (1996b), *The costs of substance abuse in Canada*, Canadian Centre on Substance Abuse (CCSA), Ottawa.

Single, E., Collins, D., Easton, B., Harwood, H., Lapsely, H., Kopp, P., Wilson, E. (2001), *International guidelines for estimating the costs of substance abuse*, Second edition, Canadian Centre on Substance Abuse (CCSA), Ottawa.

Sociaal en Cultureel Planbureau (SCP) (15 May 2002), 'Het Tijdsbestedingsonderzoek (TBO)' (http://www.tijdsbesteding.nl/).

United Nations Statistics Division. (26 June 2002), 'Time-use surveys. Improving measurement of paid and unpaid work' (http://www.un.org./Depts/unsd/timeuse/tusresource.htm).

Welte, R., König, H.-H., Leidl, R. (2000), 'The costs of health damage and productivity losses attributable to cigarette smoking in Germany', *European Journal of Public Health 10*: 31–8.

Welte, R., Jager J. C., Leidl, R. (2001), 'MICE (module for standardised indirect cost estimation) increases the transferability of study results', *Value in Health 4*: 429.

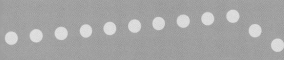

Chapter 11
Models to compute the costs to society of injecting drug use and related morbidity

Fernando Antoñanzas, Roberto Rodríguez and María Velasco

Introduction

This chapter presents a review of several studies on the calculation of the social and economic costs resulting from unhealthy consumption behaviours. We focus on the different methods used to measure these costs in order to identify similarities in the treatment of data and the measurement of costs. We also aim to formulate a general theoretical model suitable to calculate the social costs caused, in particular, by the consumption of drugs and its related diseases (hepatitis B and C and HIV).

The calculation of social cost — the cost to society — is usually based on the quantification of the effects derived from behaviours that, supposedly, have a negative impact on social welfare. The social costs are generated by the consumption of certain products (e.g. drugs) that cause externalities. Negative (or positive) externalities arise when actions taken by an economic agent impose costs (or benefits) on other economic agents. These externalities introduce a divergence between the social costs and benefits and the private ones. While the latter refer to those accruing to people involved in the activity, the former are borne by society as a whole. In general, empirical studies tend to consider only the social costs, ignoring both the social benefits (e.g. savings of future health costs due to a premature death) and the private costs and benefits. Concerning this issue, it is interesting to note that this approach is controversial. From a sickness fund perspective, it could be considered that premature deaths yield social benefits as they save future healthcare costs. Since life years have an intrinsic value 'per se', it would neither be so from a patient nor from a societal perspective. In each of these cases, a pure economic cost calculation would not be adequate, as the life years lost would have to be taken into account in some way.

The calculation of the social costs caused by the consumption of unhealthy substances (drugs) usually implies the identification and quantification of the negative (social and private) consequences derived from that behaviour both in the health sector and in others such as security, justice, etc. Decisions on the consumption of drugs are made without taking into account the costs borne by the rest of society. As a consequence, the consumption of drugs is above the amount that would be considered 'adequate' if all the costs were taken into account. To the extent that studies on the costs caused by drug use try to identify the presence and the magnitude of externalities, they must carefully separate the costs borne by the individual from those borne by society. By calculating the social costs generated by the use of drugs, the empirical studies highlight the undesirable economic effects of this consumption, suggesting that this behaviour should be restricted via public intervention. However, the desirability of such public intervention should be based not only on the potential economic gains, but also on the cost and effectiveness of the intervention itself.

In order to calculate the costs derived from the consumption of drugs, we need an epidemiological base (number of individuals facing the risk) and the costs derived from the risk (e.g. healthcare expenditures). The precision of the studies depends on the accuracy of the measurement of both elements. All the studies reviewed focus on drug addiction but differ in their objectives, theoretical models and hypotheses. In this chapter, we propose a theoretical framework within which all the reviewed studies fit. This allows us to compare them and detect whether the social costs are under- or overestimated.

Different approaches to the calculation of social costs derived from unhealthy behaviours

Lindgreen (1982) characterised three methodologies to calculate the social costs derived from an illness: prevalence costs, incidence costs and costs borne in one period. In all of them, a reference period is considered (in general, a particular year).

The prevalence approach estimates the costs caused by the prevalence or existence of the illness in the reference year. The relevant costs include: prevention, diagnosis, treatment, rehabilitation, care for chronically ill patients, and production losses due to temporary or permanent disability and mortality. When the production losses exceed the reference year, as in the cases of permanent disability and mortality, the usual practice is to discount the value of the prospective production using the human capital criterion: the actual value of the productive capacity of the individual is assigned to the year in which he or she is unable to work or died.

The approach based on the incidence assigns to the reference year the actual value of the healthcare costs generated by the incidence of the illness and the productivity losses through the whole life of the individual.

Finally, the approach based on the cost borne in a specific period takes into account the healthcare costs and production losses during that period due to the actual and previous mortality and morbidity ignoring the prospective production losses.

These methodologies yield similar results when short periods of time without further effects are considered, but, in most cases, the results are different. In general, the approach based on the costs borne in one period gives the largest estimates, followed by those obtained using the prevalence approach. The incidence approach provides the lowest estimates. The third approach includes all costs for the current period, while the incidence approach includes all the costs discounted. However, the prevalence approach only discounts some of the costs. The larger the discount rate, the larger the differences. The differences are also larger if the incidence of the disease is lower, if the costs of the treatment per period are lower or if the cost of the treatment and the losses caused by the disabilities increase with time. The third approach can be considered a particular case of the prevalence approach. For the analysis of the social costs caused by unhealthy behaviours, it could provide a more accurate measurement of the cost incurred in one period.

In search of a theoretical model to calculate social costs

Economic modelling generally assumes complete information and rational economic agents. These assumptions are not satisfied in the case of the consumption of drugs due to their addictive nature and to the lack of knowledge of the risks involved. However, the consumption of addictive products can be consistent with rational behaviour as Becker and Murphy (1988) showed. The absence of complete information and rationality implies that individuals might ignore, apart from the external costs, the private ones. In the presence of externalities and incomplete information, it is well known that a market economy does not achieve an efficient allocation of resources. In these cases, some kind of public intervention may be necessary to improve the efficiency.

The social costs can be classified as follows: (a) if the individual is aware of the risks involved, the social costs are external costs; and (b) if the individual is not aware of the risks, due to a lack of information or for other reasons, the social costs must include both the private costs derived from the unhealthy habit and the external costs. For instance, if a drunk person still keeps on drinking without deriving any utility, the costs to society should include not only the potential car-accident-related costs but also the money paid by that individual for the additional drinks that are private costs; the explanation is that some costly resources have been used to produce the alcohol that nobody is apparently enjoying, because the individual was already drunk. Most of the studies reviewed calculate a combination of private and external costs. In other words, their theoretical models assume that the individual is not fully aware of the risk.

Our analysis reviews the objectives and procedures used in the studies according to a model based on Leu (1982). The studies under consideration focus on the causes and effects of the consumption of drugs, the prevalence of the consumption, the choice of essential parameters to compare two situations (unhealthy habit versus alternative option) isolating other collateral factors (drugs, tobacco, etc.), the reduction in life expectation, the increase in healthcare costs, and the changes in other relevant costs.

The selection of the most feasible model will depend on the behavioural and informational assumptions made. If it is assumed that individuals are not aware of the risks due to a lack of information or other reasons, it is also necessary to calculate the private costs. These are very difficult to measure since the financial and the emotional impact borne by the families of drug users must be included. If, however, it is assumed that the individuals are aware of the risks, only the external costs must be considered. As we are interested in using estimates of the social costs to formulate public policies (in particular, public policies aimed at reducing the incidence of hepatitis C and other diseases among the population of drug users), we must take into account the healthcare costs stemming from the treatment of these diseases and the impact of specific public programmes on the infection rate. We think that this approach (exclusion of private costs) is the most promising one in the sense that we can obtain better estimates of the social costs. However, it should be noted that most of the studies are likely to present an underestimation of the social costs due to a lack of data.

Calculations of the social costs derived from unhealthy behaviours were first carried out for alcohol consumption. The studies by Berry (1976) and by Holtermann and Burchell (1981) in the US, and by Maynard and McDonnell (1985) in the UK marked this new line of research. Their common classification of the main cost categories became standard, even in studies focusing on unhealthy substances other than alcohol. According to the tradition, in the studies reviewed, the main cost categories can be classified as in the abovementioned pioneer studies. Until now, we have distinguished between private and social costs, since public policies are driven by the relative impact of both. However, in the studies reviewed, the authors did not explicitly classify the costs in this way, but gathered them into categories that can be defined as direct and indirect costs. The direct costs include the costs of prevention, treatment and rehabilitation of the diseases caused by the consumption of drugs (healthcare costs), together with the substantial costs related to the behaviour of the drug users (crime, property damage, research costs and social services). The indirect costs cover, apart from the costs derived from production losses, the costs of the judicial system (courts, prisons and police).

Review of relevant studies

We present seven studies that focus on the social costs caused by drug use. In order to select the studies, we consulted different databases (Medline, Francis, Socioabs, Dissertation abstract online and Articlefirst) to identify articles on the calculation of social costs, drug use and risk behaviour. From an exhaustive list, we selected a number of articles that included the cost categories mentioned in the previous section in their calculations.

Although small, the selected sample is considered to illustrate the different objectives pursued by the authors as well as the methodologies implemented. We are aware that the literature on the calculation of the social costs of the consumption of drugs has boomed in recent years. The interested reader can find additional insights in the works by Brown and Crofts (1998), Robson and Single (1995), Single (1999), and Single et al. (1996). The purpose of this chapter is to illustrate the different methodologies adopted by the authors and to highlight the cost categories they consider to be relevant to obtain accurate estimates of the social costs of the consumption of drugs. The selected articles are considered adequate to provide an understanding of the problems researchers face when calculating the social costs of drug use, as well as to identify the relevant cost categories that should be included.

In the following paragraphs, we describe the studies reviewed. The results are presented in Table 1. Table 1 shows all the calculations in euro; the exchange rates used to convert from original currency to euro are given. Although the additional introduction of a correcting inflation factor would yield better comparable results, we have disregarded this option as being beyond the scope of this chapter. As presented in Table 1, the cost figures differ substantially which is mainly due to the

Table 1: Social cost estimates (million EUR)

Cost category	García-Altés et al. (2002) (¹)	Healey et al. (1998) (²)	Heien and Salomaa (1999) (min.–max.)	Kim et al. (1995) (³)	Rice et al. (1991) (³)	Cartwright (1999) (³)	Single et al. (1998) (⁴)
Direct costs	306.01	19.20	102.00–151.99	8.25	16 820.10	30 690	63.36
Health services	264.40	4.00	61.20–91.19		2 290.20	10 890	
Hospital	53.70	0.80	9.18–13.68		627.00		
Medical visits					75.90		
Rehabilitation			43.45–64.75				
Outpatient care			8.57–12.76				
Primary care	8.86						
Long-term care	5.41						
Drugs	122.30	3.20					
Other	74.12				1 587.30		
Material costs	41.61	15.20	40.80–60.80	8.25	14 529.90	19 800	
Administration	10.76						
Crime		15.20	13.60–20.26		14 523.30	19 800	
Damage to property			4.10–6.10				
Prevention	13.54						
Social services	11.94			8.25	6.60		
Research	3.06						
Other	2.30		23.10–34.44				
Indirect costs	228.22		281–601	72.49	31 637.10	75 900	592.56
Production	122.91				9 396.20		
Absenteeism					6 576.90		
Mortality	122.91				2 819.30		
Other	105.3				22 240.90		
Institutionalisation	7.61						
Crime victims					926.20		
Imprisonment					4 877.40		
Judicial	97.68				15 373.60		
Other					1 063.70		
Total	534.23	19.20	383–753	80.74	48 457.20	106 590	655.92

(¹) Original currency ESP: EUR 1 = ESP 166.386.
(²) Original currency GBP: EUR 1 = GBP 0.625.
(³) Original currency USD: EUR 1 = USD 0.91.
(⁴) Original currency CAD: EUR 1 = CAD 1.39.

fact that the authors do not compute the same cost categories and that the population sizes differ considerably. This reduces the relevance of a strict quantitative comparison, and we have simply converted the currencies used in each study into euro to facilitate the reading of the table.

García-Altés et al. (2002) estimated the social costs caused by the consumption of illegal drugs in Spain. They performed a cost-of-illness study using the prevalence approach. The reference year was 1997. For direct costs, they included the costs of healthcare, prevention, continual education and research, together with administrative costs, the costs of non-governmental organisations, and crime-related costs (justice and criminal system). For indirect costs, the productivity losses associated with mortality and hospitalisation of drug addicts were considered.

The study determined the main health consequences of the consumption of illicit drugs and computed the associated healthcare costs. Most of the calculations (the costs of acute care, emergency care, long-term care and drugs) were made taking into account a measurement of frequency and a measurement of cost. The measurements of frequency were based on the use of healthcare services. This study contributed to the identification of the importance of the diseases related to the use of drugs by calculating the healthcare costs derived from the treatment of HIV, viral hepatitis, endocarditis, tuberculosis and mental illnesses. However, the results for the specific diseases were not reported in the study.

The minimum costs of the consumption of illegal drugs in Spain were estimated at EUR 534.23 million. Direct costs accounted for 58 % of the minimum costs, with healthcare costs amounting to 86 % of the direct costs and 50 % of the total costs. The study used very few epidemiological data as it was difficult to find accurate figures on this issue. This lack of one of the two factors for the calculation of total social costs (population and unit costs) made it impossible to obtain per capita costs.

The study by Healey et al. (1998) showed the economic and social burden associated with the use of drugs in the UK, taking 1995 as the reference year. Their estimates were based on self-reported data obtained from interviews with 1 075 drug users at intake to the 'National treatment outcome research study' and additional cost information gathered from contacts with healthcare and addiction services, the justice system and victims of drug-related crimes. They focused, in particular, on the calculation of direct costs, thereby ignoring the intangible (mainly psychological) effects as they could not be quantified. These amounted to GBP 12 million, that is approximately EUR 17 million.

Heien and Salomaa (1999) estimated the social costs of drug use in Finland between 1990 and 1995. They used the prevalence approach with data obtained from Finnish governmental bodies. The costs resulting from the use of drugs were estimated by defining the individual components affecting the costs and subsequently assigning a financial value to them. The direct costs included healthcare costs, financial compensations and disability pensions, costs of judicial and prison services, the value of property loss, and the costs of preventive activities. The indirect costs included the value of production losses due to absenteeism, costs of mortality and costs borne by victims of crime. They obtained an estimate for the total costs ranging from EUR 383 million to EUR 753 million. As in most of the studies reviewed, the healthcare costs are the most important component of the direct costs. They account for 60 % of these costs.

Kim et al. (1995) performed a cost–benefit analysis of drug use prevention programmes between 1979 and 1992 in the US. The study tried to quantify the benefits for society derived from the reduction in drug consumption achieved by drug prevention programmes. Their hypothesis, according to previous studies, was that the prevention programmes were the cause of the decrease in the drug consumption observed. By doing so, they ignored other possible causes such as risk perception. Between 1979 and 1992, there was a sustained decrease in the use of illicit drugs. While in 1979 13.7 % of the population older than 12 years reported having consumed drugs, the figure had decreased to 5.5 % in 1992. The social benefits were calculated as the costs saved by society thanks to the prevention programmes. They showed that the cost–benefit ratio was 1:15. Society saved USD 15 for each dollar spent on prevention.

Rice et al. (1991) estimated the social costs of the consumption of drugs in the US, taking 1985 as the reference year. They used a prevalence approach and calculated the costs for the years 1985 and 1988. They considered the healthcare direct costs, and the morbidity and mortality costs. They also calculated the costs of criminal activities and the value of the productivity losses due to crimes, imprisonment and family care. HIV-related costs were also taken into account. Again, the authors did not disaggregate the costs of each disease caused by the use of drugs. Their estimated social costs amounted to USD 44 052 million. Due to a lack of information, this value, as the authors recognise, must be considered as the lower limit of the real social costs.

Cartwright (1999) discussed some of the results of a study published by the National Institute on Drug Abuse, and evaluated the burden of drug use on the US economy in terms of healthcare costs, productivity costs and crime-related costs.

Drug use generated USD 4.4 billion in treatment and prevention expenditures, accounting for 4.5 % of total societal costs. Medical complications resulted in USD 5.5 billion to society. The major source of societal costs was productivity costs, which amounted to USD 69 billion (71 % of total costs). These costs included the loss of productive capacity by premature deaths due to drug use. Crime-related costs were estimated at USD 57.1 billion. Costs of USD 39.1 billion in earnings losses were due to incarceration, criminal careers and crime-related victimisation. The total social costs amounted to USD 96.9 billion.

Finally, Single et al. (1998) estimated the economic costs of the use of illicit drugs in Canada, taking 1992 as the reference year. They carried out a cost-of-illness study using the prevalence approach. Mortality and morbidity were estimated from meta-analyses to give pooled relative risk estimates and these were combined with prevalence data. The resulting estimates of attributable deaths and hospitalisations were used to calculate associated healthcare, law enforcement, productivity and other costs. Their social cost estimate amounted to CAD 0.911 billion.

Discussion

The studies reviewed show that an accurate calculation of the social costs derived from the use of illicit drugs involves a number of difficulties. Apart from deficiencies in the epidemiological data, in some circumstances, there is no precise knowledge of the causal relationships between the consumption of drugs and the associated healthcare problem. Even if the causal relationships are sometimes known, there are no quality data available.

All the studies reviewed consider similar cost categories, although they differ in the methods used to quantify them. These cost categories are the costs of production losses, the costs of health treatments, the costs of property damage, the costs of criminal activities and rehabilitation costs. The estimates differ substantially as each study applies to a specific country. The surprisingly large differences found in the estimates of the studies by Healey et al. (1998) and Cartwright (1999) can be explained by the different sizes of the populations considered. While the former study considers a sample of 1 075 drug users in the UK without further extrapolation of the results, the analysis in Cartwright (1999) is carried out at the national level for the US.

Most of the studies calculate aggregate healthcare costs with no references to specific diseases such as HIV and hepatitis B and C. This last infection has recently been the focus of several studies dealing with the calculation of its related social costs. As the studies reviewed, presented in Table 1, measure the social costs of drug use without isolating those related to specific diseases, recent studies on hepatitis C have not been included in the table. Nevertheless, we summarise their main findings below. Pollack (2001) explores the potential of NSPs to reduce the incidence and prevalence of hepatitis by using a random-mixing epidemiological model. The study predicts that the programmes have little impact on the incidence and prevalence of hepatitis C. Wong et al. (2000) estimate the future morbidity, mortality and costs resulting from HCV over the next 10 to 20 years in the US. Their projections show direct medical expenditures for HCV of USD 10.7 billion from the year 2010 to the end of 2019. Finally, Leigh et al. (2001) estimate the direct and indirect costs of HCV in the US in 1997 by using the human capital method. They estimate the total costs of HCV at USD 5.46 billion, 33 % of which were healthcare costs.

Since there are some epidemiological data available for Spain, we have calculated an approximation of the pharmaceutical costs generated by the treatments administered to IDUs with HIV and hepatitis C. According to *Boletín Epidemiológico* (2002), there were about 100 000 HIV patients in 2002. Of these patients, nearly 60 % acquired the disease through the use of drugs. If we assume that highly active antiretroviral treatment (HAART) was administered to 50 % of them and that the average cost per patient was EUR 8 000 a year, the annual pharmaceutical costs would amount to nearly EUR 240 million. The hospitalisation costs and outpatient costs as well as laboratory tests should also be included. For hepatitis C, the prevalence rate among drug users is between 50 and 90 % (Crofts et al., 1997; Stein et al., 2001). Stein et al. (2001) reported that about 50 % of the drug users with hepatitis C would be willing to use interferon therapy. The annual cost of treatment with interferon alpha and ribavirin per patient, and of medical care and laboratory tests is about EUR 8 400 and EUR 600, respectively. If we assume that 60 % of the HIV patients are drug users, and we take the lower extreme of the prevalence interval for hepatitis C, the treatment costs of hepatitis C patients would amount to EUR 135 million. Together, the pharmaceutical treatment costs of HIV and hepatitis C would be EUR 375 million. Some HIV patients are also hepatitis C infected and they need treatments for both diseases. This figure represents about 5 % of the total expenditures on prescribed drugs and nearly 1 % of the total healthcare budget in Spain. These figures are merely a preliminary, rough approximation, as there is a lack of accurate calculations of the healthcare costs of hepatitis C in the literature. Although tentative, they highlight the impact of pharmaceutical treatment of the disease on the public budget. It would have been interesting to relate these figures to the estimates found in the reviewed studies. However, the lack of specific information on the costs of HIV and hepatitis B and C in the studies does not allow such a comparison.

Recently, Godfrey et al. (2002) estimated the economic and social costs of Class A drug use in England and Wales for the year 2000. They divided the population of drug users into three types according to the intensity of use: young recreational, older regular and problem users. IDUs are a subset of problem drug users. The estimated number of aware injecting users infected with HIV is 3 694. By taking into account some expenditure estimates for combination therapy per person and per year, they come up with an estimated cost for the treatment of HIV-infected drug users of GBP 61.9 million. As regards hepatitis B, the estimated number of IDUs who have had or are currently infected with it is 53 975. By taking into account a treatment cost of GBP 143 per person per year, they obtain an annual treatment cost for hepatitis B in the order of GBP 7.8 million. The estimated number of injecting drug users infected with hepatitis C is 81 782. By assuming annual treatment costs similar to those for hepatitis B, they come up with an estimated cost of GBP 11.7 million. Infectious diseases may be costing some GBP 80 million (or EUR 115 million) per year.

In those studies that calculated indirect costs, the authors had to determine how to compute the value of production losses due to mortality. Rice et al. (1991) used the average annual income per sex and age, assuming that the prospective income of an average person will follow the pattern of the US census. However, this method to calculate the value of production losses underestimates the losses of the non-active individuals.

The unemployed are assigned an income equal to the salary for household chores without considering their potential income for out-of-home work in the future. Also, production losses have to be discounted. However, the discount rate is not mentioned and, sometimes, it is not clear whether costs have been discounted at all.

In many instances, the lack of data is a serious problem. Data on absenteeism, reduction in productivity, social services for the relatives of drug users, or criminal behaviours are almost non-existent. Moreover, these studies do not calculate the external costs the drug users cause to their relatives. The healthcare costs (depressions and stress) and the income losses due to a limited ability to work can be significant. Therefore, such a quantification of the social costs may not be very accurate.

The studies consider a fixed number of people subject to a particular risk, or to a disease caused by unhealthy behaviour, and apply to this figure a set of estimates of relevant variables (unemployment, productivity, use of healthcare services, etc.)

from other studies. Thus, the studies do not generate databases to monitor the populations.

The introduction of production losses as a component of the social costs of a disease is quite controversial. Although the human capital theory is a tool that is accepted and often used in economics (e.g. education and Grossman's microeconomic modelling of health services demand), there is no clear theoretical justification for using this approach in the macroeconomic context of cost-of-illness studies (cost of unhealthy behaviours). The decision to include production losses as a cost category, and hence as a welfare loss, discriminates against the non-active population: children, senior citizens and women. In the case of unemployed or retired persons, it is not clear how to compute the net contribution to society. In this sense, the friction cost approach by Koopmanschap et al. (1995), which considers as production losses only the training costs of the temporal replacement of the sick worker, would be more useful from a macroeconomic perspective than the human capital approach. However, this more sophisticated method has not been used in the reviewed studies.

Many of the debates within a particular scientific discipline stem from conflicting views on the objectives to be pursued and the methods to achieve them. The evaluation of the social costs derived from the use of drugs does not escape this lack of consensus. For example, a disease generates some financial flows that are not related to production (pensions and money transfers for disabilities). These financial flows are not considered to be costs of the disease as they are a mere reallocation of resources from healthy to ill people. However, although they are not economic costs, it cannot be deduced that they are immaterial for society, given their distributive effects.

None of the studies focuses on issues such as economic dependence, social isolation, the loss of promotion and education opportunities and other aspects that affect quality of life. Although difficult to measure, the costs of drug users to their families should be assessed. A database and the monitoring of individuals for 5 to 10 years would provide interesting insights that could improve future estimates of the social costs of drug consumption.

Furthermore, none of the studies distinguishes between private and external costs. This implies that the theoretical models assume that either individuals do not accurately evaluate the risks involved in the consumption of drugs or an absence of rationality.

It is difficult to compare the studies as they consider different years, countries and populations. The prevalence and incidence rates also differ across the studies. Some of the studies are more exhaustive as they disaggregate the main cost categories and provide a better understanding of the different costs caused by the use of drugs. In this sense, the studies by Rice et al. (1991) and García-Altés et al. (2002) are the most complete. Future studies should consider their cost categories and calculate the social costs of injecting drug use as accurately as possible.

The studies reviewed were aimed at making society aware of the social costs caused by unhealthy behaviours. However, if empirical studies are to be used to formulate public policies, we must conclude that we are still at a very early stage of research. In fact, the research on the evaluation of the social costs of unhealthy behaviours dates back only 20 years. What is needed is methodological standardisation, stating explicitly the theoretical assumptions on which the calculations of the social costs are based and the relevant cost categories. This will allow spatial and temporal comparisons. In the mean time, researchers should justify their methods and value judgments in detail in order to facilitate the replication of results.

In addition to the standardisation of economic calculations, further epidemiological research is needed. Health officers need precise information on both the number of patients infected and the type of treatment they receive. Once these two elements are available, better estimates of the health costs of HIV and hepatitis B and C can be obtained and better public policies can be implemented.

References

Becker, G., Murphy, K. (1988), 'A theory of rational addiction', *Journal of Political Economy* 96: 675–700.

Berry, R. (1976), 'Estimating the economic costs of alcohol abuse', *New England Journal of Medicine* 295: 620–1.

Boletín Epidemiológico (2002), Vol 10, 01, Ministerio de Sanidad y Consumo, Spain, 1–8.

Brown, K., Crofts, N. (1998), 'Health care costs of a continuing epidemic of hepatitis C virus infection among injecting drug users', *Australian and New Zealand Journal of Public Health*, 22 (3 Suppl.): 384–8.

Cartwright, W. S. (1999), 'Costs of drug abuse to society', *Journal of Mental Health Policy and Economics* 2: 133–4.

Crofts, N., Jolley, D., Kaldor, J., van Beek, I., Wodak, A. (1997), 'Epidemiology of hepatitis C virus infection among injecting drug users in Australia', *Journal of Epidemiology and Community Health* 51: 692–7.

García-Altés, A., Ollé, J. M., Antoñanzas, F., Colom, J. (2002), 'The social cost of illegal drug consumption in Spain', *Addiction* 97: 1145–53.

Godfrey, C., Eaton, G., McDougall, C. and Culyer, A. (2002), 'The economic and social cost of Class A drug use in England and Wales', Home Office Research Study 249.

Healey, A., Knapp, M., Astin, J., Gossop, M., Marsden, J., Stewart, D., Lehmann, P., Godfrey, C. (1998), 'Economic burden of drug dependency: social costs incurred by drug users at intake to the National Treatment Outcome Research Study', British Journal of Psychiatry 173: 160–5.

Heien, D., Salomaa, J. (1999), 'What are the costs of substance abuse? Alcohol and drugs', Alcologia 11: 135–43.

Holtermann, S., Burchell, A. (1981), The cost of alcohol misuse, Working Paper No 37, Government Economic Service, Economic Adviser's Office, DHSS, London.

Kim, S., Coletti, S., Williams, C., Heppler, N. (1995), 'Benefit cost analysis of drug abuse prevention programs: a macroscopic approach', Drug Education 24: 877–911.

Koopmanschap, M. A., Rutten, F. F. F., van Ineveld, M. B., van Roijen, L. (1995), 'The friction costs method for measuring indirect costs of disease', Journal of Health Economics 14: 171–189.

Leigh, J. P., Bowlus, C. L., Leistikow, B. N., Schenker, M. (2001), 'Costs of hepatitis C', Archives of Internal Medicine 161: 2231-7.

Leu, R. (1982), 'What can economists contribute?', in Grant, M., Plant, M., Williams, A. (eds), Economics and alcohol consumption and controls, Croom Helm, London and Canberra, 13–23.

Lindgreen, B. (1982), Cost of illness in Sweden 1964–1975, Institute of Health Economics, Lund.

Maynard, A., McDonnell, R. (1985), 'The cost of alcohol misuse', British Journal of Addiction 80: 27–35.

Pollack, H. (2001), 'Cost-effectiveness of harm reduction in preventing hepatitis C among injection drug users', Medical Decision Making 21: 357–67.

Rice, D., Kelman, S., Miller, L. (1991), 'Estimates of economic costs of alcohol and drug abuse and mental illness, 1985–1988', Public Health Reports 106: 280–92.

Robson, L., Single, E. (1995), Literature review of the studies on the economic costs of substance abuse, Canadian Centre on Substance Abuse, Ottawa.

Single, E. (1999), The economic implications of injection drug use, Canadian Centre on Substance Abuse, Ottawa.

Single, E., Collins, D., Easton, B., Harwood, H., Lapsey, H., Maynard, A. (1996), International guidelines for estimating the costs of substance abuse, Canadian Centre on Substance Abuse, Ottawa.

Single, E., Robson, L., Xie, X., Rehm, J. (1998), 'The economic costs of alcohol, tobacco and illicit drugs in Canada', Addiction 93(7): 991–1006.

Stein, M. D., Maksad, J., Clarke, J. (2001), 'Hepatitis C disease among injection drug users: knowledge, perceived risk and willingness to receive treatment', Drug and Alcohol Dependency 61: 211–5.

Wong, J. B., McQuillan, J. G., McHutchison, J. G., Poynard, T. (2000), 'Estimating future hepatitis C morbidity, mortality, and costs in the United States', American Journal of Public Health 90: 1562–9.

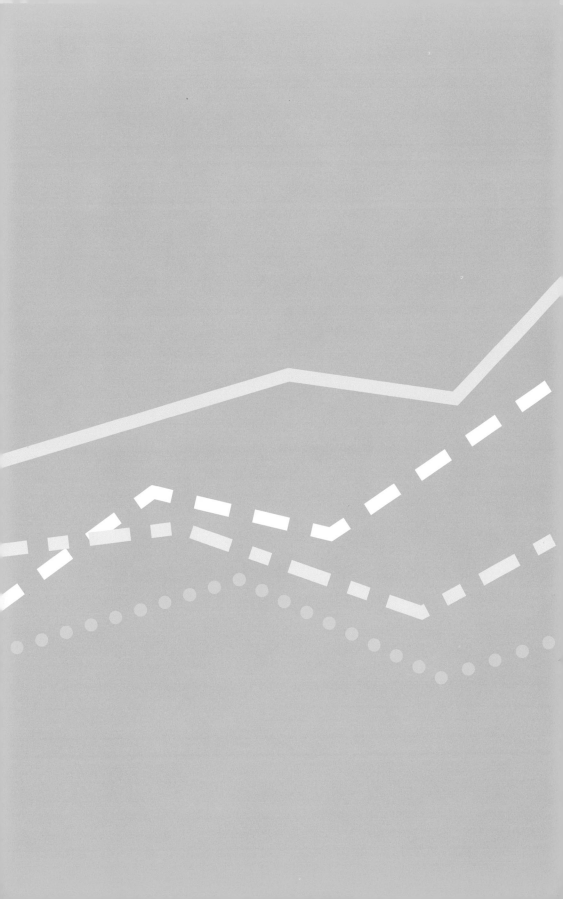

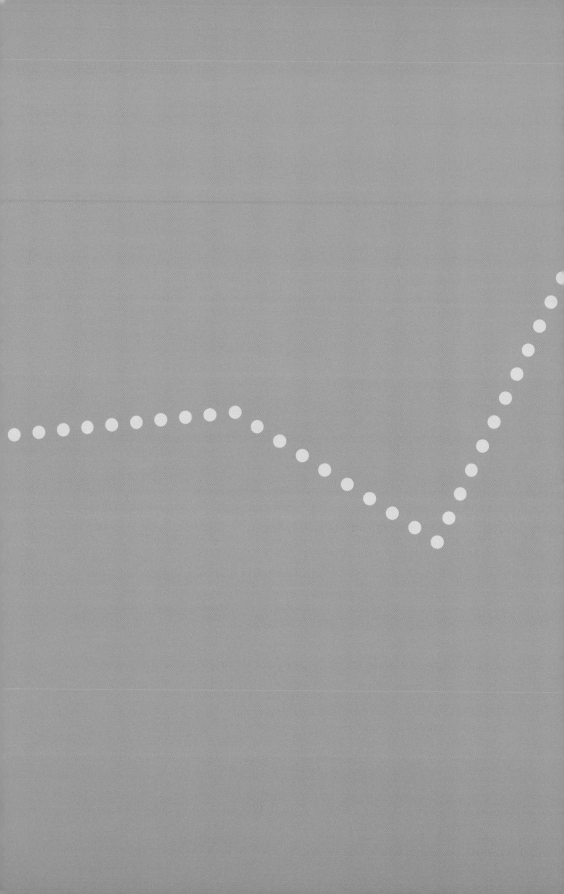

Chapter 12
Assessing the tangible and intangible costs of illicit drug use

Claude Jeanrenaud

Introduction

The purpose of this chapter is to propose a methodology that makes it possible to measure the cost of illicit drug use ([18]), including not only production losses and expenditures for medical treatment, that is indirect and direct costs, but also the effects on the quality of life of drug addicts, and the welfare of the community.

Most cost studies are restricted to the direct and indirect costs of drug use or drug trafficking using a human capital (or cost-of-illness) approach. Emphasis is placed on the areas where cost data are most easily accessible, such as direct costs of crime (justice, police and incarceration), medical treatments, and stays in institutions. The estimate of direct costs is completed by an assessment of indirect morbidity and mortality costs in terms of production losses. Mortality costs are high, since the deaths mainly affect young people — average age 31.8 years ([19]) — who would otherwise have been active for another 35 years. Estimating morbidity costs raises more questions. The only component within morbidity costs for which good data are available is the duration of work impairment during inpatient treatment at hospitals or institutions. As virtually nothing is known about the costs of drug addicts who receive outpatient treatment or no treatment at all, these costs are often neglected. Intangible costs, which are related to the reduction in quality of life for addicts, pain and grief on the part of their families, and the insecurity of those confronted with the drugs scene, are seldom included in the social costs of substance abuse estimates. Therefore, the social burden of illicit drugs remains largely underestimated, and crime-related expenses seem to constitute the most significant form of social damage.

This chapter begins with the analytical framework and a presentation of the different components making up the social costs of drug abuse. It is followed by a critical assessment of two standard valuation methods, the human capital

([18]) Cannabis, opiates, amphetamines, cocaine and hallucinogens.
([19]) OFS (1998).

approach and the willingness-to-pay approach. A new assessment method that is a compromise between the human capital and willingness-to-pay approaches is also presented. The fourth section presents a review of cost estimates carried out in Switzerland. The final section contains recommendations for carrying out estimates on the costs of substance abuse. The chapter concludes that it would be opportune to define new international guidelines that take the needs of health policy into account in a more appropriate way.

Analytical framework

The social costs of illicit drugs can be divided into three components (Figure 1). The first component corresponds to the resources that are used for medical treatment, stays in institutions, the repair of damage to property, police controls, court sentences, and law enforcement. These resources are thus diverted from other productive uses, and the costs incurred are called direct costs. The second component corresponds to the loss of resources due to the increased work impairment of drug users — reduced participation in the labour force, a higher risk of unemployment, increased absenteeism, lower work productivity — and to premature death. These costs are called indirect costs. The sum of the direct and indirect costs represents the tangible or resource costs of illicit drugs. Intangible costs due to a lower quality of life constitute a third component of social costs. Intangible costs are real in that they lead to a reduction in well-being, but they do not result in productive resources being diverted or sacrificed. If intangible costs

Figure 1: Drug-related costs

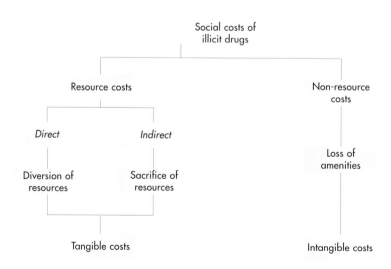

Table 1: Costs of consuming illicit drugs

Cost categories	Valuation method
Direct core costs	
Medical costs	
Treatment in specialised institutions	
Outpatient treatment centres	
Medical prescription of narcotics	
Particular pathology: AIDS, hepatitis C	HC, CV or CA
Direct non-core costs	
Drug-related crime	
Justice	
Customs controls	
Police investigation	
Incarceration	
Damage to property	
Medical costs to victims	HC, CV or CA
Indirect core costs	
Morbidity costs	
Mortality costs	
Loss of work productivity	HC, CV or CA
Indirect non-core costs	
Crime victims	
Imprisonment of drug dealers (crime careers)	
Victims of accidents	HC, CV or CA
Intangible costs	
Reduced QOL of drug users	
Reduced QOL of relatives	
Reduced QOL of victims of violent crime	
Reduced QOL of inhabitants of neighbourhoods with drug scene	CV or CA, SG or TTO with CV, HP

Abbreviations: HC = human capital; CV = contingent valuation; CA = conjoint analysis; SG = standard gamble; TTO = time–trade-off; HP = hedonic pricing; QOL = quality of life.
Sources: Jeanrenaud (2000); Jeanrenaud and Schwab Christe (1999).

were reduced, there would be no additional workforce available to meet the needs of society. Stating that resource costs are economic and intangible costs are not, however, would make little sense. It is obvious that quality of life has an economic value, since individuals are willing to sacrifice a substantial part of their income to raise it.

The physical and mental pain resulting from drug dependency and drug-related conditions dramatically reduces the quality of life of drug addicts and of their relatives. People with drug-related health problems suffer from distress and other psychological problems that change their social life and their relationship with their families.

Stating that non-resource costs cannot be measured is simply not true. The numerous studies carried out on the value of health and human life provide various methods that can be used to assess intangible costs and benefits (Jones-Lee, 1976; Johansson, 1995; Schwab Christe and Soguel, 1995a; Schwab Christe, 1995; Johannesson, 1996; Vitale et al., 1999; Jeanrenaud and Priez, 2000, 2001). Furthermore, we know that individuals spend substantial amounts of money in order to relieve pain — the world market for analgesics reached approximately USD 7.7 billion in 1999 and is growing by 7 % a year. Therefore, it can hardly be maintained that intangible costs do not represent a heavy social burden. Nevertheless, it is true that the ways in which intangibles are valued in terms of utility by standard gamble or time trade-off methods, or in monetary terms by the contingent valuation method or conjoint analysis, are quite different from the standard procedures used to assess direct or indirect costs (Table 1).

Framework: human capital versus willingness-to-pay approaches

The standard approach

An estimation of the social costs of substance abuse is generally carried out following the same procedures. Firstly, the identification of the various health implications of illicit drug use, and thus the diagnosis groups for which drug users face a higher risk. Secondly, the calculation of the proportion of deaths due to a specific drug-related condition — the so-called attributable fractions. Thus, the following information is required: the mortality risk for drug users versus the risk for the general population (relative risk), and the prevalence of drug use. Finally, the indirect morbidity costs are assessed, which requires an estimation of the effect of drug use on work impairment, the probability of unemployment, and work productivity. The lack of data is the main obstacle to valuing the social burden of illicit drug use, making the estimation process more cumbersome for illicit drugs than for addictive substances such as tobacco or alcohol.

The burden of illicit drugs can be assessed in two different ways: using the human capital approach or the willingness-to-pay approach. The two methods are based on different theoretical premisses. Human capital estimates do not reflect individuals' preferences, and the social burden corresponds to the lost production valued at market prices. The willingness-to-pay approach measures the variation in welfare based on preferences. In addition, the human capital and willingness-to-pay approaches do not consider the adverse effects resulting from substance abuse to the same extent. Human capital assesses tangible costs only; all other consequences with no direct effect on present or future consumption are ignored. These resource costs are valued at their market price and can then be compared with gross domestic product (GDP). The human capital approach is recommended in international guidelines under the label of 'cost-of-illness' approach (Single et al., 1996).

The willingness-to-pay approach makes it possible to assess the intangible costs — losses in quality of life — as well as part of the tangible costs. With a contingent valuation survey or a conjoint analysis, we can elicit the willingness to pay of the population for a better health state. For both the human capital and the willingness-to-pay approaches, we can adopt either a global or a restricted perspective. In the restricted perspective, the willingness-to-pay approach would be used only to value the components of benefits or costs for which there are no market values. In the global perspective, the willingness-to-pay approach is applied to assess all the costs borne by the community. In the same way, the human capital concept can be applied as a method of valuing only part of the costs of illicit drugs (production losses) or as a means to assess all the costs of substance abuse (Drummond et al., 1997).

Human capital: a production-based method

Human-capital-based studies only value the most visible economic consequences of illicit drugs, that is the direct and indirect costs. The direct costs reflect the resources consumed by medical treatment, damage to property, and law enforcement. Morbidity and mortality reduce a country's potential production.

Human capital studies are generally based on a prevalence framework. All individuals with drug-related diagnoses during the reference year are considered, and the medical and indirect morbidity costs are estimated for that same year. The value of production that would have been achieved by the end of an active life if the person had not died prematurely corresponds to the mortality cost. The incidence framework is used less frequently, since the required epidemiological data are often not available.

Medical and hospital costs, such as the cost of stays in institutions, correspond to treatment expenses. Premature death may reduce health costs, since health expenditure for the very elderly constitutes the main factor responsible for the increase in health expenditure in Switzerland (OECD, 2000). The question of whether the reduction in health expenditure is a benefit to be deducted from the direct cost of substance abuse is thus an ethical rather than an economic one.

The morbidity and mortality costs — indirect cost — correspond to the market value of lost production. Morbidity costs are caused by production losses due to short-term work impairment or disability for the year under consideration. In the case of premature death, the mortality costs correspond to the discounted value of lifetime production losses, which are supposed to be equal to the total of future earnings. The present value of the production losses is obtained by applying an appropriate discount rate ([20]). The human capital method does not assess the value of life, only the value of the lifetime production of an average person. It is often difficult to obtain relevant data regarding the temporary incapacity to work due to illness. The rate of impairment can, however, be estimated using an econometric model (Rice et al., 1990; Harwood et al., 1998; Vitale et al., 1999; Vitale, 2001). Health insurance statistics are another possible source of data.

When valuing production losses, it is recommended that the value of domestic activities (housekeeping, education of children) be included. If household production is disregarded, a significant part of indirect costs is ignored. Lastly, it is almost impossible to obtain data on reduced workplace productivity due to illicit drug use.

Willingness-to-pay approach: a preference-based method

The willingness-to-pay approach relies on individual preferences to estimate the value individuals assign to changes in their well-being. In order to assess the costs of substance abuse, the maximum amount an average person is willing to pay to reduce the risk of future adverse health effects (*ex ante* approach) or the maximum amount patients are willing to pay for treatment that would improve their quality of life (*ex post* approach) must be determined.

One method of obtaining this value is to ask it explicitly in a survey, by questioning individuals directly about their willingness to pay (expressed preference approach), for example. An alternative approach is to observe individuals' behaviour in order to elicit the value individuals attribute to a change in their health state (revealed preference approach) (Figure 2).

([20]) The value of lost production — and consumption — is thus underestimated, since it ignores the consumer's surplus (Collins and Lapsley, 1992).

Figure 2: Explicit or implicit values

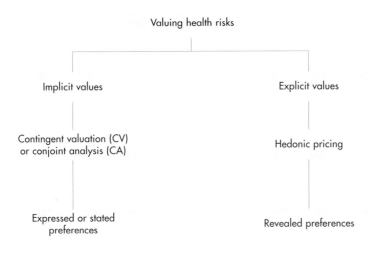

Contingent valuation is the most widely used preference-based method for valuing adverse health effects in monetary terms. The flexibility of the method makes it possible to obtain a precise breakdown of what is to be valued. Depending on the scenario, the interviewees assign values to all the consequences of the disease — resource and non-resource costs — or only to the loss in quality of life. Health may be presented as a private or public good. If the individuals who pay for it benefit from the risk reduction, health is considered a private good. If the population at large benefits, health is considered a public good. The contingent valuation questionnaire also permits us to assess the value individuals attribute to a reduction in substance abuse in the community, or elicit their willingness to pay to reduce their personal risks.

Conjoint analysis has its origin in market research, where it has been used to identify different factors influencing demand. The characteristic of conjoint analysis is that it allows the determination of the relative importance of different attributes in the provision of a service. The technique is based on the premise that the value an individual places on a product depends on the characteristics — or attributes — of that product. Conjoint analysis allows the estimation of the different aspects of care, and it helps us to understand how consumers compare health plans, or how they value the different health implications of a specific disease. If we need an estimate of both the tangible and the intangible costs, conjoint analysis seems to be a better option than contingent valuation.

Limits of the human capital approach

Some authors argue that the human capital approach strongly overestimates the magnitude of lost production. In fact, human capital relies on the assumption that non-achieved production by a person who is temporarily impaired or dies prematurely is definitively lost. This assumption is contradicted by Koopmanschap (1999), who proposed that the work of the person concerned could be carried out by other employees within the same company or by unemployed workers. The alternative method — the friction cost method — leads to lost-production estimates that are considerably lower than those obtained by the human capital method. Other critics attack the theoretical foundation of the human capital method by stating that it is not consistent with the economic theory of welfare. According to welfare economics, morbidity and mortality costs should reflect the maximum amount which individuals would find acceptable to pay for a reduced health risk (compensation criteria).

Another disadvantage of the human capital approach is that it does not permit the assessment of intangible costs such as quality of life losses for drug addicts and their relatives. The sum of direct and indirect costs provides, at best, a bottom value for the social burden due to substance abuse (Johansson, 1995). The social cost estimate does not reflect the reduction in well-being incurred by the population.

An advantage of the human capital approach is that it is easy to explain and the figures are easy to understand. Thus, it is relatively well accepted as a basis for political decision-making.

Limits of the willingness-to-pay approach

The first difficulty inherent in the willingness-to-pay approach is for an individual, who has never consumed illicit drugs, to imagine him- or herself becoming addicted and to state the maximum amount he or she would be willing to sacrifice to reduce the risk of addiction. A study carried out among the general population — the *ex ante* approach or choice under uncertainty — would probably lead to a biased estimate. Will participants consider the risk of an average person as being equivalent to their own? In the absence of information on the objective risk, it is not likely that respondents will be able to estimate a subjective risk. In an *ex ante* approach, it is better to draw up a scenario whereby the interviewee states the amount that he or she is willing to pay in order to reduce the risk for a person close to him or her rather than his or her own risk. In an *ex post* approach, the certainty scenario, a dependent consumer or a close relative would be questioned regarding his or her willingness to pay for a treatment that would halt the addiction of the person affected. This approach would almost certainly fail, as the interviewee would probably be prepared to sacrifice all his or her assets.

To overcome this obstacle, we could use a two-step valuation procedure. In the first step, we would not value the loss in quality of life in monetary terms but in QALYs, using standard gamble or time trade-off methods. In the second step, the QALY outcome would be expressed in monetary terms using studies for which both a QALY and a monetary value exist (Jeanrenaud and Priez, 2001).

A new approach: combining the human capital and willingness-to-pay approaches

Rather than choosing between the human capital approach and the willingness-to-pay approach, the two methods can also be combined. As has been said before, the human capital approach can be used to assess all the consequences of health changes as well as to value only a specific part of the social cost (Drummond et al., 1997). The intangible costs, related to the loss in quality of life, can be valued using a preference-based method. In this way, the disadvantages inherent to each approach are reduced and we get a more comprehensive picture of the social burden of illicit drugs.

The simultaneous use of a production-based and a preference-based method raises several questions, since the two approaches are not based on the same theoretical premisses. The tangible costs are the sum of the direct and the indirect costs. Adding up both cost categories poses no problem, as both are assessed in terms of market value of lost production. Greater caution is needed when adding up the values obtained by production-based and preference-based methods.

The contingent valuation method measures the maximum amount that an individual is prepared to pay in order to reduce a specific health risk and to avoid its consequences, including a drop in income or additional medical expenses. There is thus the risk of double counting, since the losses in production and income are considered twice, first via the human capital method and again when the individual's willingness to pay is at stake. We must therefore adopt a restrictive perspective and design a contingent valuation scenario whereby only the change in health-related quality of life is valued (Jeanrenaud and Priez, 1999). If the contingent valuation scenario is adequately designed, we can exclude the financial losses (drop in income, out-of-pocket payments by patients) from the cost estimate and value only the consequences of illicit drug use for health-related quality of life (see Schwab Christe and Soguel, 1995b; Vitale et al., 1998; Jeanrenaud and Soguel, 1999, for examples). Information collected when testing the questionnaires, and answers given by respondents to the follow-up questions, after interviewees have stated their willingness to pay, have shown that almost all respondents considered only their health-related quality of life when expressing their willingness to pay. The risk of encountering some embedding effect — when responses fail to meet the scope test — is thus low and can be controlled.

It is also necessary to consider whether the mortality costs include intangible costs. In fact, the indirect costs of a premature death correspond only to the additional resources that would have been available to society without any use of illicit drugs, that is the sacrificed production minus the consumption of the deceased (net production costs). The market value of the products that would have been consumed by the deceased is sometimes considered to be part of the intangible costs (Collins and Lapsley, 1991). To sum up, the social costs of illicit drugs correspond to the sum of the present value of the net production losses estimated with the human capital method, and the loss in quality of life estimated with the willingness-to-pay approach.

Costs of the consumption of illicit drugs in Switzerland

Three estimations of the social costs of illicit drug consumption have been carried out in Switzerland. The first was commissioned by the Swiss Federal Office of Public Health (Danthine and Balletto, 1990) and is based on a human capital approach. It covers only the direct and indirect costs, and provides a preliminary assessment of the social burden of illicit drugs. The second was carried out within the framework of a doctoral thesis at the University of St Gallen (Bernasconi, 1993). Its main interest is that it contains a first measurement of intangible costs for both drug addicts and their families. The third is part of the assessment studies of the programme for the medical prescription of narcotics (Frei et al., 2000) ([21]).

The authors of the first study (Danthine and Balletto, 1990) adopted a human capital approach, but without stating clearly whether the estimation covered the social or the external costs. Moreover, the study did not always make a correct distinction between the transfers or non-resource costs (fines, tax revenues) and the expenses or activities that represent a sacrifice of resources (stays in institutions, treatment costs, police control). The estimation was made for all types of illicit

---

([21]) A new estimation of the social burden resulting from the consumption of illicit drugs, which includes direct, indirect and intangible costs, is currently being carried out at the University of Neuchâtel, commissioned by the Swiss Federal Office of Public Health.

Table 2: **Costs of illicit drug consumption in Switzerland, 1988 (million EUR ([1]))**

	Lower bound	Upper bound
Medical costs	42.4	62.7
Other direct costs (crime)	92.3	93.9
Indirect costs		
Mortality	103.0	103.0
Morbidity ([2])	69.6	87.1
Social costs	307.2	346.7
As a percentage of GDP	0.2	0.2
Public policy costs	7.9	9.4

([1]) The conversion factor is the average current exchange rate for the year.
([2]) Re-estimated by IRER.
Source: Danthine and Balletto (1990).

drugs simultaneously. The methodological choices were largely dictated by the availability of data. Basing their work on a moral argument, the authors took the social value of the substances sold and consumed as zero and did not include this component in their cost estimate. However, if we accept that the production and trafficking of illicit drugs do not bring any profit to the community, the costs of their production and distribution should be included in the social costs. Persons involved in drug trafficking (crime careerists) would, in fact, have represented an economic value had they worked on the legal market (Rice et al., 1990). The question as to whether or not public policy expenses — prevention and research — should be included in the social costs is controversial (see Markandya and Pearce, 1989; Vitale et al., 1998). In our opinion, these costs should not be included in the social costs.

The social cost estimate by Danthine and Balletto (1990; Table 2) includes the direct medical costs, the gross production loss (morbidity and mortality), expenses incurred by crime and violence associated with drug trafficking, plus research and prevention costs. Medical treatment costs for drug addicts with AIDS were calculated by the Commission fédérale pour les problèmes liés au Sida (1989). The intangible costs were not assessed.

Mortality costs were estimated on the basis of the average income of the labour force in Switzerland. The average loss of productive life is supposed to be 40 years, which is certainly too high ([22]) and future earnings are discounted at 4 %. Regarding morbidity, only those individuals undergoing treatment are taken into account. The period of work incapacity is supposed to be the same, that is one year, irrespective of whether or not the drug addict is disabled or is undergoing inpatient or outpatient treatment. The morbidity cost for a drug addict receiving inpatient medical care corresponds to the income of a drug addict not receiving treatment, which is supposed to be half the average income ([23]). However, the correct procedure consists of comparing the drug addict's income, independent of whether or not the individual is undergoing treatment, with the income of an individual who does not consume illicit drugs. The estimation procedure adopted by Danthine and Balletto leads to a considerable underestimation of the morbidity costs ([24]).

The costs of crime are valued on the basis of the expenses of the police, customs authorities, courts, incarceration, and damage to property. Fines and the participation in legal expenses are deducted from the crime costs. This deduction is justified only if the objective is to obtain a measurement of the external costs of illicit drug consumption.

Bernasconi (1993) is the only researcher to have attempted a cost estimation of illicit drugs in Switzerland by means of a willingness-to-pay approach (Table 3). He is also alone in explicitly integrating the concept of rational addiction within his estimation (Becker and Murphy, 1988). Had the consumer been fully aware from the start of the risks associated with illicit drugs (including the risk of dependency), the user can be assumed to attribute a higher value to drug use than to his or her health or his or her own life. Consequently, his or her willingness to pay to reduce the risk of morbidity or premature death is nil. If so, the net costs of morbidity and mortality equal zero, i.e. the lower limit estimate. In the upper limit estimate, Bernasconi values the damage on the basis of the willingness to pay of parents or family in order to reduce the risk or mortality or illness due to the use of illicit drugs. The cost estimates rely on the following hypothesis: for each of 25 400 drug addicts, there is one person who would be prepared to sacrifice all his or her assets — on average EUR 31 270 per inhabitant — to preserve the

---

([22]) Based on an estimated average age of 25 years at death. In fact, the average age of people whose death certificate recorded heroin or cocaine as a cause of death was just below 32 (OFS, 1998).

([23]) The income of a drug user is taken to be half the average income. After the age of 30 years, the average potential income of a former drug addict progressively approaches that of the general population. The income of a former drug addict nevertheless remains 10 % lower than the average.

([24]) The average annual income is EUR 27 080 and this represents the production loss per case for inpatient treatment. The morbidity cost is the difference between the earnings of a drug addict and the average income of a worker. Using the correct estimation procedure, the morbidity cost ranges from EUR 69.6 million to EUR 87.1 million (instead of EUR 35.9 million to EUR 45.1 million).

Table 3: Cost of illicit drugs in Switzerland — tangible and intangible costs, 1990 (million EUR ([1]))

	Lower bound	Upper bound
Medical treatment	62.7	82.3
Morbidity/mortality costs ([2])	0.0	99.3
Intangible costs ([3])	1 546.5	1 546.5
Justice/police/incarceration	163.2	189.7
Miscellaneous ([4])	3.2	16.2
Total	1 775.6	1 934.0
As a percentage of GDP		
Public policy costs	16	16

([1]) The conversion factor is the average current exchange rate for the year.
([2]) Re-estimated by IRER.
([3]) *Ex post* approach in both cases.
([4]) Prevention measures, household self-insurance, loss of time due to police controls.
Source: Bernasconi (1993).

health or life of his or her family member or close friend. There is thus no distinction between morbidity and mortality costs ([25]).

The rational addiction hypothesis is also applied to the intangible costs borne by the drug user (dependency costs, drop in health-related quality of life). If the drug addict had been fully aware from the start of the risk of dependency and the effects of the substances on his or her health, the intangible costs would have been considered within his or her choice. The net intangible costs borne by the drug user would then be zero, since they are compensated by the benefits of the substances (Bernasconi, 1993). However, the intangible costs for the relatives are probably not included in the rational drug user's calculations. If so, they should be estimated and added to the social costs. The willingness to pay of families is supposed to correspond to the probability of a young person to have consumed opiates or cocaine between the ages of 17 and 25 years, multiplied by the average household assets ([26]). Other damage caused by the consumption of illicit drugs and the costs of public policies (prevention and research) are valued on the basis of resource utilisation.

([25]) Bernasconi confuses the prevalence rate and the incidence rate of hard drug use. The willingness to pay in order to reduce the health implications of hard drug use should apply to new cases only (incidence) and not to the whole population of hard drug users (prevalence). The morbidity and mortality costs would be approximately CHF 174.9 million instead of CHF 1 999.5 million as estimated by Bernasconi.

Bernasconi's approach raises several questions:

- Are consumers really capable of making a rational choice at the moment they consume illicit drugs for the first time?
- Why would the economic damage due to premature death have anything to do with family assets?
- Why would the grief and pain following the loss of a child be expressed in terms of family assets?
- Would it not be wiser to measure the intangible costs by means of an *ex ante* approach (willingness to pay for a slight variation in the risk) rather than by an *ex post* approach (willingness to pay in order to avoid the health implications of drug use)?

With a willingness-to-pay approach, it is only possible to value part of the production losses, since most of the costs are borne by the social insurance system. In studies based on human capital, the mortality and morbidity costs correspond to the value of the production that has been sacrificed. Bernasconi never raises the question of production losses, and the boundary between the economic and intangible costs is by no means clear.

An evaluation of the benefits of the programme for the medical prescription of narcotics was carried out by Frei et al. (2000; Table 4). The objective is to evaluate the programme by comparing its implementation costs with the benefits for participants and society. Only real benefits — those that reflect an increase in the population's welfare — are taken into account. Savings made due to the reduction in disability allowances, unemployment benefits or assistance subsidies are logically ignored, since they constitute mere transfers (Jeanrenaud, 2000). The valuation covers the following four areas:

- reduction in the cost of medical and hospital treatment;
- reduction in time spent in specialised institutions;
- reduction in production losses caused by morbidity;
- reduction in crime rate.

The first benefit — lower medical expenses — is obtained by comparing the number of diagnoses and the related treatment costs one month after entry into the programme with those observed one year later. The authors of the study noticed a

---

([26]) The way in which Bernasconi valued intangible costs in the lower limit estimate (*ex ante* approach) is not correct. The probability of becoming addicted to hard drugs is around 2.3 %, and not 0.13 % as stated in Bernasconi's work. For this reason, we have considered only the upper limit estimate (EUR 1 546.5).

marked reduction in the frequency of diagnoses during the first year in the programme. The hypothesis is that there is no further improvement in the health of the participants after one year in the programme, which means that the estimate is cautious. The socio-psychological care provided to the programme participants leads to a reduction in housing expenses, as it allows a substitution of private for public accommodation, and of outpatient for inpatient treatment (Frei et al., 2000). The lower crime rate and lower number of drug-related offences have reduced the police and justice expenditure, the expenses for the execution of sentences, and the damage to property.

Many potential sources of the programme's social benefits are ignored: non-market production losses (household work), lower mortality costs, and the possible conversion of dealers who take up activities that are beneficial to society. Finally, all the intangible benefits for the programme participants (improved health-related quality of life), their families and the inhabitants of neighbourhoods with a drug scene or the victims of acts of violence are not taken into account. According to the cost estimate, the victims of crimes bear only 5 % of the social cost of drug-related crime, which is hardly plausible. This low percentage is explained by the fact that the intangible costs borne by victims — the main component in the social cost of violent crimes (Miller et al., 1996) — are not included. The fact that theft is simply considered as a transfer — with no real cost to society — is a shortcut that is difficult to accept. To summarise, the Frei et al. (2000) estimate suggests that the main benefit of the programme for the medical prescription of narcotics arises from the fact that fewer judges, policemen and prison wardens are required, that these human resources could be devoted to more beneficial tasks, and that the drug-related crime rate is reduced. We believe that this suggestion results from

Table 4: **Benefits of the programme for the medical prescription of narcotics (PROVE) in Switzerland per participant and per day, 1995**

Costs	EUR (¹)	Benefits	EUR (¹)
Medical material, external services and opiates	6.1	Reduced treatment costs	11.1
Personnel costs	22.9	Reduced work impairment	2.5
Other operating costs (rent, maintenance)	3.8	Lower housing expenditures	1.6
		Reduced costs of drug-related crime	46.6
Total	32.8		61.8

(¹) The conversion factor is the average current exchange rate for the year.

methodological choices and the definition of social costs, and that it does not reflect reality. These choices lead to an underestimation of the benefits of the programme: instead of a benefit of EUR 1.14 for each euro invested in the programme, we believe that a cost–benefit ratio of between 2 and 3.5 is more realistic (Jeanrenaud, 2000).

Conclusion

The adequate framework for measuring the costs of illicit drugs is that of a cost–benefit analysis rather than a cost-of-illness approach. One could ask whether restricting the scope of the study to production losses without considering the consequences of using drugs on the quality of life makes any real sense. In order to evaluate the tangible and intangible social costs, the most appropriate method consists of combining a human capital type of approach with an evaluation of costs based on the willingness-to-pay approach. In both cases, this is a matter of adopting a restrictive perspective. The human capital approach serves to evaluate only the direct and indirect costs, and a contingent valuation survey is used only to value the intangible components, that is those components that have no monetary market value. We therefore consider that the guidelines for the estimation of the costs of substance abuse should be redesigned to include intangibles as well as production losses.

Estimating morbidity costs is a difficult exercise. The assessment method generally used to measure work incapacity due to alcohol or tobacco consumption is based on an econometric model (Rice et al., 1990; Harwood et al., 1998; Jeanrenaud et al., 2001). The dependent variable is either the income or the number of days during which the subject is impaired over a reference period. The independent variables are the consumption of the substance and the socioeconomic characteristics of the population. The data used to construct this type of model are obtained by large-scale health surveys, such as the health survey (*Enquête suisse sur la santé*) carried out by the Swiss Federal Statistical Office every five years (OFS, 1997). However, in the case of illicit drugs, the Swiss health survey cannot be used because most hard drug users do not take part in it.

The estimation of the costs of drug addiction usually involves all illicit drugs rather than a single substance. A separate estimate for each substance would be preferable if the aim is to provide support to policy decision-making. Yet the lack of data and the fact that drug addicts often consume more than one product render such an exercise difficult, if not impossible.

We do not think that the costs of prevention and research should be included in the social costs. These expenses first and foremost constitute an indication of the efforts made by the public authorities to prevent drug addiction. This, however, is a controversial issue; some authors add the public policy costs — education, research and prevention — to the social costs. Comparing them with the economic consequences of substance abuse may reveal a problem. The sums allocated to prevention by the public authorities in Switzerland only represent 1.8 % of the direct and indirect costs. A comparison of the prevention efforts with the expenditure on repression is quite revealing: Switzerland spends almost 20 times more money on fighting drug-trafficking-related criminality than on the prevention of drug use.

References

Becker, G. S., Murphy, K. M. (1988), 'A theory of rational addiction', *Journal of Political Economy* 96: 675–700.

Bernasconi, D. (1993), 'Ökonomische Ansätze zur Ausgestraltung der Drogenpolitik in der Schweiz', Dissertation der Hochschule St Gallen für Wirtschafts-, Rechts und Sozialwissenschaften, Difo-Druck GmbH, Bamberg.

Collins, D. J., Lapsley, H. M. (1991), *Estimating the economic costs of drug abuse in Australia*, Monograph Series No 15, Australian Government Publishing Service, Canberra.

Collins, D. J., Lapsley, H. M. (1992), 'Drug abuse economics: cost estimates and policy implications', *Drug and Alcohol Review* 2: 379–88.

Commission fédérale pour les problèmes liés au Sida and Office fédéral de la santé publique (1989), Le sida en Suisse. *L'épidémie, ses conséquences et les mesures prises*, Office fédéral de la santé publique, Berne.

Danthine, J.-P., Balletto, R. (1990), 'Le coût de la consommation des drogues illégales', in ISPA (ed.), *Le problème de la drogue — en particulier en Suisse — considéré sous son aspect social et préventif*, Report drawn up on the request of the Swiss Federal Office of Public Health, Swiss Institute for the Prevention of Alcoholism, Lausanne.

Drummond, M. F., O'Brien, B., Stoddart, G. L., Torrance, G. W. (1997), *Methods for the economic evaluation of health care programmes*, Oxford University Press, Oxford.

Frei, A., Greiner, R. A., Mehnert, A., Dinkel, R. (2000), 'Socioeconomic evaluation of heroin maintenance treatment', in Gutzwiller, F., Steffen, T. (eds), *Cost–benefit analysis of heroin maintenance treatment*, Volume 2, Karger, Basle.

Harwood, H., Fountain, D., Livermore, G. (1998), *The economic costs of alcohol and drug abuse in the United States, 1992*, National Institute on Drug Abuse/National Institute on Alcohol Abuse and Alcoholism, Bethesda.

Jeanrenaud, C. (2000), 'Commentary', in Gutzwiller, F., Steffen, T. (eds), *Cost–benefit analysis of heroin maintenance treatment*, Karger, Basle.

Jeanrenaud, C., Priez, F. (1999), 'Human costs of chronic bronchitis in Switzerland', *Revue Suisse d'économie politique et de statistique* 3: 287–301.

Jeanrenaud, C., Priez, F. (2000), *Valuing intangible costs of lung cancer*, Working Papers 00-01, IRER, Neuchâtel.

Jeanrenaud, C., Priez, F. (2001), 'Introduction', *Revue suisse d'économie politique et de statistique* 1: 1–6.

Jeanrenaud, C., Schwab Christe, N. (1999), 'Bewertung der sozialen Kosten des Suchtmittelkonsums', in Uchtenhagen, A., Zieglgänsberger, W. (eds), *Suchtmedizin. Konzepte, Strategien und therapeutisches Management*, Urban & Schwarzenberg, Munich.

Jeanrenaud, C., Soguel, N. (eds) (1999), *Valuing the cost of smoking*. Assessment methods, risk perception and policy options, Kluwer Academic Publishers, Boston.

Jeanrenaud, C., Priez, F., Vannotti, M. (2001), 'Valuing the intangible costs of cirrhosis of the liver: a two step procedure', *Revue suisse d'économie politique et de statistique* 1: 87–102.

Johanesson, M. (1996), *Theory and methods of economic evaluation of health care*, Kluwer Academic Publishers, Dordrecht.

Johannsson, P. O. (1995), *Evaluating health risks: an economic approach*, Cambridge University Press, Cambridge.

Jones-Lee, M. W. (1976), *The value of life*, Martin Robertson, Oxford.

Koopmanschap, M. A. (1999), 'Estimating the indirect costs of smoking using the friction cost method', in Jeanrenaud, C., Soguel, N. (eds), *Valuing the cost of smoking*. Assessment methods, risk perception and policy options, Kluwer Academic Publishers, Boston.

Markandya, A., Pearce, D. W. (1989), 'The social costs of tobacco smoking', *British Journal of Addiction* 84: 1139–50.

Miller, T. R., Cohen, M. A., Wiersema, B. (1996), *Victim costs and consequences: a new look*, Research report, US Department of Justice, National Institute of Justice, Washington.

Office fédéral de la statistique (OFS) (1997), 'Enquête suisse sur la santé', Office fédéral de la statistique, Neuchâtel.

Office fédéral de la statistique (OFS) (1998), 'Statistique des causes de décès', Office fédéral de la statistique, section santé, Neuchâtel.

Organisation for Economic Cooperation and Development (OECD) (2000), *Études économiques de l'OCDE — Suisse*, OECD, Paris.

Rice, D. P., Kelman, S., Miller, L. S., Dunmeyer, S. (1990), *The economic costs of alcohol and drug abuse and mental illness: 1985*, Institute for Health and Ageing, University of California, San Francisco.

Schwab Christe, N. (1995), 'The valuation of human costs by the contingent method: the Swiss experience', in Schwab Christe, N., Soguel, N. C. (eds), *Contingent valuation, transport safety and the value of life*, Kluwer Academic Publishers, Boston.

Schwab Christe, N., Soguel, N. C. (1995a), *Le prix de la souffrance et du chagrin*, EDES, Neuchâtel.

Schwab Christe, N., Soguel, N. C. (1995b), *Contingent valuation, transport safety and the value of life*, Kluwer Academic Publishers, Boston.

Single, E., Collins, D., Easton, B., Harwood, H., Lapsley, H., Maynard, A. (1996), *International guidelines for estimating the costs of substance abuse*, Canadian Centre on Substance Abuse, Ottawa.

Vitale, S. (2001), 'L'estimation du coût indirect de la maladie: méthodes d'évaluation et application à la consommation excessive d'alcool', Doctoral thesis, University of Neuchâtel, Neuchâtel.

Vitale, S., Priez, F., Jeanrenaud, C. (1998), *Le coût social de la consommation de tabac en Suisse*, IRER, University of Neuchâtel, Neuchâtel.

Vitale, S., Jeanrenaud, C., Priez, F. (1999), *Le coût social de la consommation d'alcool dans le canton de Genève*, Les cahiers de l'action sociale et de la santé, 12, Direction générale de la santé, Geneva.

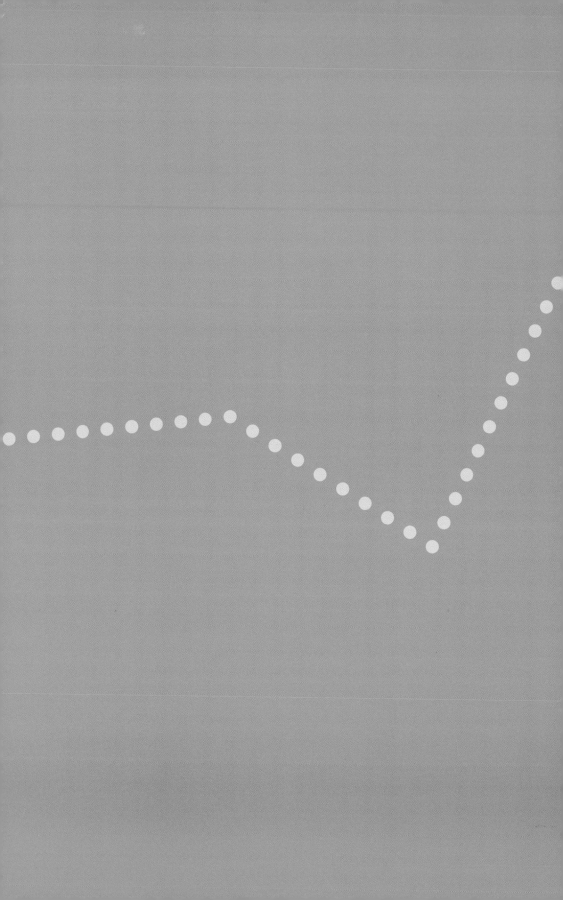

Chapter 13
Social costs of drug use in France

Pierre Kopp and Nicolas Blanchard

Introduction

Illegal drug use imposes a variety of expenses on our society. The purpose of this study is to quantify the adverse consequences of drug use in monetary terms in order to render them comparable. We hope that this information will contribute to a better understanding of the nature and magnitude of drug use implications and that this understanding will help policy-makers to identify appropriate strategies for reducing the undesirable consequences of drug use.

Political analysts and researchers interested in the costs and consequences of drug use can use this study. It should be noted that the data presented in this chapter should not be overinterpreted. However, this work provides an indication of the optimal reduction of social costs attainable by public policies (cost–benefit).

This chapter does not present an evaluation of the effectiveness of a given intervention, but may serve as a basis for assessing potential policy changes, and may help in testing the results of theoretical models.

The main reason for undertaking an evaluation of costs of drugs for society, other than those stated above, is to make policy-makers aware of the need to make political choices regarding legislation relating to drug use and other psychoactive substances.

Methodology

This chapter presents an estimate of the costs of illicit drug use in France in 1997 using cost-of-illness methodology. The guiding principle of the cost-of-illness approach is that the costs incurred by an illness or a social problem require the allocation of resources that would otherwise have been allocated elsewhere.

Two assumptions are retained: firstly, the full use of production factors is realised, that is all existing resources are used in order to produce goods and services and,

305

secondly, that the reallocation of resources eliminating drugs will not affect the level of benefit to society. These two assumptions allow us to consider the consequences of drug use as 'social costs'.

This reasoning is based on the concept of 'opportunity cost', which implies the possibility of using the resources allocated to an activity in an alternative, and more advantageous manner. We then speak of a 'counterfactual' scenario that describes an alternative state of affairs.

Our study is limited to tangible costs, which correspond to monetary losses (e.g. loss of income), and we exclude intangible costs, which correspond to monetary valuation of subjective damage (e.g. pain and suffering), from the framework.

Costs, as measured by a cost-of-illness study, cover all tangible costs related to drug consumption and trafficking (excluding purchase) borne by society. Society includes private agents (private costs) and public organisations (public costs).

Private costs include costs borne by the substance consumer, for example loss of revenue linked to premature death and non-reimbursable medical expenses, and indirect or external private costs borne by non-consuming private individuals and organisations. The second category includes costs inflicted by consumers on other private non-consumers, such as the cost borne by companies associated with production losses due to absenteeism of drug consumers as well as the expenses of private agents (mainly associations).

Public costs cover three types of expense linked to drug consumption and trafficking. The first category consists of public spending at a national level as included in the State's budget for the various ministries. The second category represents all resources involved at regional and local levels. The third category consists of social transfers, in particular those in the healthcare sector. These transfers are considered to be public costs, although neither the French national accounting system nor those of most European countries do so, as these costs are financed by society as a whole, including those households or companies which are 'private agents'. Nevertheless, in order to permit comparability of different international studies, we conform to American and British usage and incorporate all social transfers into public spending. In doing so, we follow Single et al.'s (1995) and Collins and Lapsey's (1995) recommendation that cost of illness should include only the 'gross' social cost and not the possible 'net' positive side effects of the consumption of certain substances. Table 1 presents both the nature of the costs considered and the repartition of these costs between individuals and/or institutions.

Factors	Consumers	+ Non-consumers	+ State and public authorities	+ Social security	= Society
Direct costs	Purchasing costs	—	Public spending for prevention and maintenance programmes	Hospitalisation and other healthcare costs	
Costs of direct consequences	Non-reimbursed healthcare costs and judicial services	Non-reimbursed healthcare costs (transmissible drug-related pathologies) and other costs	Healthcare costs on administration budgets; judicial costs	Healthcare costs (reimbursed part)	Total cost to society
Costs of indirect consequences	Income losses	Productivity and income losses	Lost taxes	Lost obligatory deductions	
Costs of intangible consequences	Welfare loss due to drug-related pathologies, death and incarceration	Welfare loss concerning families of drug users and victims of drug-related violence	—	—	

Table 1: The social cost of drug use in cost-of-illness studies

The study is prevalence based, that is, it estimates the costs of problems that exist during the course of one year, in this case 1997.

Lost income and productivity due to premature death are estimated using the human capital method with the help of the present value of future revenue. This more frequently used approach differs from the willingness-to-pay method (Hodgson and Meiners, 1979) in that the latter values human life as the price individuals are prepared to pay to change their life expectancy. As a general rule, the results obtained with the human capital method are not as pronounced as those calculated with the willingness-to-pay technique.

The human capital method involves calculating the present value of future revenue lost due to premature mortality attributable to drug consumption. The results presented will be calculated using a discount rate of 6 %. However, before making any estimate of costs resulting from drug consumption, we present drug use figures for France as well as drug use patterns.

French drug use

Unlike tobacco or alcohol use, there are no reliable data on the quantity of drugs sold and/or consumed, nor is there a feasible method for producing such data. To gain insight into the drug consumption and drug consuming behaviour of the French population, a representative sample would be required. However, the illicit nature of the products used is likely to introduce two major biases: firstly, because the honesty of interviewees may be doubtful and, secondly, because of difficulties in following up marginalised people, who are over-represented in the drug consumer population and tend to be excluded from study samples. Despite these imperfections, the Observatoire français des drogues et des toxicomanies (OFDT) (OFDT, 1999) gives some indication of drug consumption and its structure in France.

In 1995, 6.5 million (15.8 %) individuals aged 18 to 75 had consumed an illegal substance and 1.8 million people (4.4 %) during the last 12 months. This admitted consumption of illegal drugs concerns primarily cannabis and those under 45 years old. Thus, in 1995, around one quarter of the population aged 18 to 44 years had experimented with cannabis, and 1.76 million people (7.7 %) had used it more often (occasionally or regularly).

Confessed experimentation with products other than cannabis proved to be distinctly more marginal. Still, it was estimated that the number of people who admitted having experimented with hallucinogens varied between 340 000 and 750 000. As under-declaration is highly probable, the actual numbers are far from negligible.

Little information is available on the breakdown of consumers by gender. Nonetheless, it appears that men admit to being consumers more often than women, at least of cannabis, although this gap is reduced among the 18–24-year-olds. This gap doubles among the 25–34-year-olds and again among the 35–44-year-olds.

It is estimated that one third of adolescents have experimented with drugs, usually cannabis. Other products are rarely mentioned, and, if they are, they most often concern hallucinogens or ecstasy. Almost 25 % of the 15–19-year-olds admit to taking drugs at least once a year.

It is as difficult to estimate drug users' annual investment in drugs as it is to assess the number of consumers. We therefore limit ourselves to a very general estimate of the turnover of illegal drugs based on prevalence data. The figures for cannabis consumption are based on several hypotheses: the average price of the resin is FRF 35/g (EUR 5.34); daily smokers use an average of 0.5 g/day; those who smoke at least once a week use 1.5 g/week; those who smoke at least once a month use 0.5 g; and the average consumption of those smoking less than once a month is 0.5 g every two months (Table 2).

Table 2 presents the annual consumption of cannabis. The total expenditure is estimated at EUR 671.61 million. For heroin, expenditure is estimated at EUR 701.27 million, and for cocaine the total spent is estimated at EUR 457.35 million to EUR 1 524.49 million.

In conclusion, according to the OFDT, the total spent on illegal drug consumption in France is somewhere between EUR 1.831 billion and EUR 3 billion.

Table 2: Turnover of cannabis

Frequency of consumption	Percentage of consumers over the year	Number of consumers	Grams consumed each time	Chances to consume during the year	Tonnes consumed	Expenditure (million EUR)
Daily	17	374 000	0.5	365	68.26	364.19
Once or more a week (not daily)	31	682 000	1.5	52	53.20	283.83
Once a month	15	330 000	0.5	12	1.98	10.56
Less than once a month	37	814 000	0.5	6	2.44	13.02
Total	100	2 200 000	—	—	125.87	671.61

Cost of drugs to the French economy

This section deals with the elements that make up the economic costs associated with drug use in France:

• cost of healthcare associated with drug consumption;

• public administration expenses for prevention and repression measures;

• income and production lost;

• lost taxes;

• privately funded organisations involved in prevention and research;

• other costs, in particular fines for violations of legislation on illegal drugs (Ilid).

Drug-related healthcare costs

Healthcare costs attributable to drug consumption are much more complicated to evaluate than those associated with tobacco or alcohol consumption. This is due to a lack of data on the drug-related pathologies themselves as well as on the risks attributable to the risk factor 'drugs' for these pathologies. It appears, therefore, that one of the priorities in calculating healthcare statistics on drugs would be to draw up a list of pathologies related to drug use, and to produce figures that allow a more reliable evaluation of healthcare statistics imputable to drugs.

However, it appears that only costs related to AIDS treatment and those involved in drug addiction treatment with Subutex® can be used in a tentative evaluation.

Cost of AIDS due to drug use

Hospital costs are estimated on the basis of simulated data of 55 000 people receiving hospital care because of HIV (73.5 %) or AIDS (26.5 %); 75.5 % of those with AIDS and 26 % of those with HIV got the virus through drug addiction. In 1995 the costs of hospital treatment were assessed at EUR 25 070 for an AIDS patient and at EUR 5 066 for an HIV patient.

Hospital costs amounted to EUR 87.69 million for patients with AIDS and EUR 53.25 million for HIV-positive patients. In 1995, the total hospital costs for treating HIV and AIDS in drug consumers amounted to EUR 140.94 million.

Subutex® and its cost

Since 1996, Subutex® has been on the market in France as a substitution treatment for opioid dependence. According to Kopp et al. (accepted), Subutex® is a long-acting, highly dosed form of buprenorphine, supposedly without the risk of respiratory depression. The Siamosis (an information system on the accessibility of sterile injecting material) estimates that from June 1996 onwards 14 000 to 18 000 patients have been treated per month, and nearly 40 000 patients in June 1997. A Centre de recherches économiques, sociologiques et de gestation study (Paree et al., 1997) assessed the cost of medical treatment with Subutex® at EUR 2 332.47 per person per year. Thus, with 40 000 persons on substitution treatment with Subutex®, the direct medical cost would be EUR 93.30 million.

Healthcare expenses for substitution treatment with Subutex® and treatment of drug-related HIV and AIDS in hospital would then amount to EUR 234.24 million.

Public administration costs

In this section, we first discuss the costs incurred by public administration, the main activities of which centre around repression (justice, police, gendarmerie, customs), secondly, the administration responsible for implementing health and social measures, and thirdly, the administration responsible for the design and implementation of preventive measures.

The Ministry of Justice

A first cost category relates to the activities of magistrates and judges involved in criminal court proceedings. These costs are presented under the heading of judicial services. A second category concerns the incarceration of those charged and convicted; these are the costs of the prison administration.

Judicial services: Judicial services encompass the activities of criminal and civil jurisdiction. The common method of calculating the cost of infractions of Ilid is firstly to determine the total expenditure of the criminal sector and, secondly, to determine the proportion spent on infractions.

About 5 847 magistrates (excluding magistrates in the appeal courts) devote nearly 3.59 % of their time to Ilid cases, or 210 full-time equivalent (FTE) magistrates. The average budgetary cost of a magistrate is estimated at EUR 53 190, the total cost of 210 FTE magistrates amounts to EUR 11.17 million.

Other personnel categories to be considered in judicial services are court clerks and other civil servants. We estimate that these involve close to 327.25 FTE at an average of EUR 29 000 per year, which amounts to EUR 9.49 million on a yearly basis. In the appeal courts, it is estimated that 64 civil servants devote all their time to Ilid-related cases, at a total cost of EUR 1.86 million. In all, budgetary employment costs for court clerks and justice civil servants amount to

EUR 8.04 million. The costs of other judicial services, such as infrastructure and legal assistance, are estimated at EUR 15.23 million. By adding all personnel costs (8.04 + 11.17 million) to the costs of other judicial services (15.23 million), we obtain the total costs of judicial services involved in drug-related activities, that is EUR 34.44 million.

Prison administration: Prison statistical data allow us to estimate the total incarceration time of persons convicted in 1995. This time amounts to 845 504.4 months made up of crimes (93 927 months), offences (751 576.8 months) and fifth-class violations (0.6 months). The number of months of incarceration associated with Ilid amounts to 194 122.5 or 22.96 % of the total incarceration time. By analogy, Ilid-related prisoners do 22.96 % of the total time of the entire incarcerated population. Thus, with a budget of EUR 873.22 million for the prison administration in 1995, the costs of detention for Ilid-related crimes reached EUR 200.49 million.

Directorate-General for Customs and Excise

In 1995, the customs service had a little over 20 000 budgetary posts. A total of 500 customs officers, without being officially assigned to the battle against drug trafficking, are considered to devote all their time to this task. With the average personnel cost of a post in 1995 being estimated at EUR 24 086, 500 customs officers cost nearly EUR 12 million. As operational costs per officer are about EUR 5 411.94, the total expenditure associated with 500 customs officers amounted to EUR 14.76 million in 1995. In that same year, another 9 000 agents carried out surveillance tasks for 25 % of their time amounting to 2 250 FTE. With the same personnel costs and operating expenses, 2 250 customs officers cost about EUR 66.39 million. In all, almost EUR 81.15 million was allocated in 1995 to customs and excise for their engagement in the fight against drugs.

National Gendarmerie

The Gendarmerie (under the control of the French Ministry of Defence) is involved in three distinct Ilid-related activities. Firstly, according to the Gendarmerie's statistics, 7.4 % are involved in repressive Ilid-related activities. Added to the total activity of the Gendarmerie's 'judicial police', we estimate that just over 2 million hours were allocated to Ilid in 1995. According to the Gendarmerie, the cost of a gendarme-hour was EUR 23.48 (figure communicated by the Gendarmerie), so the global costs of the Gendarmerie's repressive activities related to Ilid were EUR 47.51 million. Secondly, according to Gendarmerie estimates, public safety claimed another 23.7 million gendarme-hours, 3 % of which were estimated to concern Ilid. Thus, the total costs for Gendarmerie Ilid activities targeted at public safety were EUR 16.69 million. Finally, expenses such as remuneration of trainers or dog-handlers amounted to EUR 5.82 million. In all, in 1995, the national Gendarmerie spent almost EUR 70 million on Ilid-related activities.

National police

Of the entire national police force, 2 000 active civil servants spent all their time on the fight against drugs. Another 195 policemen were also indirectly involved in Ilid activities. In all, the budget allotted to police services specialised in the fight against drugs amounted to EUR 76.76 million.

In addition, 82 000 public safety civil servants were partly involved in the fight against drugs. Combining national police statistics on Ilid-related convictions with the number of civil servants working in the penal sector, we estimate that 3 469 FTE civil servants were involved in repressive activities and 867 FTE were allocated to preventive activities. Therefore, nearly 4 336 civil servants working in the public safety sector devoted all their time to Ilid. Keeping the personnel costs and the operating costs in mind, we arrive at a total expenditure of EUR 111.64 million for the civil servants of the public safety sector.

In all, the national police allocated nearly EUR 188.40 million to Ilid-related activities.

Ministry of Social, Health and City Affairs

Concerning the fight against drugs, the Ministry of Social, Health and City Affairs focuses particularly on prevention and treatment. Most costs associated with health/medical treatment are absorbed by the Directorate-General for Health (DGH) and the budget allocated to drugs amounted to EUR 106.15 million. The Administration of Social Affairs (ASA) and the Inter-Ministerial Delegation of the City (IMDC) spent EUR 2.13 million and EUR 3.35 million on treatment and prevention, respectively. Finally, activities of government personnel concern the coordination and management of the Departmental and Regional Administrations of Sanitary and Social Affairs (DASSA and RASSA) for a total amount of EUR 2.48 million. In total, the Ministry of Social, Health and City Affairs spent EUR 114.13 million on the fight against drugs.

Other ministries involved

The Ministry of National and Higher Education and Research is estimated to allocate EUR 6.66 million per year to prevention campaigns and research programmes in the fight against drug addiction. Doping as a form of drug addiction costs the Ministry of Youth and Sports a minimum of EUR 1.34 million per year. Finally, through the Ministry of Foreign Affairs and the Ministry of International Cooperation, France contributes EUR 8.63 million to international organisations against drug trafficking on an annual basis.

France's contribution to the EU budget

The EU budget for the fight against drugs amounted to EUR 27.938 million in 1995, in particular EUR 13.3 million for programmes within the Union and EUR 14.59 million in south and east European countries. France's contribution consisted of 17 % of the entire budget, or EUR 4.74 million in 1995.

Table 3 summarises the expenditure of public administration on the fight against drugs.

Income and production losses attributable to drugs

Income and production losses correspond to a fraction of the cost calculated within a larger context called 'human capital'. This corresponds globally to past, present and future costs borne by society and the individual due to premature death.

However, we are not interested in this human capital approach as our major concern is future income lost by an individual who died prematurely and the actual sum of lost production attributable to an early death, and other income and production losses attributable to drugs.

Loss of individual income

The calculation of income lost because of drug use firstly requires identification of the category of the individuals concerned and, secondly, requires a definition of the steps to be taken in the monetary valuation of the time lost by these individuals. Two groups of individuals are distinguished: those who died prematurely due to drug consumption either directly (overdose) or indirectly (HIV infection), and those who were incarcerated for Ilid. People hospitalised or on sick leave were excluded from this study because no relevant data were available.

Lost income due to premature death

The assessment of lost income in monetary terms involves two steps: firstly, the calculation of the number of years lost due to premature death, and, secondly, the calculation of the present value of future income lost using a certain discount rate.

Table 3: Costs of public administration attributable to drugs (million EUR)

Nature of the expense	Expenditure (budget)	Expenditure (inter-ministerial credits)	Total expenditure
Ministry of Justice	234.94	2.52	237.47
Of which:			
• Judicial services	34.45	—	34.45
• Prison administration	200.49	—	200.49
Customs and excise	81.15	3.09	84.22
Gendarmerie	70.02	1.58	71.60
Of which:			
• Judicial police	47.51	—	47.51
• Public safety	16.69	—	16.69
• Other expenditure	5.82	—	5.82
Police	188.41	3.79	192.20
Ministry of Social, Health and City Affairs	114.13	7.64	121.77
Of which:			
• DGH	106.15	3.98	110.13
• ASA	2.13	2.22	4.35
• IMDC	3.35	1.44	4.79
• DASSA and RASSA	2.48	—	2.48
MILDT	n.a.	6.92	6.92
Ministry of National Education, Higher Education and Research	6.66	1.88	8.54
Ministry of Youth and Sports	1.34	1.26	2.60
Ministries of Foreign Affairs and International Cooperation	8.63	1.37	10.00
Contribution to EU drugs budget	4.74	—	4.74
Work, jobs and professional training	—	0.12	0.12
Total	710.00	30.17	740.17

Abbreviations:
n.a. = not available
DGH = Directorate-General for Health
ASA = Administration of Social Affairs
IMDC = Inter-Ministerial Delegation of the City
DASSA = Departmental Administration of Sanitary and Social Affairs

RASSA = Regional Administration of Sanitary and Social Affairs
MILDT = Mission interministérielle de lutte contre la drogue et la toxicomanie

| Table 4: Lost income due to drug-related premature deaths | | | | | | |
</br>

Medical	Lost years		Number of deaths		Lost income	
causes of death	men	women	men	women	men (¹)	women (¹)
Overdose (²)	45		228		11.22	
AIDS and HIV	36	42	259	60	16.87	3.22

(¹) Million EUR.
(²) Overdose data refer to men and women.

The two major medical causes of death attributable to drugs are overdose and HIV infection. The OFDT estimates the number of deaths due to overdose at 228. The average age at time of death is assumed to be 35 years. The Institut national de la santé et de la recherche médicale (Inserm) estimated that, in 1997, 1 017 men aged 20 to 79 and 237 women aged 20 to 84 died of AIDS. As 25.47 % of all AIDS and HIV cases are attributable to drug use, it follows that 259 men and 60 women died of drug use. In all, nearly 547 people died because of drugs. With an available annual gross income of EUR 14 789.38 and a discount rate of 6 %, it can easily be calculated that close to EUR 31.31 million is lost to drug-related deaths. Table 4 gives the lost income for both causes of death of individuals prematurely deceased.

Lost income due to incarceration

On the basis of the prison administration's expense data, the number of months of incarceration associated with Ilid equals 194 122.5 months. The average sentence is 18.1 months (a period too short to require a discount rate), and the gross monthly income is EUR 14 789.38/12 = 1 232.44. If we combine the gross monthly income with the total time of incarceration, we arrive at a total lost income of EUR 239.24 million.

In all we can estimate lost income attributable to drugs at EUR 270.55 million. Naturally, this estimate does not represent all losses as only those losses relating to death by overdose or AIDS have been taken into consideration. Therefore, this figure should be used with extreme caution, as a large portion of lost income is not included in this estimate.

Production losses

Loss of production due to premature death or incarceration is by no means easy to estimate, as no satisfactory indicator is available. However, the construction of an aggregate measuring the value added over the course of a year when compared with the hours worked annually by the total population would provide an estimate of losses. This corresponds to the 'apparent added value work schedule'.

According to Institut national de la statistique et des études économiques (INSEE) data, the average working week consisted of 39.8 hours, giving a total of 39.8 x 47 = 1 870.6 hours in 1996. Considering that the number of jobs in 1997 was estimated at 22.337 million and assuming that the number of working hours did not change between 1996 and 1997, we estimated that the number of hours worked by the total working population at 41 783.6 million. Using an amount of EUR 1 142 058.7 million (INSEE) for the global added value for 1997, we calculated that the added value created by one hour of work equals EUR 27.33 (EUR 217.57 per day or EUR 51 131.26 per year). Based on these figures, we can assess the loss of production due to premature death and incarceration.

Lost production due to premature death

The number of premature deaths must be recalculated in relation to the age of retirement. As the retirement age is 65 years, and 547 people a year die of drug-related causes, the number of premature deaths is 533. Based on this figure, we can attempt a preliminary assessment relative to the cause of death and gender and the difference between retirement age and the average age of death (number of potential work years lost). Based on the average amount of annual added value created by interior jobs (EUR 51 131.26) and a discount rate of 6 %, it is possible to assess monetarily the total loss of added value attributable to drug-related premature deaths. The figures are presented in Table 5.

Thus, in total, EUR 150.21 million of added value was lost due to drug-related AIDS and overdose death.

It should, however, be noted that this estimate does not entirely correspond to production losses because part of the added value is paid directly to the State and

Table 5: Added value losses attributed to drug-related premature deaths

Medical	Lost years		Number of deaths		Lost income	
causes of death	men	women	men	women	men ([1])	women ([1])
Overdose ([2])	30		228		60.89	
AIDS and HIV	25	28	249	56	73.73	15.59

([1]) Million EUR.
([2]) Overdose data refer to men and women.

Medical causes of death	Lost years		Number of deaths		Lost income	
	men	women	men	women	men ([1])	women ([1])
Overdose ([2])	30		228		39.98	
AIDS and HIV	25	28	249	56	48.41	10.23

Table 6: Lost production due to drug-related premature deaths

([1]) Million EUR.
([2]) Overdose data refer to men and women.

another part is paid to employees in the form of income. It is therefore necessary to calculate the loss of primary income due to premature deaths and then to deduct the lost added value, which will yield an approximation of the monetary value of lost production. According to our estimates, which are based on INSEE figures, the total loss of primary income of both men and women due to premature deaths by overdose equals EUR 20.91 million. The loss due to AIDS-related premature deaths is EUR 25.32 million and EUR 5.35 million for men and women, respectively. The difference between the loss of added value and the loss of primary income equals the loss of production due to premature death. The results are presented in Table 6.

In all, EUR 98.62 million of lost production was attributable to drugs because of people dying prematurely from overdose or AIDS.

Lost production due to incarceration

The same method can be applied to prisoners; first the loss of added value was calculated and from the outcome, the lost primary income was subtracted. By substituting the years of life lost by the total term of incarceration, we reached an estimate of lost added value in the order of EUR 844.74 million for those incarcerated for Ilid. From this, we then deducted the primary income, which is EUR 284.10 million. We thus obtained an estimate of production loss for Ilid-related incarcerations amounting to EUR 560.64 million. In all, income and production losses due to drug-related premature death or incarceration were estimated at nearly EUR 929.82 million per year.

Lost obligatory deductions attributable to drugs

Income and production losses due to drug-related premature deaths or incarceration do not constitute the sole costs emerging from drug-related premature deaths and incarcerations. Incarcerations, premature deaths and hospitalisations attributable to drugs reduce the amount of taxes and, de facto, effect the resources available for the community. As such, it seems pertinent and legitimate to include lost taxes in the calculation of the economic cost of illegal drugs. Calculation of these losses requires the same data as used earlier, but tax rates need to be transposed to an individual level. With a gross available income of EUR 14 789.39 and a total of taxes reaching EUR 7 218.01, we calculated a rate of deduction of income of 48.81 % (14 789.38/7 218.01). In applying this rate to the loss of income calculated above, we found the amount of lost taxes linked to premature deaths and incarcerations. As calculated above, the loss of income amounts to EUR 31.31 million, and with a tax rate of 48.81 %, the tax losses equalled EUR 15.28 million. For the people incarcerated, whose income amounted to EUR 239.24 million, the tax losses equal EUR 116.77 million.

In so far as data on drug-related crimes and infractions and on hospitalisations are not available, we assess the total loss of taxes attributable to drugs at EUR 132.06 million, a figure that concerns only drug-use-related premature deaths and Ilid-related incarcerations.

Other costs borne by private agents

Lastly, other costs attributable to drugs may be mentioned. These costs correspond to fines for individuals who violate drug legislation, to sentences for Ilid-related convictions and to the cost of lawyers. Unfortunately, only data on fines are available. According to the Ministry of Justice, 2 139 fines, at an average of EUR 375.02, were given in 1996. In total, those convicted for Ilid-related crimes paid nearly EUR 802 177.58 in fines.

Conclusion

Table 7 summarises all the costs discussed. Obviously, these costs, as well as the final estimate, are subject to discussion, particularly since certain aspects have not been taken into account. However, bearing in mind the limitations mentioned (i.e. a lack of information preventing us from evaluating certain drug-related costs), in our estimation, the costs to the community amount to EUR 2 035.24 million (excluding the cost of purchase). This amount does not include the cost of purchasing drugs because the methodology used (i.e. the counterfactual scenario) presumes that, in the absence of drugs, the consumer would spend his or her money on other goods without generating the costs incurred by drug consumption.

Table 7: Synthesis of expenditure attributable to drugs (million EUR)

	Social costs
Consumption	1 831 to 3 000
Healthcare expenses	234.24
Of which:	
AIDS	140.94
Subutex®	93.30
Public administration expenditure	740.15
Of which:	
Ministry of Justice	237.47
Customs and excise	84.22
Gendarmerie	71.60
Police	192.20
Ministry of Social, Health and City Affairs	121.77
MILDT	6.92
Ministry of National and Higher Education and Research	8.54
Ministry of Youth and Sports	2.60
Ministries of Foreign Affairs and International Cooperation	10.0
Contribution to the EU drugs budget	4.74
Professional training	0.12
Losses of income and production	929.82
Of which:	
Income loss of private agents	270.56
For medical cause of death	*31.31*
For imprisonment	*239.24*
Production loss	659.26
Due to medical cause of death	*98.62*
Due to incarceration	*560.64*
Loss of taxes	132.06
Of which:	
Medical causes of death	15.28
Incarceration	116.78
Other costs borne by private agents (fines)	0.80
Total (excluding purchase cost)	2 037.07
Total (including purchase cost)	From 3 868.07 to 5 037.07

Abbreviation: MILDT = Mission interministérielle de lutte contre la drogue et la toxicomanie.

With a gross national product (GNP) of EUR 1 240 480.00 billion in 1997, the costs borne by the community due to drug use corresponded to approximately 0.16 % of GNP in that year. Another figure, which permits a better understanding of the volume of this expenditure, is the average cost per capita attributable to drugs. If we use the figure of 58.7 million inhabitants at 1 January 1998 (INSEE), each French citizen has to bear an average cost of EUR 34.67 per year as a consequence of drug consumption. It must be concluded that, in economic terms, illegal drugs are by no means the social curse they are said to be. In comparison, Kopp and Fenoglio (2000) estimate the cost of alcohol and tobacco at nearly EUR 17 595.80 million and EUR 9 929.34 million, respectively. In other words, alcohol and tobacco cost society nearly nine and five times as much, respectively, as illegal drugs on an annual basis.

References

Collins, D., Lapsey, H. M. (1995), *The social costs of drug abuse in Australia in 1988 and 1992*, Monograph No 30, Commonwealth Department of Human Services and Health, Australian Government Printing Services.

Hodgson, T. A., Meiners, M. (1979), *Guidelines for cost of illness studies in public health*, Task Force on Cost of Illness Studies, US Public Health Service, Washington, DC.

Kopp, P., Fenoglio, P. (2000), *Le coût social des drogues licites (alcool et tabac) et illicites en France*, Étude N° 22, OFDT, Paris.

Kopp, P., Rumeau-Pichon, C., Le Pen, C. (accepted), 'Les enjeux financiers des traitements de substitution dans la toxicomanie: le cas de Subutex®', *Revue Française d'Epidémiologie* (accepted).

Observatoire français des drogues et des toxicomanies (OFDT) (1999), *Drogues et toxicomanies; indicateurs et tendances*, OFDT, Paris.

Paree, F., Allenet, B., Lebrun, T. (1997), *Subutex® dans l'arsenal thérapeutique de prise en charge des héroïnomanes: environnement et estimation du coût de prise en charge médicale*, Centre de recherche économiques, sociologiques et de gestion, Lille.

Single, E., Easton, B., Collins, D., Harwood, H., Lapsey, H., Maynard, A. (1995), *International guidelines for estimating the costs of substance abuse*, Canadian Centre on Substance Abuse, Ottawa.

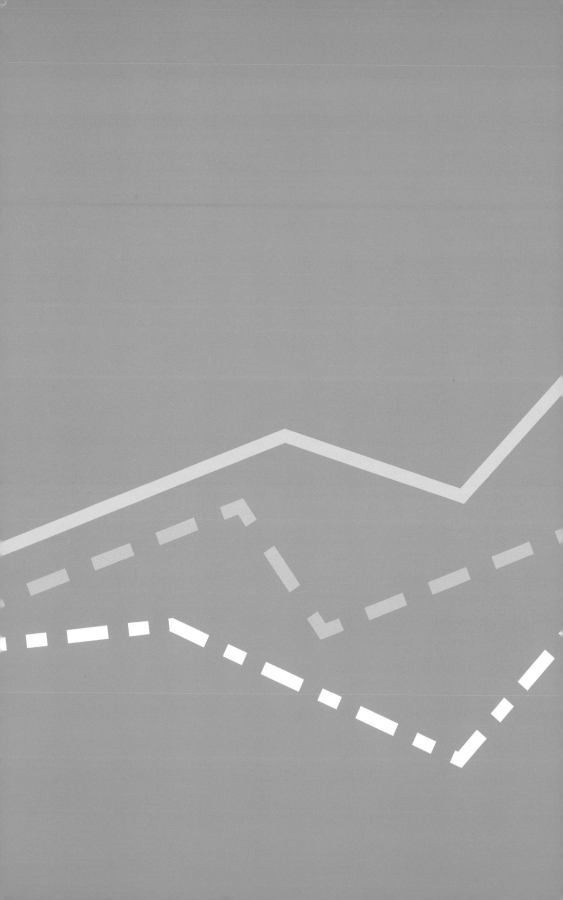

Cost-effectiveness of needle and syringe programmes and methadone maintenance

PART **V**

Introduction

This final section focuses on one of the major questions of the monograph: '(How) can further HCV transmission in IDUs be prevented?' Two key interventions for IDUs, needle and syringe programmes (NSPs) and methadone maintenance treatment (MMT), are analysed with regard to their cost-effectiveness in reducing incidence of HCV.

De Wit and Bos present a literature review of economic analyses of NSPs. In previous reviews there is consensus that NSPs are cost-effective for the prevention of HIV, but much less so if only hepatitis C is regarded. The authors find seven studies with a full economic analysis of NSPs, all of these focusing on averted HIV infections as the measure of effectiveness, while only one included an analysis of HCV infection. Although several of the reviewed studies show methodological shortcomings, often in the form of incomplete assessments of especially the costing part, the authors also conclude that NSPs are cost-effective in preventing the spread of HIV. One additional study is discussed that did not meet the inclusion criteria of the review of being full economic evaluation and which suggests that NSPs are not cost-effective with regard to HCV alone (Pollack, 2001). Several potential sources of bias exist. NSPs often provide much broader services to IDUs than only clean needles and syringes and they may serve as an important point of (first) contact with IDUs. This causes potentially more favourable outcomes than if an isolated analysis of the pure NSP component were possible. Similarly, even if NSPs may not be cost-effective with regard to HCV in isolation, the potential additional effects, such as hepatitis prevention, referrals to other services, gaining access to a hidden population etc. are obtained with no or small additional costs. Ideally, and most relevant for practical policy-making, an intervention-oriented economic evaluation integrating both HIV and HCV is required.

Pollack and Heimer use mathematical modelling to compare the cost-effectiveness of MMT to other public health interventions. They analyse both a dynamic situation where prevalence is rising strongly, and a steady-state model within a stable endemic situation, as is currently observed among IDUs in the EU. The dynamic analyses show the high importance of optimising treatment quality (i.e. to reduce relapses so that exits from the IDU population are increased and to increase treatment adherence so that injecting and needle sharing are reduced). They also show that efficiency of further prevention is reduced once sharing goes down in the MMT population. They conclude that MMT is highly cost-effective for preventing HIV and potentially cost saving. For HCV, costs per averted infection are estimated at USD 180 000 in the baseline scenario indicating that prevention through MMT is not cost saving if compared to discounted average lifetime HCV treatment costs (see also Chapter 8). The steady-state analyses suggest that very high coverage of the IDU population with MMT may result in low costs per averted infection, due to herd immunity effects. In addition, the effects of other interventions such as NSPs have not been taken into account and these may lower the minimum coverage level needed for MMT to achieve relevant herd immunity and favourable cost-effectiveness. The modelling results further suggest that increasing MMT coverage is more cost-effective at the higher end of the coverage scale: increasing coverage from 50 % to 60 % is done at lower costs than for a rise from 10 % to 20 %.

Recent criticism has been put forward on cost-effectiveness analyses of treatment and prevention interventions (Piot et al., 2002, see also the introduction to Part III). Can they be safely compared within a strict public health perspective, or may cost-effectiveness analysis in some cases provide endorsement for overall under-investment? What if costs of programmes and treatments are not stable, but highly volatile, as is currently the case for HIV? Strong changes in medication prices will severely affect cost–benefit estimates of any intervention that is compared to life-long treatment costs. Moreover, the standard comparison to discounted lifetime treatment costs (estimated on USD 195 000 for HIV) as a basis for decision-making may not always be suitable. For example, if lifetime treatment costs of HCV are about a factor 10 lower than for HIV, this could in the extreme case lead to a policy decision of not funding HCV prevention just because treatment costs are low. It seems therefore important that economic analyses include a cost–utility component, where the benefits of an intervention are also estimated in terms of discounted QALYs or DALYs gained. A threshold value of USD 50 000 has been proposed per QALY gained (Owens, 1998). As discussed earlier in this volume, from a societal perspective, an exclusive focus on direct healthcare costs, excluding other costs to society or the individual, is likely to underestimate the cost-effectiveness ratio of an intervention.

Lucas Wiessing

References

European Monitoring Centre for Drugs and Drug Addiction (EMCDDA) (2002), *Annual report on the state of the drugs problem in the European Union and Norway 2002*, Office for Official Publications of the European Union, Luxembourg. Available at http://ar2002.emcdda.eu.int/en/page54-en.html.

Owens, D. K. (1998), 'Interpretation of cost-effectiveness analyses', *Journal of General Internal Medicine* 13: 716–7.

Piot, P., Zewdie, D., Turmen, T. (2002), HIV/AIDS prevention and treatment', *The Lancet* 360: 86.

Pollack, H. A. (2001), 'Cost-effectiveness of harm reduction in preventing hepatitis C among injection drug users', *Medical Decision Making* 21: 357–67.

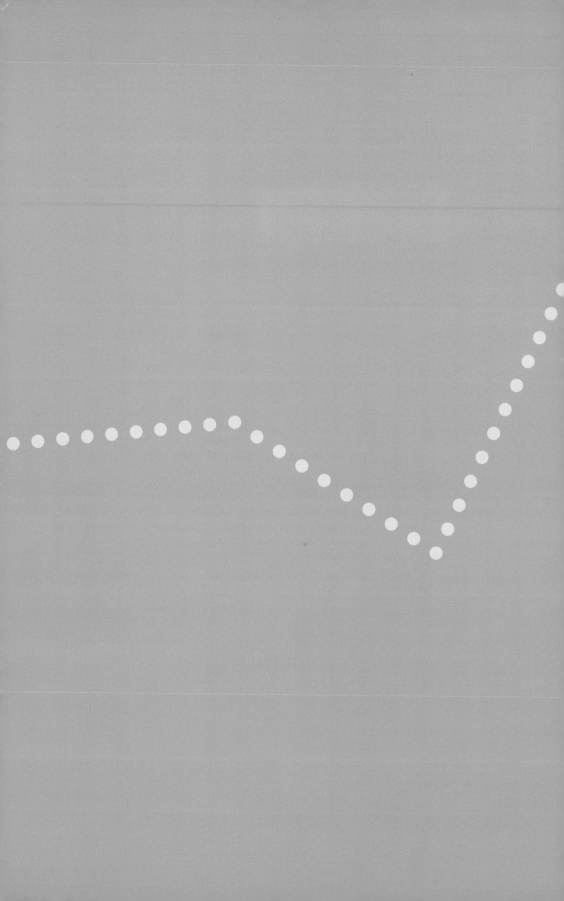

Chapter 14
Cost-effectiveness of needle and syringe programmes: a review of the literature

Ardine de Wit and Jasper Bos

Introduction

The sharing of injecting equipment is associated with the transmission of blood-borne pathogens, such as HIV and hepatitis B and C viruses. In non-endemic countries, the highest incidence of these blood-borne viruses is usually found in IDUs. As a consequence, IDUs are one of the driving forces in sustaining epidemic levels of these infectious diseases. Moreover, due to mixing of IDUs with other groups in the population, the disease could potentially become endemic in the general population. At low levels of an epidemic, an infectious disease can sustain itself only in subgroups of the general population, differing from the general population by having a larger number of sexual partners, injecting drug use or other risk factors for transmission. Thus, these subgroups play a disproportionate role in the maintenance and transmission of the epidemic (Anderson and May, 1991). After establishing themselves in these populations, the viruses may spread quickly to other sectors of the community. For instance, HIV may first spread to sexual partners of IDUs and later by sexual transmission to other parts of the population. This is partly due to the fact that a relatively large proportion of IDUs are involved in commercial sex work. Also, the high incidence of concurrent viruses, such as the herpes simplex virus (HSV), facilitates the sexual transmission of HIV (Burrows, 2000). HCV is spread less easily through sexual contact than HIV, but due to its much higher parenteral infectivity it spreads very easily among IDUs. Therefore, most IDU populations experience HCV prevalence exceeding 50 % (CDCP, 1998).

It is assumed that, in the early phase of a blood-borne epidemic, one of the main routes of transmission is through the sharing of contaminated needles. Other routes of transmission become predominant when the epidemic has sustained itself in the general population. This emphasises the role that harm reduction programmes targeted at IDUs can play in the reduction of the negative consequences associated with injecting drug use. This chapter is concerned with one specific form of harm reduction, namely needle and syringe programmes

(NSPs). The first NSP was launched in Amsterdam, the Netherlands, in 1984 (Coutinho, 1995). At the instigation of the local junkie union, but with financial and organisational assistance of the Amsterdam Municipal Health Service, the programme was introduced without any political interference or discussion. Within the NSP, sterile syringes were provided to IDUs and used equipment was subsequently collected to be disposed of. In 1986, several pilot programmes in the UK followed the Amsterdam initiative, and, a few years later, these programmes were extended throughout the UK, other European countries and Australia. In the US, however, the federal government banned the use of its funds to support NSPs in 1988, and this ban still holds today. It is argued that providing needles to addicts lends a certain degree of validation to their illegal behaviour. As a consequence of the ban mentioned above, as many as half of all US programmes are operating in a semi-legal or illegal environment (Ferrini, 2000). Most of the over 100 existing US programmes are funded locally, privately or by the State.

Many NSPs have expanded their services with the provision of other sterile equipment that facilitates safer injection, such as cottons, cookers, water and bleach (Bastos and Strathdee, 2000). In addition, NSPs may distribute condoms, provide HIV counselling, hepatitis B immunisation, offer screening for sexually transmitted diseases and refer users to specialised drug abuse treatment centres. Some of these extended NSPs have developed into comprehensive 'harm reduction centres', offering a complete range of services to prevent the transmission of infectious diseases, both within the group of IDUs and among their sexual partners, relatives and the public at large.

Major reviews (summarised in Vlahov and Junge, 1998; Bastos and Strathdee, 2000; Ferrini, 2000) suggest that NSPs may reduce rates of seroconversion to HIV and hepatitis by one third or more, without negative side effects on the number of IDUs or injection frequency among IDUs (Vlahov and Junge, 1998). A landmark study from Hurley et al. combined HIV seroprevalence data from 81 cities with ($n = 52$) or without ($n = 29$) NSPs (Hurley et al., 1997). They showed that the average annual seroprevalence was 11 % lower in cities with an NSP than in cities without an NSP, providing important evidence on the effectiveness of NSPs in reducing the spread of HIV. Regarding hepatitis viruses, however, the effectiveness of NSPs in reducing the incidence and/or prevalence of infection is still highly controversial. A prospective cohort study found that NSPs were not effective in the reduction of hepatitis C incidence among users (Hagan et al., 1999) while ecological and cross-sectional analyses suggest the opposite: a reduction of hepatitis C prevalence among users of NSPs (McDonald et al., 2000; Taylor et al., 2000; Goldberg et al., 2001; Hahn et al., 2001). On the other hand, in a recent report by the Commonwealth Department of Health and Ageing (2002) in Australia, the study approach of Hurley et al. was repeated, collecting data on both HIV seroprevalence and HCV seroprevalence. The results of these studies strongly suggest the effectiveness of NSPs in reducing the spread of HIV and, to a lesser extent, also the spread of HCV.

Many of the currently available effectiveness studies may be criticised because of inadequate statistical control for all factors that simultaneously influence the incidence and/or prevalence of HIV and hepatitis (Bastos and Strathdee, 2000). However, even those case studies that showed a decline in hepatitis C prevalence among IDUs agree that hepatitis C prevalence is still too high, with prevalence exceeding 50 % in most IDU populations. There seems to be consensus that NSPs are more successful in preventing HIV spread than in the prevention of transmission of hepatitis viruses (Coutinho, 1998; Crofts et al., 2000; Commonwealth Department of Health and Ageing, 2002).

The purpose of this study is to review and compare current knowledge about the cost-effectiveness of NSPs. Although the principal aim of most NSPs has been the reduction of HIV spread, they may also play a role in the prevention of transmission of hepatitis B and C viruses. However, most economic studies have assessed the cost-effectiveness of NSPs with regard to HIV prevention only. Only one study (Commonwealth Department of Health and Ageing, 2002) incorporated effects on HCV prevention as well. As a consequence of the prevailing focus on HIV, this chapter focuses mainly on HIV prevention. Whenever available, information on the (cost-)effectiveness of NSPs with regard to hepatitis viruses is specifically discussed.

Methods

We performed a review of the literature. Inclusion criteria for the review were: (i) full economic evaluation (to be explained later in this section) considering NSPs; and (ii) publication in English, French, German or Dutch. The period under review was 1984 (first NSPs initiated) until June 2002.

Studies were identified by searches of the following databases:

1. Medline, a database of medical literature maintained by the US National Library of Medicine.
2. Health technology assessment database, a database of publications by members of the International Network of Agencies of Health Technology Assessment (Inahta).

3. NHS-EED (NHS economic evaluation database). This database is maintained by the National Health Service Centre for Reviews and Dissemination, University of York.

The search strategy that was used for the searches included one of the following terms as a MESH term: Needle exchange programs/all, Intravenous substance abuse/all, Needle-sharing/all, in combination with either Cost or cost-analysis/all or Cost–benefit analysis/all. Furthermore, titles and abstracts of publications indexed in Medline were searched using a combination of 'needle exchange' or 'syringe exchange' or 'intravenous drug' or 'substance abuse' or 'needle sharing' or 'syringe sharing' with either 'cost benefit' or 'cost effectiveness' of 'cost utility' or 'economic evaluation'. Similar terminology was used to search the Inahta database and the NHS-EED. The references of all articles that were assessed were also checked for relevant articles.

A full economic evaluation is a study describing all necessary input and all relevant outcomes of healthcare interventions (Drummond et al., 1997). This definition immediately distinguishes cost studies from full economic evaluations, since effect measures are lacking in cost studies. One basic principle of economic evaluation is that at least one intervention is compared to another: either a status quo intervention or doing nothing. Four basic types of full economic evaluations may be distinguished (Drummond et al., 1997):

- cost-minimisation analysis (CMA), which assumes that two or more interventions are equally effective, and thus aims at the determination of the cheapest intervention;
- cost–benefit analysis (CBA), which requires that all costs and benefits are expressed in monetary terms;
- cost-effectiveness analysis (CEA), which aims to find the cost per unit of outcome, e.g. the cost per life year gained;
- and cost–utility analysis (CUA), an extension of cost-effectiveness analysis that also includes the effects of an intervention on quality of life. The output parameter is called the cost per quality-adjusted life year (QALY) gained.

From the inclusion criterion that studies should be full economic evaluations, it follows that all other studies, including theoretical models, reviews and cost studies only, were not selected for this review.

Results

The Medline search as described in the 'Methods' section identified 107 references. From the NHS-EED and the Inahta database, a total of 28 references were found. Often, it was immediately clear from the content of the abstract, or the publication type (e.g. editorial), that the paper was not suitable for further assessment. Ultimately, six papers that covered both the costs and effects of NSPs were identified through the Medline search. Unselected studies appeared to concentrate on other harm reduction measures or to be partial economic evaluations, although they were sometimes incorrectly labelled as full economic evaluation studies in either the title or the abstract. Also, studies often appeared to be cost studies only. Via reference tracking, one further full economic evaluation study was added to the six studies already selected (Commonwealth Department of Health and Ageing, 2002).

Table 1 shows a comprehensive overview of the seven selected studies with the following key features: first author and year of publication, interventions compared, study design, number of patients, economic study design, viewpoint of study, type of costs included, valuation of costs, year of study, timespan of study, discounting of costs and effects with discount rate, (type of) sensitivity analysis, and main outcomes. In the remainder of the 'Results' section, we discuss some of the findings of the selected studies.

Epidemiological modelling

Because experimental study designs have so far not been used in the evaluation of NSP effectiveness, all the selected studies applied more or less sophisticated models to predict the effectiveness of NSPs in terms of reduction in virus transmission. These models translate (changes in) behavioural risk data, for example the percentage of needles that is shared with other users, into estimates of the number of infections (averted by an intervention). The seven economic evaluations that were selected for this review use either more (Pinkerton et al., 2000) or less (Laufer, 2001) sophisticated epidemiological models. The main outcome of all the studies was the number of HIV infections averted. One study also focused on the number of HCV infections averted (Anonymous, 2002). Published data from the literature were used as the main source of evidence in all the studies. Some of the studies also used empirical data observed from one or more NSPs (Jacobs et al., 1999; Pinkerton et al., 2000).

Table 1: Summary of the main characteristics of studies selected for review

First author/year of publication	Intervention(s) assessed	Study design	Economic design (¹)
Commonwealth Department of Health and Ageing, 2002	NSP versus doing nothing	Modelling of annual rate of change of seroprevalence	CEA/CUA
Gold (1997)	NSP (mobile van) versus doing nothing	Decision analytical model	CEA
Holtgrave (1998)	Increasing access to sterile needles through NSPs + pharmacy sales versus status quo	Mathematical modelling in hypothetical cohort of 1 million IDUs	CEA
Jacobs (1999)	NSP versus doing nothing	Mathematical modelling study using data from one intervention cohort	CEA
Laufer (2001)	NSP versus doing nothing	Calculations of infections averted in seven NSP sites	CEA
Lurie (1997)	NSP versus doing nothing	Modelling study in hypothetical cohort of IDUs	CEA
Pinkerton (2000)	A combination of interventions directed at injecting drug use and sexual risk behaviour versus doing nothing	Mathematical modelling study using data from eight different intervention cohorts	CEA/CUA

First author/year of publication	Country of study and year to which data apply	Viewpoint	Main effects included	Source of effectiveness data
Commonwealth Department of Health and Ageing, 2002	Australia, 1990–2000	Healthcare payer	Number of HIV and HCV infections averted	Review of literature
Gold (1997)	Canada, 1992–97	Society	Number of HIV infections averted	Review of literature
Holtgrave (1998)	US, 1995–97	Society	Number of HIV infections averted	Published studies + assumptions
Jacobs (1999)	Canada, 1997	Society	Number of HIV infections averted	Published studies + interviews with IDUs

Table 1 (continued)

First author/year of publication	Country of study and year to which data apply	Viewpoint	Main effects included data	Source of effectiveness
Laufer (2001)	US, 1996	Society	Number of HIV infections averted	Published studies
Lurie (1997)	US, 1991–95	Not stated	Number of HIV infections averted	Published studies
Pinkerton (2000)	US, 1987–end year not stated	Not stated, but probably societal viewpoint	Number of HIV infections averted, QALYs	Published studies + behavioural data from cohort studies

First author/year of publication	Costs included in study ([2])	Valuation of costs ([3])	Time span of study	Discounting	Incremental analysis
Commonwealth Department of Health and Ageing, 2002	2, 3	1, 2, 3	Lifetime	5 % cost and effects	No
Gold (1997)	1, 4	1, 2, 4	5 years	5 % costs only	No
Holtgrave (1998)	1, 3	4	1 year	—	Yes
Jacobs (1999)	1, 3, 4	1, 4	1 year	—	No
Laufer (2001)	1, 3	1, 4	1 year	3 % (future treatment costs only)	No
Lurie (1997)	2	3, 4	9 years	Yes, costs, but % not mentioned	No
Pinkerton (2000)	2	3, 4	Lifetime	3 % costs, unclear (effects)	No

First author/year	Sensitivity analysis	Main conclusions
Commonwealth Department of Health and Ageing, 2002	Yes: discount rate, effect of NSP on HIV incidence, treatment costs costs of NSP, quality of life adjustments	NSP is cost saving in all circumstances tested and is associated with gains in quality and quantity of life
Gold (1997)	Yes: HIV incidence, number of users, discount rate	NSP is cost saving in all circumstances tested
Holtgrave (1998)	Yes: HIV incidence, new infections attributable to injecting behaviour, cost of syringe provision	Increasing access to sterile syringes with a one-year programme is cost saving, even at high levels (88 %) of coverage

Table 1 (continued)

First author/year	Sensitivity analysis	Main conclusions
Jacobs (1999)	Yes: extreme value analysis for HIV prevalence among IDUs and behavioural data	The NSP results in net savings and is therefore a dominant strategy in base case analysis, but not in all extreme value sensitivity analyses
Laufer (2001)	Yes: number of shared injections per IDU/year, HIV incidence among non-NSP users	NSP is cost saving in all circumstances tested
Lurie (1997)	No	NSP is dominant strategy, i.e. cost saving. However, programme costs were not studied
Pinkerton (2000)	Yes, extreme value analysis for behavioural data, lifetime costs and QALYs	Intervention is most likely cost saving, in all circumstances tested

(¹) CMA = cost-minimisation analysis; CBA = cost–benefit analysis; CEA = cost-effectiveness analysis; CUA = cost–utility analysis; LYG = life years gained; QALY = quality-adjusted life years gained.
(²) 1 = direct healthcare costs (complete); 2 = direct healthcare costs (partially); 3 = direct non-healthcare costs; 4 = indirect non-healthcare costs (productivity costs); 5 = indirect healthcare costs.
(³) 1 = real (opportunity) costs; 2 = charges/tariffs; 3 = unclear, not stated; 4 = cost figures quoted from other studies.

Economic evaluation methodology

All seven studies followed a cost-effectiveness approach, while two studies also used a cost–utility framework to evaluate NSPs. The cost per HIV infection averted was the main outcome in all the studies. The cost–utility study provided the cost per QALY gained as an outcome measure (Pinkerton et al., 2000).

Viewpoint

The viewpoint of the study is important because an intervention may be attractive from one perspective, but not from another. For instance, influenza vaccination on healthy working adults may be attractive from the employer's perspective, but not from a healthcare payer's perspective. Most of the studies claimed to take a societal perspective, implying that all relevant costs and effects to the society at large are included, irrespective of who pays for the costs or who receives the benefits. In some studies (Lurie and Drucker, 1997; Pinkerton et al., 2000), the perspective was not stated, but most likely here, the perspective is the societal as well. One study was performed with a healthcare-payer perspective (Commonwealth Department of Health and Ageing, 2002). However, none of the studies incorporated all the relevant costs to society (see later).

Costs incurred and valuation method used for costing

All the studies incorporated direct healthcare costs, although not all of them reported on all relevant direct healthcare costs. For instance, the study by Lurie and Drucker (1997) ignored the cost of the NSP itself. Some papers lacked own-costing studies, but quoted cost data (i.e. charges) from the literature. All the studies but one (Commonwealth Department of Health and Ageing, 2002) relied on external sources for the estimation of lifetime costs of treating HIV infection and AIDS. None of the studies succeeded in applying the opportunity cost principle for the entire cost study. At best, the studies combined partial valuation of costs with cost data from previously published sources. Indirect non-healthcare costs (productivity costs) were included in only two studies. In general, the studies may be characterised as weak on the costing part.

Discounting

Discounting is a basic principle of economic evaluation methodology. It accommodates for the differences in timing of costs and effects in economic analyses that include future events. For instance, NSPs require investments today, while effects may occur in the future, resulting in savings on future treatment costs. By the application of a discount rate to these future costs and effects, the present value of these future costs and effects is calculated. Discounting of costs was applied in most of the studies with a timespan of more than one year. However, discounting of effects was either not performed (Gold et al., 1997; Lurie and Drucker, 1997; Laufer, 2001) or it was unclear what discounting percentage was used (Pinkerton et al., 2000). The discount rates applied varied between 3 and 5 %.

Sensitivity analysis

Economic analyses should include sensitivity analyses to provide evidence on the robustness of the conclusions reached. Six of the seven selected studies performed such sensitivity analyses. All of them considered the effects of changes in HIV incidence/prevalence. The two studies that used behavioural data from IDUs performed extreme value analysis to provide worst- and best-case scenarios for the cost-effectiveness of NSPs. In general, it is concluded that the outcome that NSPs are cost saving is stable in all the circumstances tested.

Discussion

The conclusion to be drawn from the studies summarised in Table 1 is that NSPs seem to be cost-effective in preventing the spread of HIV. All the studies have employed some sort of modelling technique to estimate the effectiveness of NSPs in terms of number of averted HIV infections. The future savings on the cost of treatment of HIV/AIDS cases that are prevented are then compared with the average operating cost of an NSP, resulting in a statement that NSPs are cost saving. However, the modelling approaches as applied in the different cost-effectiveness analyses are, in general, simplified approaches to the dynamics of HIV spread, ignoring heterogeneous patterns of HIV spread among subgroups of the IDU community differing in risk behaviour. More enhanced models are generally expected to confirm conclusions drawn from simple modelling approaches, by taking into account secondary effects of reduced HIV spread to populations other than IDUs. One modelling study that approaches the subject of costs and effects of HIV prevention programmes from an operations research perspective has not been included in our review (Kaplan, 1995). However, this study contributes to the conclusions drawn from the studies in our review, by making it likely that the average cost per averted infection is far below the lifetime treatment cost of HIV infection. Also, one analysis, excluded from our review because it was not a full economic evaluation, demonstrates that five different syringe provision programmes are cost-neutral to society when local annual HIV seroincidence rates exceed 0.3 % (for direct syringe sale) to 2.1 % (for an NSP) (Lurie et al., 1998). As the annual seroconversion rates are higher in many IDU populations, this adds to the evidence that the provision of syringes is cost-effective.

The studies described in the 'Results' section reveal several methodological problems. These may both over- and underestimate the cost-effectiveness of NSPs. Some reasons for the overestimation of the cost-effectiveness of NSPs may be as follows:

• All studies have linked the NSP cost to an estimate of the number of HIV infections averted, thus calculating the cost per averted infection. Subsequently, the cost per averted infection is linked to (previously published) estimates of lifetime costs of average HIV treatment from other sources. Then, it is concluded that the NSP is cost saving, while ignoring the fact that many IDUs will never have access to the full range of possible treatments and, as a consequence, that costs averted for HIV treatment are not as high as estimated (Reitemeijer et al., 1993). By ignoring this, the cost-effectiveness of NSPs is systematically overestimated. Only in the studies of Pinkerton et al. (2000) and Laufer (2001) has this effect been taken into account. However, the overestimation of cost-effectiveness in most studies may be moderated by the fact that the cost figures for lifetime HIV/AIDS treatment that are quoted in the studies will be (much) higher at present, due to recent additions to HIV treatment, such as protease inhibitors.

• As a secondary function, NSPs may refer IDUs to services with which they may otherwise not come into contact. In evaluative studies, it is difficult to study the cost-effectiveness of all harm reduction policies separately (Pinkerton et al., 2000). Because HIV and other blood-borne pathogens may be transmitted due to injecting risk behaviour and sexual risk behaviour, and both risks may be addressed by NSP-associated services, the overall impact of interventions is less than suggested by summing the separate estimates. As a consequence, the cost-effectiveness of syringe exchange as an isolated harm reduction instrument is difficult to measure, but may be less positive than current studies have shown.

On the other hand, some methodological choices may result in an underestimation of the cost-effectiveness of NSPs.

• The majority of the studies reviewed only consider the effects of NSPs on HIV prevention, while the effects of transmission of the hepatitis B and C viruses are largely ignored. The combined effect of an NSP on all viruses' transmission should be larger than the effect of the NSP on HIV transmission alone, thereby underestimating the effectiveness and cost-effectiveness of the NSP.

• The effects of secondary exchange of clean needles from NSP visitors to IDUs who do not directly access the NSP themselves have not been assessed in any of the studies under review. Likewise, only one study incorporated the effect of interventions on reducing secondary transmission of HIV to sex partners (Pinkerton et al., 2000). Lurie and Drucker (1997) have estimated that 100 primary HIV infections among IDUs result in 13 secondary infections among IDUs' partners and children. Hence, the effects of NSPs on infectious disease transmission may be more profound than shown in the studies so far if secondary effects were to be taken into account, with subsequent positive results for the cost-effectiveness ratio.

• Most of the studies quote effectiveness data (i.e. HIV incidence rates) based on observations of cohorts of IDUs over a certain timespan. Those IDUs who are successfully referred to addiction treatment disappear from follow-up, with subsequent underestimation of the effectiveness (and cost-effectiveness) of the programme.

- The savings that were incorporated into most of the studies only relate to the direct healthcare costs of treating HIV/AIDS. Incorporation of potential savings into averted productivity losses could have further improved the cost-effectiveness of programmes (i.e. could have augmented the future savings level).

- Although the studies assess the cost-effectiveness of NSPs with regard to their primary purpose, the prevention of blood-borne viral infections, the cost-effectiveness may be improved if the effect of gaining access to a hidden population with multiple health concerns is taken into account. Without the NSP, major parts of this population would not be reached by regular health and social services.

It is difficult to predict what the overall influence of the combined over- and underestimation described above will be. A further problem in the interpretation of study results is that the majority of programmes evaluated have a highly local character. NSPs vary in the amount of ancillary services they offer, hampering the transfer of study conclusions to other sites, within the same country or across countries. Indeed, the study of Pinkerton et al. (2000) showed substantial variability in the effectiveness of interventions across study sites, with the cost-effectiveness ratio from one site being almost 20 times as high as the ratio from another site.

There is increasing evidence that sterile needles and syringes are not sufficient as harm reduction tools, especially in the case of prevention of hepatitis C, which is much more infectious than HIV or hepatitis B (Hankins, 1998; Caflisch et al., 1999). HCV has the capacity to survive for a long time. IDUs may use sterile needles and syringes, but still share other equipment, such as cookers, spoons and filters. This other equipment is found to have high presence of the HCV (van Beek et al., 1998; Crofts et al., 2000). One theoretical modelling study that concentrated on the cost-effectiveness of NSPs as a tool to prevent hepatitis C concluded that NSPs are relatively ineffective and thus not cost-effective for this purpose (Pollack, 2001). The costs per case and mortality rate of HCV also affect the relative cost-effectiveness of NSPs for HCV prevention. In general, the costs per case and mortality rate of HCV are lower than for HIV, leading to less monetary and health benefits when compared to HIV prevention. Hence, despite the apparent effectiveness in reducing the spread of HCV, NSPs for HCV are not necessarily a cost-effective intervention.

All articles reviewed in this chapter use a short-term incidence analysis. Pollack has shown that this may overestimate the benefits of programmes in high prevalence (> 60 %) populations, simply because the majority of the target population has already acquired the infection. This is also the case with HCV, because, due to its high infectivity, most IDUs acquire HCV infection shortly after the onset of injecting drug use; by the time of first contact between the IDU and the NSP, HCV infection has already occurred. In the IDU population still free from HCV at entrance to an NSP, infection may be delayed for some time, but within the average duration of injecting drug use (assumed to be 11 years in Pollack's paper), almost every IDU will be infected. So, it is presumable that NSPs are not cost-effective in a real-world setting with respect to HCV prevention alone (Pollack, 2001). The articles reviewed in this chapter all focus on a short time-horizon, and therefore do not take these effects into account.

The omission of the above-discussed effects by short-term incidence analyses makes it difficult to draw firm conclusions with respect to the cost-effectiveness of NSPs for HCV prevention. We therefore recommend that formal transmission models for HCV be developed that account for realistic levels of prevalence and incidence as currently observed in epidemiological studies.

The economic evaluations identified in general show NSPs to be cost-effective or even cost saving in HIV prevention. Future cost-effectiveness analyses should be employed to determine how to prevent the most infections with limited funding. This encompasses the simultaneous study of a whole array of (combined) interventions targeted at HIV prevention with budget allocation models, as was attempted in the study of Zaric and Brandeau (2001). Most likely, the most cost-effective prevention strategy uses a combination of preventive interventions.

References

Anderson, R. M., May, R. M. (1991), *Infectious diseases of humans: dynamics and control*, Oxford University Press, New York.

Bastos, F. I., Strathdee, S. A. (2000), 'Evaluating effectiveness of syringe exchange programmes: current issues and future prospects', *Social Science and Medicine* 51: 1771–82.

Burrows, D. (2000), 'Starting and managing needle and syringe programs: a guide for central and eastern Europe and the independent States of the former Soviet Union', International Harm Reduction Development, New York (available at: http://www.harm-reduction.org/ch1.htm).

Caflisch, C., Wang, J., Zbinden, R. (1999), 'The role of syringe filters in harm reduction among injection drug users', *American Journal of Public Health* 89: 1252–4.

Centers for Disease Control and Prevention (CDCP) (1998), 'Recommendations for prevention and control of hepatitis C (HCV) infection and HCV-related chronic diseases', *MMWR* 47 (RR19).

Commonwealth Department of Health and Ageing (2002), *Return on investment in needle and syringe programs in Australia — Report*, Commonwealth of Australia (available at: http://www.health.gov.au/pubhlth/publicat/document/roireport.pdf).

Coutinho, R. (1995), 'Annotation: needle exchange programs — do they work?', *American Journal of Public Health* 85: 1490–1.

Coutinho, R. (1998), 'HIV and hepatitis C among injecting drug users. Success in preventing HIV has not been mirrored for hepatitis C', *British Medical Journal* 317: 424–5.

Crofts, N., Caruana, S., Bowden, S., Kerger, M (2000), 'Minimising harm from hepatitis C virus needs better strategies', *British Medical Journal* 321: 899.

Drummond, M. F., O'Brien, B. J., Stoddart, G. L., Torrance, G. W. (1997), *Methods for the economic evaluation of health care programmes*, Oxford University Press, Oxford.

Ferrini, R. (2000), 'American College of Preventive Medicine public policy on needle-exchange programs to reduce drug-associated morbidity and mortality', *American Journal of Preventive Medicine* 18: 173–5.

Gold, M., Gafni, A., Nelligan, P., Millson, P. (1997), 'Needle exchange programs: an economic evaluation of a local experience', *Canadian Medical Association Journal* 157: 255–62.

Goldberg, D., Burns, S., Taylor, A., Cameron, S., Hargreaves, D., Hutchinson, S. (2001), 'Trends in HCV prevalence among injecting drug users in Glasgow and Edinburgh during the era of needle/syringe exchange', *Scandinavian Journal of Infectious Diseases* 33: 457–61.

Hagan, H., McGough, J. P., Thiede, H., Weiss, N. S., Hopkins, S., Alexander, E. R. (1999), 'Syringe exchange and risk of infection with hepatitis B and C viruses', *American Journal of Epidemiology* 149: 203–13.

Hahn, J. A., Page-Shager, K., Lum, P. J., Ochoa, K., Moss, A. R. (2001), 'Hepatitis C virus infection and needle exchange use among young injection drug users in San Francisco', *Hepatology* 34: 180–7.

Hankins, C. (1998), 'Syringe exchange in Canada: good but not enough to stem the HIV tide', *Substance Use and Misuse* 33: 1129–46.

Holtgrave, D. R., Pinkerton, S. D., Jones, T. S., Lurie, P., Vlahov, D. (1998), 'Cost and cost-effectiveness of increasing access to sterile syringes and needles as an HIV prevention intervention in the United States', *Journal of Acquired Immune Deficiency Syndromes and Human Retrovirology* 18 (Suppl. 1): S133–8.

Hurley, S. F., Jolley, D. J., Kaldor, J. M. (1997), 'Effectiveness of needle-exchange programmes for prevention of HIV infection', *The Lancet* 349: 1797–800.

Jacobs, P., Calder, P., Taylor, M., Houston, S., Saunders, L. D., Albert, T. (1999), 'Cost-effectiveness of Streetworks' needle exchange program of Edmonton', *Canadian Journal of Public Health*: 168–71.

Kaplan, E. H. (1995), 'Economic analysis of needle exchange', *AIDS* 9: 1113–9.

Laufer, F. N. (2001), 'Cost-effectiveness of syringe exchange as an HIV prevention strategy', *Journal of Acquired Immune Deficiency Syndromes* 28: 273–8.

Lurie, P., Drucker, E. (1997), 'An opportunity lost: HIV infections associated with lack of a national needle-exchange programme in the USA', *The Lancet* 349: 604–8.

Lurie, P., Gorsky, R., Jones, T. S., Shomphe, L. (1998), 'An economic analysis of needle exchange and pharmacy-based programs to increase sterile syringe availability for injection drug users', *Journal of Acquired Immune Deficiency Syndromes and Human Retrovirology* 18 (Suppl. 1): S126–32.

McDonald, M. A., Wodak, A. D., Dolan, K. A., van Beek, I., Cunningham, P. H., Kaldor, J. M., for the Collaboration of Australian NSPs (2000), 'Hepatitis C virus antibody prevalence among injecting drug users at selected needle and syringe programs in Australia, 1995–1997', *Medical Journal of Australia* 172: 57–61.

Pinkerton, S. D., Holtgrave, D. R., DiFranceisco, W., Semaan, S., Coyle, S. L., Johnson-Masotti, A. P. (2000), 'Cost-threshold analysis of the national AIDS demonstration research HIV prevention interventions', *AIDS* 14: 1257–68.

Pollack, H. A. (2001), 'Cost-effectiveness of harm reduction in preventing hepatitis C among injection drug users', *Medical Decision Making* 21: 357–67.

Reitemeijer, C. A., Davidson, A. J., Foster, C. T., Cohn, D. L. (1993), 'Cost of care for patients with human immunodeficiency virus infection', *Archives of Internal Medicine* 153: 219–25.

Taylor, A., Goldberg, D., Hutchinson, S., Cameron, S., Gore, S. M., McMenamin, J., Green, S., Pithie, A., Fox, R. (2000), 'Prevalence of hepatitis C virus infection among injecting drug users in Glasgow 1990–1996: are current harm reduction strategies working?', *Journal of Infection* 40: 176–83.

van Beek, I., Dwyer, R., Dore, G. J., Luo, K., Kaldor, J. M. (1998), 'Infection with HIV and hepatitis C virus among injecting drug users in a prevention setting: retrospective cohort study', *British Medical Journal* 317: 433–7.

Vlahov, D., Junge, B. (1998), 'The role of needle exchange programs in HIV prevention', *Public Health Reports* 113 (Suppl. 1): 75–80.

Zaric, G. S., Brandeau, M. L. (2001), 'Optimal investment in a portfolio of HIV prevention programs', *Medical Decision Making* 21: 391–408.

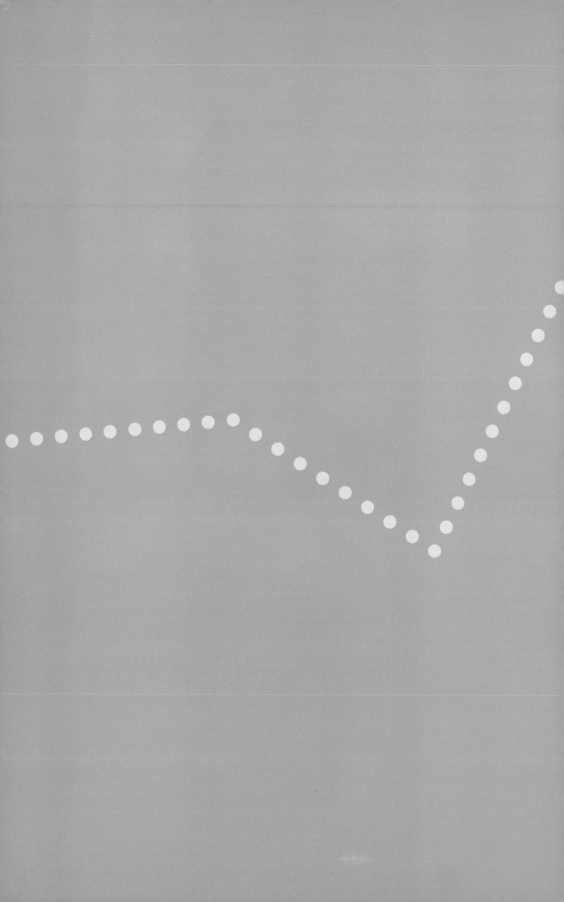

Chapter 15
The impact and cost-effectiveness of methadone maintenance treatment in preventing HIV and hepatitis C

Harold Pollack and Robert Heimer

Many studies indicate that MMT for illicit drug users can reduce long-term medical expenditures, antisocial behaviour, and post-treatment drug use. As blood-borne pathogens such as HIV and HCV become prevalent among IDUs, the ability of substance abuse treatment to reduce infectious disease spread becomes an important public health question. The cost-effectiveness of substance abuse treatment in achieving this goal is also a pertinent concern, given the variety of diverse interventions designed to slow the spread of infectious disease. This chapter contains a simplified but pertinent epidemiological model designed to address both these questions. Our analysis allows us to compare the cost-effectiveness of methadone outpatient treatment with that of other, widely accepted, public health interventions. We explore the cost per averted infection of a representative methadone outpatient treatment regime in preventing HIV and HCV among IDUs.

In the area of HIV prevention, analytical models are made necessary by the scarcity of epidemiological data which demonstrate the impact of MMT on incident HIV infections (Moss et al., 1994; Broers et al., 1998; Metzger et al., 1998; Moss and Hahn, 1999). Such models help health officials and planners to identify the key parameters associated with infectious disease transmission.

Analytical models are particularly necessary in the area of HCV prevention. In 1995, a consortium of experts presented evidence from five cities which demonstrated that early and substantial interventions in response to the HIV epidemic could maintain low seroprevalence among IDUs (Des Jarlais et al., 1995). However, the available data indicate that the epidemic spread of HCV was not slowed by these preventive interventions. After interventions in Sydney, Australia, Lund, Sweden, and Seattle, US, HCV incidence among IDUs exceeded 20 % per person-year (Mansson et al., 2000; Hagan et al., 2001; van Beek et al., 1998). Mathematical models such as that described in this chapter help to indicate if and when expanded provision of MMT can be expected to effectively and economically reduce HCV transmission.

Background and significance

Interventions designed to control the spread of blood-borne disease among IDUs include primary prevention to deter initiation into drug use, harm reduction interventions designed to make drug use less dangerous, and substance abuse treatment. The last strategy, substance abuse treatment, seeks, ideally, to achieve complete cessation of injecting drug use. Unfortunately, data from many treatment settings indicate that most clients fall short of this aspiration, and that the majority relapse into continued drug use. Many US studies have found that 80 % or more of current MMT clients relapse (Ball and Ross, 1991). Within the EU, data from Germany indicate that 20 to 30 % of MMT clients achieve complete abstinence after treatment intervention (Farrell, 1995). Results from the Amsterdam cohort study are more favourable, but still indicate that the substantial majority of MMT clients resume injecting drug use (Langendam et al., 2000).

Although complete cessation is not typically achieved, many drug treatment clients reduce their frequency of drug use, and may eventually (perhaps with repeated treatment interventions) halt their injecting drug use. Many studies have examined the impact of drug treatment on the well-being and social performance of IDUs. Best-practice MMT has been shown to significantly reduce opiate use (McGlothin and Anglin, 1981; Kosten et al., 1986; Anglin and Fisher, 1987; Hubbard,1989; Gerstein and Harwood, 1990; Hser et al., 1990–91; Ball and Ross, 1991; Kleiman, 1993; Rydell, Caulkins and Everingham, 1996; Egertson et al., 1997). Even if relapse eventually occurs, methadone is associated with significant periods of halted or reduced drug use. In-treatment IDUs often relapse or attend a sequence and variety of treatment interventions over a drug using career.

Drug treatment may also slow infectious disease spread by including harm reduction elements, such as warnings against syringe sharing and instruction on the proper use of bleach, that reduce the risks of drug use. Treatment clients are less likely than out-of-treatment IDUs to share needles and to practise other high-risk behaviours (Ball et al., 1988). Treatment clients inject drugs less frequently, thereby reducing accompanying risk. An important study by Metzger and colleagues found a sixfold difference in HIV seroconversion rates between steady methadone clients and an out-of-treatment group (Metzger et al., 1993). Results from the Amsterdam cohort study also support the efficacy of MMT in reducing HIV risk (Langendam et al., 2000).

Research on HCV transmission is less extensive. As described elsewhere in this monograph, HCV is spread through the sharing of infected syringes, and perhaps through other items used in drug preparation and injection such as cookers and filters (Battjes et al., 1995; McCoy et al., 1998). HCV is more efficiently transmitted than HIV (Short and Bell, 1993; Alter and Moyer, 1998). Studies of hospital needle-stick accidents suggest that more than 3 % of hospital workers exposed to HCV subsequently contracted the virus (Short and Bell, 1993; MacDonald et al., 1996; Alter and Moyer, 1998). The comparable risk from HIV-infected needle-sticks is tenfold lower (Zaric et al., 2000a, b). Because HCV is so readily transmitted, treatment and prevention interventions appear far less successful in containing HCV than in containing HIV (Crofts et al., 1994, 1997; Alter and Moyer, 1998; CDC, 1998; Coutinho, 1998; Garfein et al., 1998; Mather and Crofts, 1999).

Many IDU populations with low HIV prevalence display epidemic prevalences of HCV (Garfein et al., 1998). A review of the published literature on HCV prevalence among European IDUs indicates marked diversity across countries, with prevalences between 65 and 85 % in most populations. Only 4 of the 40 studies examined indicated an HCV prevalence below 50 %. Some studies suggest that prevalences in younger injectors, in some locations after the commencement of harm reduction programmes, and in England, have remained low (Broers et al., 1998; Taylor et al., 2000; Goldberg et al., 2001; Hope et al., 2001). However, other studies are less sanguine (van Ameijden et al., 1993; Mansson et al., 2000). These reports suggest that, for our analysis, we need to look at prevalences in the range of 40 to 90 %, focusing on prevalences between 75 and 80 % (Trepo and Pradat, 1999; Touzet et al., 2000).

Prevalence comparisons between in-treatment and out-of-treatment IDUs have yielded mixed results. Although out-of-treatment IDUs are often found to have lower HCV prevalence rates, this result is probably confounded by the older age of the treatment population. More limited data exist regarding HCV incidence, reflecting the greater difficulty in assembling and following cohorts when compared with simpler cross-sectional studies.

We have identified only four European studies that report HCV incidence rates among IDUs. These show a very wide range, between 4 and 29 % per year (van den Hoek et al., 1990; Rezza et al., 1996; Broers et al., 1998; Mansson et al., 2000). The higher rates reported in these studies are consistent with what has been seen outside Europe in communities which have instituted NSPs and other harm reduction services (Selvey et al., 1997; Brunton et al., 2000).

Existing research is particularly clear in identifying the sharp contrast between HIV and HCV prevalence among IDUs generally, and in particular among MMT clients. HCV prevalence exceeds 60 % in most populations, even those in which HIV prevalence is quite low (Crofts et al., 1994, 1997; Selvey et al., 1997). Within the EU, the review conducted by Farrell and colleagues suggests a similar contrast within many countries where HIV and HCV prevalence is reported (Farrell, 1995). Early 1990s data from Antwerp, Belgium, indicate that less than 4 % of IDUs were reported to be HIV positive, but 56 % tested positive for HCV. In Ireland, only 8 % of new treatment clients were estimated to be HIV positive, while 84 % of IDUs tested seropositive for HCV. In Glasgow, Scotland, HCV prevalence exceeded 70 % among IDUs, whereas HIV prevalence has never exceeded 5 % (Goldberg et al., 1998a, b; Taylor et al., 2000).

Epidemiological studies and analytical models of NSPs are consistent with these reports. Using data from Seattle, Washington, Hagan and collaborators found no protective benefits of NSPs against HCV (Hagan et al., 1999). Pollack similarly found little impact and poor cost-effectiveness for typical NSPs in HCV prevention (Pollack, 2001a, b). Moreover, policy analysis based on the short-term impact of syringe exchange would greatly overstate long-term programme effectiveness in reducing highly infectious agents.

The effectiveness and cost-effectiveness of MMT complementary services remain unclear. Kraft and colleagues examined the cost-effectiveness of such approaches (Kraft et al., 1997). They reported median costs per abstinent client-year of USD 11 887 for methadone treatment with minimal services, USD 7 932 for methadone plus intensive psychological counselling, and USD 9 471 for an enhanced service model. Although the enhanced service model produced slightly greater abstinence, this did not justify the additional cost.

More recently, Avants and collaborators examined the cost-effectiveness of intensive day treatment for unemployed, inner-city methadone patients (Avants et al., 1999). Both modalities of care appeared to improve patient well-being. Although intensive day treatment cost USD 55 per day (compared with USD 18 for enhanced standard care), it appeared to produce little improvement in drug abstinence initiation and maintenance, or in HIV risk behaviours.

These authors indicated that their results were consistent with other large-scale studies, which also failed to identify improved outcomes associated with intensive interventions. Such poor results may reflect poor matching of specific clients with treatment modalities or patient dissatisfaction with intensive services among first-time MMT patients.

Epidemiological model

Although analytical models have been used to analyse NSPs (Kaplan, 1995; Kaplan and Heimer, 1994; Kahn, 1996), models of substance abuse treatment have been less extensively explored. Zaric and collaborators have published two explicit cost-utility analyses of MMT for HIV prevention (Zaric et al., 2000a, b). Pollack (2002) examined the cost per averted HIV infection associated with MMT, finding a cost per averted infection of USD 100 000 to USD 300 000. These papers documented that MMT is highly cost-effective when compared with lifetime HIV treatment costs or the costs of other interventions that policy-makers value to extend life and improve health. None of these papers considered HCV.

By necessity, models are based on a highly simplified depiction of both injecting drug use and treatment interventions. Individuals vary in the manner, frequency, and social context of their injecting drug use. Because injecting is a covert behaviour, patterns of HIV/HCV risks are imperfectly known. Transmission through needle sharing may depend upon viral load and other complex characteristics of infected and uninfected persons. MMT itself is not a uniform product delivered to uniform consumers; its content and quality vary greatly.

Our analysis of the impact of MMT uses a relatively simple epidemiological model. In particular, we use a standard, random-mixing model of infectious disease transmission to explore the impact and cost-effectiveness of methadone treatment (Anderson and May, 1991). This approach necessarily excludes some important factors in disease spread. However, simplification has its merits. First, it illuminates basic trade-offs that confront policy-makers, and it helps to identify critical parameters that determine likely policy success. Second, by explicitly computing costs per averted infection for both HIV and HCV, this model provides a simplified, but useful yardstick to compare MMT with other prevention efforts.

We consider a self-contained population of some number (N) of active IDUs. New (uninfected) drug users enter the population at a constant rate of θ per day. Drug users leave the population at random at some constant rate of δ per person per day. This implies that the average duration of an individual's drug use 'career' is $1/\delta$. The parameter δ is assumed to be independent of disease status and independent of one's previous experience as a drug user. Mean drug careers vary across places and populations. Averaging estimates from Kaplan's 'needles that kill' analysis and those reported from among Baltimore's 'Alive' cohort yields $\delta = 1/(3\,994\ \text{days})$ (Kaplan et al., 1989; Vlahov et al., 1995).

These duration data reflect the observation of IDUs within the US. Analyses for specific communities within the EU require empirically grounded parameters that match specific local patterns of drug use. The values used here are extremely close to the 10.5-year average duration of heroin use reported in recent Swiss research (Steffen et al., 2001).

To simplify a complex pattern, we collapse all injecting equipment into a single entity — syringes — and assume that all IDUs share syringes. It is easy to modify the model to allow for some fraction of drug users who do not place themselves at risk. This complicates the algebra but does not alter the essential conclusions. A more realistic model would allow more varied behaviours from extremely low-risk to extremely high-risk behaviour (Battjes et al., 1995).

We suggest that drug users freely share syringes at shooting galleries and similar venues that promote random mixing. Even when not sharing syringes directly, IDUs often share cookers and filters, use water sources contaminated by syringe mixing, use previously used syringes to introduce water for dissolving the drug, or apportion drug solutions with previously used syringes. All these practices may have the same result as syringe sharing (Koester et al., 1990, 1996; Grund et al., 1991; Jose et al., 1993; Shah et al., 1996; Stark et al., 1996; Hagan et al., 2001). These circumstances promote rapid disease spread as susceptible IDUs encounter contaminated, potentially infectious, injecting paraphernalia in many forms.

From a sociological perspective, other approaches such as social network models may provide a more realistic framework, particularly in low-prevalence populations (Kretzschmar and Wiessing, 1998). Although random mixing is a worst-case assumption, mathematical models indicate that it provides a good approximation to non-random models for highly infectious diseases, given some overlap across disparate sharing networks (Kaplan et al., 1989; Kaplan and Lee, 1990; Watts, 1999).

Drug users are assumed to frequent these locations with a constant arrival rate of λ per unit time. Following earlier research, we assume that IDUs share syringes once per week (Kaplan et al., 1989; Kaplan and Heimer, 1992). Although recent data suggest that IDUs in some locales now share less frequently, individuals may under-report the extent of sharing (Des Jarlais et al., 1999). Infectious disease transmission can occur when an uninfected person shares a syringe first used by someone carrying a virus. When such sharing occurs, we assume a constant probability of κ that the virus is actually transmitted. Rather than pick a specific point estimate, we examine a range of values from a low of $\kappa = 0.5\ \%$ to a high value of $\kappa = 7.5\ \%$. The low value corresponds to published analyses of HIV transmission, while the high value is extrapolated from data from needle-stick accidents involving healthcare workers (Alter and Moyer, 1998; CDC, 1998; Zaric et al., 2000a).

At any given time t, there are $N(t)$ active IDUs, including some $I(t)$ infected individuals. The proportion of infected individuals is then the ratio $\pi(t) = I(t)/N(t)$.

A random-mixing model can be extended to overlapping subgroups in which an individual routinely shares syringes within his or her subgroup, with only occasional contact with members of other groups. This model is most appropriate for drug cultures with widespread sharing (Battjes et al., 1995). More elaborate contact patterns and social networks can also be modelled using graph-theoretic approaches (Des Jarlais and Friedman, 1990; Kretzschmar and Wiessing, 1998).

Table 1 summarises the relevant parameters and simulation values.

Table 1: Model parameters and baseline values

Parameter	Definition	Baseline value
$N(t)$	IDU population	(see text)
$I(t)$	Number infected	(see text)
$\pi(t)$	HIV or HCV prevalence	(see text)
θ	Arrival rate into IDU population	0.5/day
λ	Rate of needle sharing among IDUs	1/week
κ	Infectivity	0.005 to 0.075
δ	Exit rate from active IDU population	1 per 4 000 days
Treatment parameters		
M	Number of treatment slots	(see text)
c	Treatment cost/day	USD 14.00
β	Reduction in injection rate during treatment	75 %
μ	Exit rate from treatment	1 per 400 days
$V(M)$	Present discounted value of infections given M slots	(see text)

The impact of methadone treatment

This section develops a simple model that incorporates methadone treatment. Treatment programmes vary greatly in content, quality, and client population. Moreover, drug treatment influences drug behaviour in many ways. Drug treatment leads individuals to exit the population of active drug users. Even if a methadone client eventually relapses into injecting drug use, he or she may reduce the frequency or the risk associated with his or her drug use. Treatment may link clients with important social and medical services that influence infection risk, drug use, and general well-being (D'Aunno et al., 1999). This is especially true for treatment programmes which follow harm reduction principles in teaching clients about the dangers of needle sharing, and provide instruction in the proper cleaning of injecting equipment (IOM, 2000). Treatment may also encourage condom use, though programmes report mixed success in influencing sexual risks.

This model abstracts from a complex reality by presuming that MMT induces a constant exit rate from the drug using population of μ per person per unit time, over and above the 'natural' exit rate of δ from the drug using population.

Methadone treatment also has a secondary effect, by reducing the rate of hazardous syringe sharing among clients who would otherwise use illicit drugs. Instead of sharing syringes at a rate of λ times per week, MMT clients share at the rate of $\lambda(1 - \beta)$. Complete adherence corresponds to a value of $\beta = 1.0$.

The analysis ignores the complex matching process that links individuals with different forms of substance abuse treatment. This is a good approximation in locations where MMT is the major form of drug treatment. Matching is more important in settings in which MMT is extremely scarce, or where many IDUs receive less effective forms of therapy such as short-term detoxification therapy alone. It is assumed that some number, M, of MMT treatment 'slots' are provided, and that drug users are randomly assigned to these slots regardless of disease status. Clients do not self-select and are not carefully sorted into the treatment population.

We assume that disease prevalence among treatment participants mirrors prevalence within the entire drug using population. This assumption may understate the value of MMT in reducing disease spread. MMT clients tend to be older than other IDUs, and hence may have a higher prevalence of blood-borne disease.

Each treatment slot costs USD c per person per day in pharmaceutical costs, labour, and other expenses. Treatment slots are always in use. This assumption of excess demand matches conditions in many US and European cities, in which long waiting lists exist.

Treatment services are embedded in the epidemiological model developed above. This simplified model captures important qualitative features of infectious disease spread, and allows approximate calculation of the cost-effectiveness of drug services, linking a plausible simplified treatment model with the underlying epidemiology of HIV.

On any given day, $N(t) - I(t) = N(t)[1 - \pi(t)]$ uninfected drug users remain susceptible to infection. However, uninfected MMT clients who adhere to treatment do not share needles. Assuming that disease prevalence among methadone clients mirrors prevalence in the broader drug using population, and that treatment reduces syringe sharing by the proportion β, we must subtract $M\beta[1 - \pi(t)]$ from the population of those at risk, leaving $(N(t) - \beta M)[1 - \pi(t)]$ susceptible drug users who are actively at risk.

Each IDU shares at a rate of λ per day. Given random mixing, the probability that one shares a needle with an infected drug user is the same as the overall proportion of infected persons ($\pi(t)$) throughout the drug using population. When a susceptible person shares with an infected person, he or she has a probability, κ, of becoming infected.

Combining these terms, infectious disease incidence — the number of new infections per day — is

$$\iota(t) = \kappa\lambda\pi(t)\big[1 - \pi(t)\big]\big(N(t) - \beta M\big).$$

The epidemic spreads most rapidly when half of the population is infected. At this prevalence, the number of sharing pairs that involve one infected and one uninfected person is maximised.

In cost-effectiveness analysis, the important quantity is the number of averted infections associated with treatment intervention. However, the timing of infections also matters. An averted infection five years from now is less valuable than an averted infection today. Given the time value of money, future averted infections must be discounted by precisely the same factor as the funds expended to finance the intervention. Given M treatment slots and a discount rate, r, mathematically minded readers will recognise that the present discounted value of new infections is

$$V(M) = \int_0^\infty \iota(t)e^{-rt}dt = \int_0^\infty \kappa\lambda\pi(t)\big[1 - \pi(t)\big]\big(N(t) - \beta M\big)e^{-rt}dt.$$

In similar fashion, the present discounted cost of maintaining M treatment slots in perpetuity is USD Mc/r. If, considering treatment costs, the reduced lifespan and the reduced well-being of infected persons, one values an averted infection at some monetised level of USD S, the optimum policy is to choose the number of slots M that minimises $SV(M) - Mc/r$, the present monetary value of disease incidence minus the overall treatment cost.

Average costs per averted infection

In comparing MMT with other prevention efforts or other competing uses of public funds, it is especially illuminating to calculate the average cost of MMT per averted infection. If there are no treatment slots, the present discounted value of new infections is some (larger) quantity $V(0)$. So the average cost per averted infection,

$$\frac{Mc}{r\big[V(0) - V(M)\big]},$$

can be determined for MMT in preventing HCV and HIV infections (Pollack, 2002). These analyses presume that MMT cannot be exclusively targeted at active syringe sharers.

Tables 2 and 3 show the sensitivity analyses that result from these models. These models demonstrate the value of treatment adherence β and treatment-related exits, μ, as a function of relapse rates from substance abuse treatment. One obvious implication of this model is that optimising MMT to improve treatment adherence and to reduce relapse can significantly reduce the costs of preventing infection.

In the case of HIV, costs per averted infection are USD 113 000 in the baseline specification of 75 % treatment adherence, 80 % relapse, and 30 % needle sharing. This estimate is far below reasonable valuations of the social and individual costs of HIV infection. Lifetime treatment costs provide a useful and commonly cited valuation of social costs. Holtgrave and Pinkerton (1997) estimate USD 195 000 for the present discounted lifetime treatment costs associated with

Relapse (%)	Treatment adherence		
	50 % (β = 0.5)	75% (β = 0.75)	100 % (β = 1.0)
30 % of MMT clients share needles			
90	USD 321 304	USD 278 720	USD 240 166
80	USD 140 655	USD 113 083	USD 103 634
70	USD 114 072	USD 104 695	USD 99 540
60	USD 107 140	USD 101 912	USD 98 419
20 % of MMT clients share needles			
90	USD 481 932	USD 418 062	USD 360 236
80	USD 210 983	USD 169 625	USD 155 458
70	USD 171 108	USD 157 042	USD 149 306
60	USD 160 710	USD 152 868	USD 147 630
10 % of MMT clients share needles			
90	USD 963 556	USD 836 151	USD 720 491
80	USD 421 966	USD 339 249	USD 310 917
70	USD 342 217	USD 314 085	USD 298 613
60	USD 321 421	USD 305 736	USD 295 260

Table 2: Average cost per averted HIV infection (60 % of IDUs in methadone treatment): κ = 0.01, varying rates of needle sharing and treatment adherence rates

HIV infection. It is therefore possible that MMT is cost saving within high-risk IDU populations because it successfully prevents new cases of HIV (Holtgrave and Pinkerton, 1997). Note that this method provides a lower-bound estimate of the value of HIV prevention. It does not include many pertinent social costs, and it does not consider the impact of infection on patient well-being. Most pertinent, Holtgrave and Pinkerton (1997) estimate that HIV infection is associated with a loss of 7.10 QALY. Across a wide range of public health interventions, interventions costing between USD 50 000 and USD 150 000 per QALY are widely regarded to be cost-effective by policy-makers and the public (Hirth et al., 2000). By this cost–utility standard, MMT appears highly cost-effective for virtually all of our specifications when compared with other public health interventions.

These results are especially notable because they presume highly imperfect treatment interventions in which 80 % of MMT clients eventually relapse into injecting drug use. These results also presume higher infectivity (κ = 0.01), and high associated HIV prevalence. Lower values of κ, such as those used by Zaric

Table 3: Average cost per averted hepatitis C infection (60 % of IDUs in methadone treatment): $\kappa = 0.03$, varying rates of needle sharing and treatment adherence rates

Relapse (%)	Treatment adherence		
	50 % ($\beta = 0.5$)	75% ($\beta = 0.75$)	100 % ($\beta = 1.0$)
30 % of MMT clients share needles			
90	USD 724 851	USD 580 067	USD 450 781
80	USD 314 433	USD 180 162	USD 81 548
70	USD 210 434	USD 118 877	USD 76 188
60	USD 163 421	USD 95 055	USD 75 809
20 % of MMT clients share needles			
90	USD 1 087 180	USD 870 020	USD 676 163
80	USD 471 641	USD 270 239	USD 122 321
70	USD 315 647	USD 178 314	USD 114 376
60	USD 245 130	USD 142 582	USD 113 697
10 % of MMT clients share needles			
90	USD 2 174 360	USD 1 740 102	USD 1 351 685
80	USD 943 270	USD 540 473	USD 244 641
70	USD 631 283	USD 356 626	USD 228 733
60	USD 490 258	USD 285 163	USD 227 426

et al. (2000a, b), yield more favourable cost-effectiveness of the MMT intervention.

Results are more discouraging for the prevention of HCV infection. Given the suggested sharing rate of once per week, MMT is estimated to have a small impact on both incidence and prevalence. In most specifications, costs per averted HCV infection were substantially higher than those corresponding to HIV. When the present discounted value of lifetime treatment costs for HCV is far below that of HIV, it appears difficult to justify MMT based solely on its role in HCV prevention (Brown and Crofts, 1998; Wong et al., 1998).

Given imperfect adherence by MMT patients, plausible analytical models indicate that most IDUs will seroconvert to HCV even when the majority of IDUs are provided with MMT treatment. This is precisely the experience in Australia and in some European IDU populations where widespread MMT provision is part of a comprehensive effort to successfully contain HIV while having a small impact on HCV.

Steady-state calculations

The above analyses are based on differential equations and computer simulations, and are therefore difficult to interpret from an intuitive perspective. A long-run, or steady-state, analysis provides a useful approximation for the case of a highly infectious agent (Pollack, 2001a). The steady-state approach is only appropriate to a stable environment where an epidemic quickly approaches equilibrium incidence and prevalence. This analysis is quite useful for HCV, but is less applicable to HIV because of the slow convergence to steady-state prevalence.

In steady state, there will be N^* active drug users, with steady-state prevalence π^*. Every day, some θ uninfected individuals initiate drug use, while $(N^*\delta + M\mu)$ IDUs leave the population. In steady state, these flows balance each other, which happens at a population size

$$N^* = \frac{\theta - M\mu}{\delta}.$$

Therefore, one benefit of treatment is to reduce the overall population of active drug users.

In steady state, there are $N^*[1 - \pi^*]$ uninfected IDUs who may still become infected. However, some fraction, β, of uninfected MMT clients will abstain from use and not face infection risk. We assume that prevalence among treatment clients mirrors prevalence in the broader drug using population. We must therefore subtract $M\beta[1 - \pi^*]$ from the population of those at risk, leaving $(N^* - \beta M)[1 - \pi^*]$ susceptible IDUs who are actively at risk.

Over time, the rate of new infections will come to match the exit rate of infected individuals from the population of active IDUs. Without drug treatment there would be $N_0 = \theta/\delta$ active drug users. When steady-state prevalence is positive, one can show, using algebra, that

$$\pi^* = 1 - \frac{\delta}{\kappa\lambda}\left(\frac{N_0\delta}{N_0\delta - M[\mu + \beta\delta]}\right).$$

The steady-state prevalence is between 0 and 1.0. When the above expression is negative, π^* goes to zero. The quantity $(\delta/\kappa\lambda)$ is the reciprocal of the reproductive rate of infection, or R_0. Absent drug treatment, R_0, is the expected number of individuals who would be infected by a single infected drug user introduced into an entirely susceptible population.

The quantity $(N_0\delta)/[N_0\delta - M(\mu + \beta\delta)]$ reflects the reduction in disease prevalence attributable to treatment. The quantity $(\mu + \beta\delta)$ includes the effect of treatment to hasten exit from the drug using population (μ), and also the effect of treatment to reduce needle sharing while individuals are in treatment $(\beta\delta)$.

In similar fashion, when prevalence is positive, steady-state disease incidence is given by

$$\iota^*(M) = \theta\left[1 - \frac{1}{R_0}\left(\frac{N_0\delta}{N_0\delta - M[\mu + \beta\delta]}\right)\right].$$

Since treatment costs USD c per client per day, the total cost of drug treatment is USD Mc per day. At positive steady-state prevalence, average cost per averted infection is therefore [27]

$$AC = \frac{cM}{\iota^*(0) - \iota^*(M)} = \left(\frac{c}{\mu + \beta\delta}\right)R_0\left(1 - \frac{M[\mu + \beta\delta]}{N_0\delta}\right).$$

Sometimes, but not always, broad provision of MMT can drive steady-state prevalence to zero. Given low adherence, an epidemic can survive even when all IDUs are enrolled into MMT. Setting $M = N^*$, one can show that eradication is possible when $\mu > \delta[R_0(1 - \beta) - 1]$.

Simulation results

Using the values in Table 1, we then explore the implications of this model for steady-state cost-effectiveness. Figure 1 shows average costs per averted infection as a function of infectivity κ and the number of treatment slots M. In all cases, we assume that $\lambda = 1$/week, that drug treatment is 75 % effective ($\beta = 0.75$), and that $\delta = \mu = 1/4\,000$.

Average costs increase proportionally with κ. This implies that the impact and cost-effectiveness of MMT are sensitive to changes in infectivity, even at very high values of steady-state prevalence. Moreover, complementary interventions such as

[27] If steady-state prevalence goes to zero, the average cost per averted infection is given by
$AC = cMR_0 / [N_0\delta(R_0 - 1)]$.

Figure 1: Average cost per averted infection: steady-state analysis

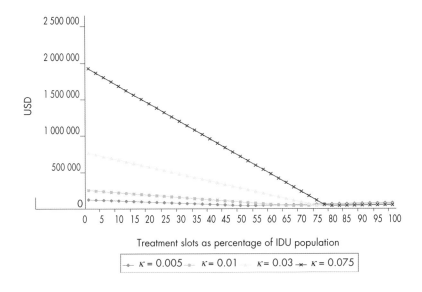

Treatment slots as percentage of IDU population

$\kappa = 0.005$ $\kappa = 0.01$ $\kappa = 0.03$ $\kappa = 0.075$

harm reduction for out-of-treatment IDUs produce important spillovers by reducing steady-state incidence and prevalence. These spillovers increase the benefits associated with MMT.

Note also the economies of scale associated with MMT. For the chosen parameters, broad provision of MMT assists clients, but it also reduces overall disease prevalence among all IDUs. Because MMT generates herd immunity, providing MMT to half the drug using population is far more cost effective than the provision of MMT to a small minority of active injectors. These scale economies are proportional to the reproductive rate of infection R_0, and are therefore especially pertinent to highly prevalent epidemics.

Because average costs per averted infection decline linearly with M, increasing coverage where it is already high — say moving from 50 % to 60 % coverage of the IDU population — may be more cost-effective than increasing coverage from 10 % to 20 % of a population with scarce access to drug treatment.

Discussion

This chapter reviewed the impact and cost-effectiveness of methadone treatment in preventing HIV and hepatitis C. Building upon simplified but informative epidemiological models, it draws five main conclusions:

- MMT appears to be highly cost-effective as a means of HIV prevention in high-risk populations. In our baseline specification, the costs of even highly imperfect MMT interventions compare favourably to the lifetime treatment costs associated with HIV infection. MMT appears especially cost-effective when one considers the reduced lifespan and well-being of HIV-infected individuals. If MMT brought no improvement in mental health and physical well-being, no reduced rates of criminal offending, and no improved social integration, MMT would remain highly cost-effective based solely upon its ability to reduce HIV infection (Gerstein and Harwood, 1990).

- Typical MMT programmes appear less effective (and therefore less cost-effective) in the control of hepatitis C. Because HCV is so efficiently transmitted, typical programmes have a smaller impact on HCV incidence than on reducing HIV. This result is predicted by epidemiological models, and it is consistent with practical observation within the EU and in other settings. Such results underscore the reality that treatment and harm reduction interventions proven effective in HIV prevention may be less effective against HCV.

- MMT treatment quality is more important to the success of HCV prevention than to the prevention of HIV. When an infectious agent such as HCV is efficiently transmitted, the impact and cost-effectiveness of MMT become especially sensitive to treatment quality. The rate of treatment-related exits and the proportion of treatment-adherent MMT clients both play critical roles in the impact and cost-effectiveness of MMT treatment.

These sensitivity analyses suggest reasons to hope that our discouraging main findings do not apply to some communities of IDUs. We assume high rates of relapse and non-adherence among MMT patients. Simulations indicate that MMT programmes with extremely low rates of relapse and non-adherence can have a strong effect on HCV spread.

We also assume random mixing among IDUs. This appears reasonable within high-prevalence communities of IDUs. This framework is especially suited to the US context in which paraphernalia laws and other law enforcement strategies encourage use of shooting galleries and other high-risk behaviours. Random mixing may be overly pessimistic in describing some EU settings that include effective harm reduction and public health interventions.

Perhaps for these reasons, some recent reports describe declining HCV incidence in Glasgow and other locations (e.g. Goldberg et al., 2001). Such findings may reflect more favourable environmental conditions than are assumed in the present chapter.

- MMT is most cost-effective when broadly applied to a large fraction of active IDUs. Because many current and former MMT clients share (or would share, if they were active injectors) syringes with other IDUs, broad coverage creates substantial benefits, even for active drug injectors who are not currently in treatment interventions. Treatment upon request — as advocated by the US Institute of Medicine (IOM, 2000), and as provided in many EU settings (Des Jarlais et al., 1995) — provides substantial protection against HIV and other blood-borne diseases. Inferences drawn from populations in which few IDUs are enrolled in drug treatment are likely to understate the potential impact of MMT in reducing the incidence and prevalence of blood-borne disease.

- Effective harm reduction interventions can increase the impact and cost-effectiveness of concomitant treatment interventions. Costs per averted infection of MMT are proportional to the reproductive rate of infection R_0. Interventions that reduce steady-state prevalence, for example those that encourage bleach provision or that shorten drug using careers, augment the cost-effectiveness of MMT. Prevention of highly infectious agents is a cooperative enterprise, in which each intervention is likely to be more effective when others are in place. Empirical studies support this contention (Des Jarlais et al., 1995; Watters, 1996; Watters et al., 1995). The converse also holds. Broad availability of MMT to slow the spread of blood-borne disease increases the cost-effectiveness of harm reduction interventions (Pollack, 2001a).

Harm reduction components of MMT, though the object of less extensive research, may further increase the cost-effectiveness of MMT. The current analysis does not consider components of MMT designed to reduce the risk that an infected client who relapses will go on to infect other IDUs. If current and former clients practise safer injecting behaviours even after they resume drug use, the experience of substance abuse treatment may prevent many future cases.

Although this chapter explores the cost-effectiveness of MMT, several important factors that influence treatment-effectiveness were not considered. Targeted treatment interventions for high-risk individuals may be especially important in controlling disease spread. Treatment strategies for homeless IDUs, and those with criminal justice involvement or psychiatric disorders are likely to prove especially important (Hammett et al., 1998; Magura et al., 1998; Thompson et al., 1998).

Measures to reduce polydrug use may also improve treatment cost-effectiveness. MMT has proved markedly less effective in reducing injecting and non-injecting cocaine use. There is some evidence that MMT may aggravate cocaine abuse among treatment clients (Preston et al., 1996). Indeed, methadone has been shown to increase the pleasure associated with cocaine use. Continued cocaine use is an important risk factor for HIV seroconversion among MMT clients, and is associated with increased frequency of continued heroin use (Hartel. et al., 1995; Preston et al., 1998).

Recent attention to prevention strategies among HIV-positive injectors suggests a second important opportunity to improve typical MMT interventions. The US Institute of Medicine notes that HIV-infected men and women are in a unique position to prevent further disease spread (IOM, 2000). Incorporating this insight within the daily realities of methadone treatment would greatly increase the impact and cost-effectiveness of treatment intervention.

References

Alter, M. J., Moyer, L. A. (1998), 'The importance of preventing hepatitis C virus infection among injection drug users in the United States', *Journal of Acquired Immune Deficiency Syndromes and Human Retrovirology* 18(S1): S6–S10.

Anderson, R. M., May, R. M. (1991), *Infectious diseases of humans*, Oxford University Press, Oxford.

Anglin, M. D., Fisher, D. G. (1987), 'Survival analysis in drug program evaluation. Part II. Partitioning treatment effects', *International Journal of Addictions* 22: 377–87.

Avants, S. K., Margolin, A., Sindelar, J. L., Rounsaville, B. J., Schottenfeld, R., Stine, S., Cooney, N. L., Rosenheck, R. A., Li, S. H., Kosten, T. R. (1999), 'Day treatment versus enhanced standard methadone services for opioid-dependent patients: a comparison of clinical efficacy and cost', *American Journal of Psychiatry* 156: 27–33.

Ball, J. C., Ross, A. (1991), *The effectiveness of methadone maintenance treatment: patients, programs, services, and outcome*, Springer-Verlag, New York.

Ball, J. C., Lange, W. R., Myers, C. P., Friedman, S. R. (1988), 'Reducing the risk of AIDS through methadone maintenance treatment', *Journal of Health and Social Behaviour* 29: 214–26.

Battjes, R. J., Pickens, R. W., Brown, L. S., Jr (1995), 'HIV infection and AIDS risk behaviours among injection drug users entering methadone treatment: an update', *Journal of Acquired Immune Deficiency Syndromes and Human Retrovirology* 10: 90–6.

Broers, B., Junet, C., Bourquin, M., Deglon, J. J., Perrin, L., Hirschel, B. (1998), 'Prevalence and incidence rate of HIV, hepatitis B and C among drug users on methadone maintenance treatment in Geneva between 1988 and 1995', *AIDS* 12: 2059–66.

Brown, K., Crofts, N. (1998), 'Health care costs of a continuing epidemic of hepatitis C virus infection among injecting drug users', *Australian and New Zealand Journal of Public Health* 22 (3 Suppl.): 384–8.

Brunton, C., Kemp, R., Raynel, P., Harte, D., Baker, M. (2000), 'Cumulative incidence of hepatitis C seroconversion in a cohort of seronegative injecting drug users', *New Zealand Medical Journal* 113: 98–101.

Center for Disease Control (CDC) (1998), 'Recommendations for prevention and control of hepatitis C virus (HCV) infection and HCV-related chronic disease', *Monthly Millbank Weekly Reviews* 47 (RR19).

Coutinho, R. (1998), 'HIV and hepatitis C among injecting drug users: success in preventing HIV has not been mirrored for hepatitis C', *British Medical Journal* 317: 424–5.

Crofts, N., Hopper, J. L., Milner, R., Breschkin, A. M., Bowden, D. S., Locarnini, S. A. (1994), 'Blood-borne virus infections among Australian injecting drug users: implications for spread of HIV', *European Journal of Epidemiology* 10: 687–94.

Crofts, N., Nigro, L., Oman, K., Stevenson, E., Sherman, J. (1997), 'Methadone maintenance and hepatitis C virus infection among injecting drug users', *Addiction* 92: 999–1005.

D'Aunno, T., Vaughn, T. E., McElroy, P. (1999), 'An institutional analysis of HIV prevention efforts by the nation's outpatient drug abuse treatment units', *Journal of Health and Social Behaviour* 40: 175–92.

Des Jarlais, D. C., Friedman, S. R. (1990), 'Shooting galleries and AIDS: infection probabilities and "tough" policies', *American Journal of Public Health* 80: 142–4.

Des Jarlais, D. C., Hagan, H., Friedman, S. R., Friedmann, P., Goldberg, D., Frischer, M., Green, S., Tunving, K., Ljungberg, B., Wodak, A. (1995), 'Maintaining low HIV prevalence in populations of injecting drug users', *Journal of the American Medical Association* 274: 1226–31.

Des Jarlais, D. C., Paone, D., Milliken, J., Turner, C. F., Miller, H., Gribble, J., Shi, Q., Hagan, H., Friedman, S. R. (1999), 'Audio-computer interviewing to measure risk behaviour for HIV among injecting drug users: a quasi-randomised trial', *The Lancet* 353: 1657–61.

Egertson, J. A., Fox, D. M., Leshner, A. I. (eds) (1997), *Treating drug abusers effectively*, Blackwell, Malden, MA.

Farrell, M. (ed.) (1995), *Drug prevention: a review of the legislation, regulation and delivery of methadone in 12 Member States of the European Union*, National Addiction Centre, London.

Garfein, R. S., Doherty, M. C., Monterroso, E. R., Thomas, D. L., Nelson, K. E., Vlahov, D. (1998), 'Prevalence and incidence of hepatitis C virus infection among young injection drug users', *Journal of Acquired Immune Deficiency Syndromes and Human Retrovirology* 18(S1): S11–S19.

Gerstein, D. R., Harwood, H. J. (1990), *Treating drug problems*, National Academy Press, Institute of Medicine, Washington, DC.

Goldberg, D., Allardice, G., McMenamin, J., Codere, G. (1998a), 'HIV in Scotland — the challenge ahead', *Scottish Medical Journal* 43: 168–72.

Goldberg, D., Cameron, S., McMenamin, J. (1998b), 'Hepatitis C virus antibody prevalence among injecting drug users in Glasgow has fallen but remains high', *Communicable Diseases of Public Health* 1: 95–7.

Goldberg, D., Burns, S., Taylor, A., Cameron, S., Hargreaves, D., Hutchinson, S. (2001), 'Trends in HCV prevalence among injecting drug users in Glasgow and Edinburgh during the era of needle/syringe exchange', *Scandinavian Journal of Infectious Diseases* 33: 457–61.

Grund, J. P., Kaplan, C. D., Adriaans, N. F., Blanken, P. (1991), 'Drug sharing and HIV transmission risks: the practice of frontloading in the Dutch injecting drug user population', *Journal of Psychoactive Drugs* 23: 1–10.

Hagan, H., McGough, J. P., Thiede, H., Weiss, N. S., Hopkins, S., Alexander, E. R. (1999), 'Syringe exchange and risk of infection from hepatitis B and C viruses', *American Journal of Epidemiology* 149: 203–13.

Hagan, H., Thiede, H., Weiss, N. S., Hopkins, S. G., Duchin, J. S., Alexander, E. R. (2001), 'Sharing of drug preparation equipment as a risk factor for hepatitis C', *American Journal of Public Health* 91: 42–6.

Hammett, T. M., Gaiter, J. L., Crawford, C. (1998), 'Reaching seriously at-risk populations: health interventions in criminal justice settings', *Health Education and Behaviour* 25: 99–120.

Hartel, D. M., Schoenbaum, E. E., Selwyn, P. A., Kline, J., Davenny, K., Klein, R. S., Friedland, G. H. (1995), 'Heroin use during methadone maintenance treatment: the importance of methadone dose and cocaine use', *American Journal of Public Health* 85: 83–8.

Hirth, R. A., Chernew, M. E., Miller, E., Fendrick, A. M., Weissert, W. G. (2000), 'Willingness to pay for a quality-adjusted life year: in search of a standard', *Medical Decision Making* 20: 332–42.

Holtgrave, D. R., Pinkerton, S. D. (1997), 'Updates of cost of illness and quality of life estimates for use in economic evaluations of HIV prevention programs', *Journal of Acquired Immune Deficiency Syndromes and Human Retrovirology* 16: 54–62.

Hope, V. D., Judd, A., Hickman, M., Lamagni, T., Hunter, G., Stimson, G. V., Jones, S., Donovan, L., Parry, J. V., Gill, O. N. (2001), 'Prevalence of hepatitis C among injection drug users in England and Wales: is harm reduction working?', *American Journal of Public Health* 91: 38–42.

Hser, Y. I., Anglin, M. D., Liu, Y. (1990–91), 'A survival analysis of gender and ethnic differences in responsiveness to methadone maintenance treatment', *International Journal of Addictions* 25(11A): 1295–315.

Hubbard, R. L. (1989), *Drug abuse treatment: a national study of effectiveness*, University of North Carolina Press, Chapel Hill, NC.

Institute of Medicine (IOM) (2000), *No time to lose: making the most of HIV prevention*, National Academy Press, Washington, DC.

Jose, B., Friedman, S. R., Neaigus, A., Curtis, R., Grund, J. P., Goldstein, M. F., Ward, T. P., Des Jarlais, D. C. (1993), 'Syringe-mediated drug-sharing (backloading): a new risk factor for HIV among injecting drug users', *AIDS* 7: 1653–60.

Kahn, J. G. (1996), 'The cost-effectiveness of HIV prevention targeting: how much more bang for the buck?', *American Journal of Public Health* 86: 1709–12.

Kaplan, E. H. (1995), 'Economic analysis of needle exchange', *AIDS* 9: 1113–9.

Kaplan, E. H., Heimer, R. (1992), 'A model-based estimate of HIV infectivity via needle sharing', *Journal of Acquired Immune Deficiency Syndromes and Human Retrovirology* 5: 1116–8.

Kaplan, E. H., Heimer, R. (1994), 'A circulation theory of needle exchange', *AIDS* 8: 567–74.

Kaplan, E. H., Lee, Y. S. (1990), 'How bad can it get? Bounding worst case endemic heterogeneous mixing models of HIV/AIDS', *Mathematical Biosciences* 99: 157–80.

Kaplan, E. H., Cramton, P. C., Paltiel, A. D. (1989), 'Non-random mixing models of HIV transmission', in Castillo-Chavez, C. (ed.), *Lecture notes in biomathematics*, Springer-Verlag, New York, 218–41.

Kleiman, M. (1993), *Against excess*, Basic Books, New York, NY.

Koester, S., Booth, R. E., Wiebel, W. (1990), 'The risk of HIV transmission from sharing water, drug mixing containers and cotton filters among intravenous drug users', *International Journal of Drug Policy* 1: 28–30.

Koester, S., Booth, R. E., Zhang, Y. (1996), 'The prevalence of additional injection-relation HIV risk behaviours among injection drug users', *Journal of Acquired Immune Deficiency Syndromes and Human Retrovirology* 12: 202–7.

Kosten, T. R., Rounsaville, B. J., Kleber, H. D. (1986), 'A 2.5 year follow-up of depression, life crises, and treatment effects on abstinence among opioid addicts', *Archives of General Psychiatry* 43: 733–8.

Kraft, M. K., Rothbard, A. B., Hadley, T. R, McLellan, A. T., Asch, D. A. (1997), 'Are supplementary services provided during methadone maintenance really cost-effective?', *American Journal of Psychiatry* 154: 1214–9.

Kretzschmar, M., Wiessing, L. G. (1998), 'Modelling the spread of HIV in social networks of injecting drug users', *AIDS* 12: 801–11.

Langendam, M. W., van Brussel, G. H., Coutinho, R. A., van Ameijden, E. J. (2000), 'Methadone maintenance and cessation of injecting drug use: results from the Amsterdam cohort study', *Addiction* 95: 591–600.

MacDonald, M. A., Crofts, N., Kaldor, J. (1996), 'Transmission of hepatitis C virus: rates, routes, and cofactors', *Epidemiologic Reviews* 18: 137–48.

Magura, S., Nwakeze, P. C., Demsky, S. Y. (1998), 'Pre- and in-treatment predictors of retention in methadone treatment using survival analysis', *Addiction* 93: 51–60.

Mansson, A. S., Moestrup, T., Nordenfelt, E., Widell, A. (2000), 'Continued transmission of hepatitis B and C viruses, but no transmission of human immunodeficiency virus among intravenous drug users participating in a syringe/needle exchange program', *Scandinavian Journal of Infectious Diseases* 32: 253–8.

Mather, D., Crofts, N. (1999), 'A computer model of the spread of hepatitis C virus among injecting drug users', *European Journal of Epidemiology* 15: 5–10.

McCoy, C. B., Metsch, L. R., Chitwood, D. D., Shapshak, P., Comerford, S. T. (1998), 'Parenteral transmission of HIV among injection drug users: assessing the frequency of multiperson use of needles, syringes, cookers, cotton, and water', *Journal of Acquired Immune Deficiency Syndromes and Human Retrovirology* 18(S1): S25–S29.

McGlothlin, W. H., Anglin, M. D. (1981), 'Shutting off methadone. Costs and benefits', *Archives of General Psychiatry* 38: 885–92.

Metzger, D. S., Woody, G. E., McLellan, A. T., O'Brien, C. P., Druley, P., Navaline, H., DePhilippis, D., Stolley, P., Abrutyn, E. (1993), 'Human immunodeficiency virus seroconversion among intravenous drug users in- and out-of-treatment: an 18-month prospective follow-up', *Journal of Acquired Immune Deficiency Syndromes and Human Retrovirology* 6: 1049–56.

Metzger, D. S., Navaline, H., Woody, G. E. (1998), 'Drug abuse treatment as AIDS prevention', *Public Health Reports* 113 (Suppl. 1): 97–106.

Moss, A. R., Hahn, J. A. (1999), 'Invited commentary: needle exchange — no help for hepatitis?', *American Journal of Epidemiology* 149: 214–6.

Moss, A. R., Vranizan, K., Gorter, R., Bacchetti, P., Watters, J., Osmond, D. (1994), 'HIV seroconversion in intravenous drug users in San Francisco, 1985–1990', *AIDS* 8: 223–31.

Pollack, H. A. (2001a), 'Cost-effectiveness of harm reduction in preventing hepatitis C among injection drug users', *Medical Decision Making* 21: 357–67.

Pollack, H. A. (2001b), 'Ignoring "downstream infection" in the evaluation of harm reduction interventions for injection drug users', *European Journal of Epidemiology* 17: 391–5.

Pollack, H. A. (2002), 'Methadone treatment as HIV prevention', in Kaplan, E., Brookmeyer, R. (eds), *Quantitative analysis of HIV prevention programs*, Yale University Press, New Haven.

Preston, K. L., Sullivan, J. T., Strain, E. C., Bigelow, G. E. (1996), 'Enhancement of cocaine's abuse liability in methadone maintenance patients', *Psychopharmacology* 123: 15–25.

Preston, K. L., Silverman, K., Higgins, S. T., Brooner, R. K., Montoya, I., Schuster, C. R., Cone, E. J. (1998), 'Cocaine use early in treatment predicts outcome in a behavioural treatment program', *Journal of Consultation Clinical Psychology* 66: 691–6.

Rezza, G., Sagliocca, L., Zaccarelli, M., Nespoli, M., Siconolfi, M., Baldassarre, C. (1996), 'Incidence rate and risk factors for HCV seroconversion among injecting drug users in an area with low HIV seroprevalence', *Scandinavian Journal of Infectious Diseases* 28: 27–9.

Rydell, C. P., Caulkins, J. P., Everingham, S. S. (1996), 'Enforcement or treatment? Modelling the relative efficacy of alternatives for controlling cocaine', *Operations Research* 44: 687–95.

Selvey, L. A., Denton, M., Plant, A. J. (1997), 'Incidence and prevalence of hepatitis C among clients of a Brisbane methadone clinic: factors influencing hepatitis C serostatus', *Australian and New Zealand Journal of Public Health* 21: 102–4.

Shah, S. M., Shapshak, P., Rivers, J. E., Stewart, R. V., Weatherby, N. L., Xin, K. Q., Page, J. B., Chitwood, D. D., Mash, D. C., Vlahov, D., McCoy, C. B. (1996), 'Detection of HIV-1 DNA in needle/syringes, paraphernalia, and washes from shooting galleries in Miami: a preliminary laboratory report', *Journal of Acquired Immune Deficiency Syndromes* 11: 301–6.

Short, L. J., Bell, D. M. (1993), 'Risk of occupational infection with blood-borne pathogens in operating and delivery room settings', *American Journal of Infection Control* 21: 343–50.

Stark, K., Muller, R., Bienzle, U., Guggenmoos-Holzmann, I. (1996), 'Frontloading: a risk factor for HIV and hepatitis C virus infection among injecting drug users in Berlin', *AIDS* 10: 311–7.

Steffen, T., Blattler, R., Gutzwiller, F., Zwahlen, M. (2001), 'HIV and hepatitis virus infections among injecting drug users in a medically controlled heroin prescription programme', *European Journal of Public Health* 11: 425–30.

Taylor, A., Goldberg, D., Hutchinson, S., Cameron, S., Gore, S. M., McMenamin, J., Green, S., Pithie, A., Fox, R. (2000), 'Prevalence of hepatitis C virus infection among injecting drug users in Glasgow 1990–1996: are current harm reduction strategies working?', *Journal of Infection* 40: 176–83.

Thompson, A. S., Blankenship, K. M., Selwyn, P. A., Khoshnood, K., Lopez, M., Balacos, K., Altice, F. L. (1998), 'Evaluation of an innovative program to address the health and social service needs of drug-using women with or at risk of HIV infection', *Journal of Community Health* 23: 419–40.

Touzet, S., Kraemer, L., Colin, C., Pradat, P., Lanoir, D., Bailly, F., Coppola, R. C., Sauleda, S., Thursz, M. R., Tillmann, H., Alberti, A., Braconier, J. H., Esteban, J. I., Hadziyannis, S. J., Manns, M. P., Saracco, G., Thomas, H. C., Trepo, C. (2000), 'Epidemiology of hepatitis C virus infection in seven European Union countries: a critical analysis of the literature. Hencore Group (Hepatitis C European Network for Cooperative Research)', *European Journal of Gasteroenterology and Hepatology* 12: 667–78.

Trepo, C., Pradat, P. (1999), 'Hepatitis C virus infection in western Europe', *Journal of Hepatology* 31(S1): 80–3.

van Ameijden, E. J., van den Hoek, J. A., Mientjes, G. H., Coutinho, R. A. (1993), 'A longitudinal study on the incidence and transmission patterns of HIV, HBV and HCV infection among drug users in Amsterdam', *European Journal of Epidemiology* 9: 255–62.

van Beek, I., Dwyer, R., Dore, G. J., Luo, K., Kaldor, J. M. (1998), 'Infection with HIV and hepatitis C virus among injecting drug users in a prevention setting: retrospective cohort study', *British Medical Journal* 317: 433–7.

van den Hoek, J. A., van Haastrecht, H. J., Goudsmit, J., de Wolf, F., Coutinho, R. A. (1990), 'Prevalence, incidence, and risk factors of hepatitis C virus infection among drug users in Amsterdam', *Journal of Infectious Diseases* 162: 823–6.

Vlahov, D., Khabbaz, R. F., Cohn, S., Galai, N., Taylor, E., Kaplan, J. E (1995), 'Incidence and risk factors for human T-lymphotropic virus type II seroconversion among injecting drug users in Baltimore, Maryland, USA', *Journal of Acquired Immune Deficiency Syndromes and Human Retrovirology* 9: 89–96.

Watters, J. K. (1996), 'Impact of HIV risk and infection and the role of prevention services', *Journal of Substance Abuse Treatments* 13: 375–85.

Watters, J. K., Bluthenthal, R. N., Kral, A. H. (1995), 'HIV seroprevalence in injection drug users', *Journal of the American Medical Association* 273: 1178.

Watts, D. (1999), *Small worlds: the dynamics of networks between order and randomness*, Princeton University Press, Princeton, NJ.

Wong, J. B., Bennett, W. G., Koff, R. S., Pauker S. G. (1998), 'Pretreatment evaluation of chronic hepatitis C: risks, benefits, and costs', *Journal of the American Medical Association* 280: 2088–93.

Zaric, G. S., Barnett, P. G., Brandeau, M. L. (2000a), 'HIV transmission and the cost-effectiveness of methadone maintenance', *American Journal of Public Health* 90: 1100–11.

Zaric, G. S., Brandeau, M. L., Barnett, P. G. (2000b), 'Methadone maintenance and HIV prevention: a cost-effectiveness analysis', *Management Science* 46: 1013–31.

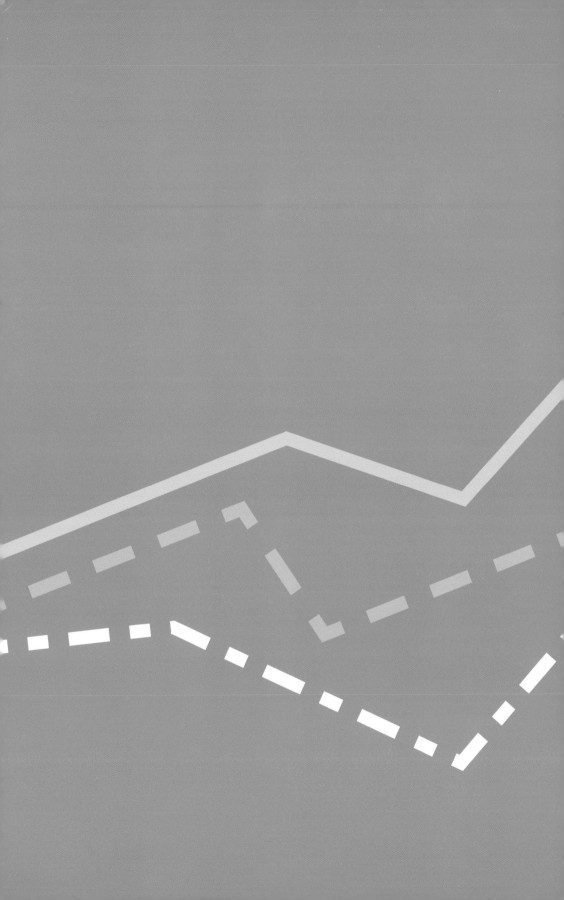

General conclusions

General conclusions

General conclusions

Lucas Wiessing, Wien Limburg and Johannes Jager

In this monograph, several themes emerge as important entries for intervention and policy around hepatitis C and injecting drug use. There are two broad areas for public health policy: prevention and treatment. Current options to specifically prevent hepatitis C infection among drug injectors are limited, and two main interventions for IDUs, methadone maintenance therapy and NSPs, are analysed. Treatment of HCV infection is examined in detail and with regard to IDUs, through both an overview of recent developments in diagnostics and antiviral therapy, and a cost-effectiveness analysis of antiviral therapy for IDUs with at least moderate liver disease. The recent debate on improving access of IDUs to HCV treatment is also pointed out. The monograph presents a comprehensive overview of the scientific literature regarding hepatitis C in IDUs as well as (in some cases, preliminary) results of original research. The main tools used for the original analyses are mathematical models and costs and cost-effectiveness estimation methods.

In these general conclusions, we first summarise each chapter with a focus on opportunities for intervention. In the final section, we list a set of main areas that might deserve specific attention with regard to current decision-making around HCV and injecting drug use. We do not strictly follow the order of the monograph, but start with the chapters that deal directly with the prevention and treatment of HCV in injectors, followed by the chapters on mathematical modelling, the economic evaluations of both HCV in injectors and (injecting) drug use.

Options for the prevention of hepatitis C infection in IDUs

Two main interventions are analysed in-depth in this monograph: MMT and NSPs.

Based on the literature, Pollack and Heimer (Chapter 15) state that MMT reduces injecting frequency and needle sharing among opiate injectors and may halt injecting drug use, depending on dose and treatment policy, while it is a cheap and cost-effective measure to prevent HIV infection. However, evidence suggests that it may not slow the spread of HCV. The original analyses presented by the authors are based on simple and transparent mathematical models and indeed suggest MMT is not cost-effective for HCV prevention, as the estimated costs per averted HCV infection are much higher than discounted lifetime HCV treatment costs. This is highly dependent on treatment quality, and the outcome might become positive if extremely high MMT coverage and therapy adherence rates and low relapse rates could be achieved. MMT was set up to curtail the spread of HIV/AIDS. As such, it proved highly effective as well as cost-effective. Any preventive effect it has on the spread of other infectious diseases like HCV is therefore an added bonus. The effect of MMT on the HCV epidemic among IDUs is probably small because most injectors are infected prior to MMT entry and even low levels of residual risk behaviour will soon lead to infection even if most IDUs are in MMT. Steady-state analyses suggest that, in the case of HCV, the coverage of the IDU population with MMT is crucial, and the effect of MMT increases strongly with high coverage due to herd immunity effects, also protecting those who are not in MMT. At high levels of coverage, different interventions will act in synergy and mutually reinforce one another's effects. Therefore, it remains critical to implement different prevention measures (including NSPs, HCV counselling and testing, and other drug treatment modalities) simultaneously and to attain high coverage with them all. Interestingly, these analyses also suggest that the impact and cost-effectiveness of MMT are highly sensitive to changes in infectivity, even at high values of prevalence. Changes in infectivity might be achieved by substantial uptake of HCV treatment resulting in strong reductions of viral load. Likewise, complete elimination of the virus through successful HCV treatment would reduce the average duration that infected IDUs spend in the population as a virus carrier, which is expected to have strong effects on HCV prevalence as well (see also Kretzschmar and Wiessing, Chapter 5).

A second main prevention tool analysed in this monograph is NSPs, which exchange or distribute clean needles and syringes to IDUs in order to reduce the use of contaminated materials. De Wit and Bos (Chapter 14) present a review of the literature regarding the cost-effectiveness of NSPs for both HIV and HCV prevention. While the effectiveness and cost-effectiveness of NSPs in reducing the spread of HIV seem beyond doubt, the effects for HCV are inconclusive and different studies report conflicting results. Regarding cost-effectiveness, their formal literature review identified only one study that covered both the costs and effects of NSPs for HCV prevention with a full economic evaluation, and they found only seven studies on HIV prevention. All seven studies concluded that NSPs are cost-effective in preventing HIV spread. With respect to the cost-effectiveness of NSPs for HCV prevention, the single full economic analysis that was found in the literature concluded that the introduction of NSPs reduced the incidence and prevalence of HCV (Commonwealth Department of Health and Ageing, 2002). This study concluded that NSPs, considering these effects on HCV and HIV, are a cost-effective intervention. However, De Wit and Bos report that a theoretical modelling study, not included in the review, concluded that NSPs are likely to be relatively ineffective in preventing HCV and would thus not be cost-effective for this purpose alone (Pollack, 2001), while different epidemiological studies also found conflicting evidence regarding the effects of NSPs on HCV incidence. The cost-effectiveness of NSPs for the prevention of HCV might further be hampered by the relatively low mortality rates and low lifetime costs per infection when compared with HIV. However, the combined cost-effectiveness of NSPs in reducing the transmission of HIV, hepatitis and other blood-borne viruses is beyond doubt. In addition to these effects on the transmission of infectious agents, NSPs can also play an important role as a main point of contact for IDUs who are not in contact with other services. They can be instrumental in referring IDUs to supplementary services, thereby greatly extending the coverage of the IDU population by those services. While these effects should enhance the health benefits (and cost-effectiveness) associated with NSPs, they were not considered in all of the studies reviewed. Future economic analyses may attempt to simultaneously analyse all relevant costs and effects and not be limited to one effect (e.g. HIV prevention) while disregarding other potentially important effects such as HCV prevention or referrals.

In a literature overview, Limburg (Chapter 1) states that prevention of HCV is difficult, as no vaccine exists. Screening has proven very successful in the case of blood and blood products. Screening of risk groups is indicated, especially for IDUs, but maybe also for non-IDUs and partners of HCV-positive persons. This may be done through health services in contact with IDUs, and through outreach programmes or special studies with street recruitment where testing is offered. Testing should always include counselling and education, and referral in the case of a positive test result. Ideally, IDUs should stop injecting and enter treatment; however, this is difficult to achieve. Substitution therapy is often more realistic and should include education to reduce risk behaviour, while peer education and counselling may be especially effective. Methadone substitution therapy is important and has become widely available in the EU. If provided in the right dosage, methadone substitution reduces injecting and needle sharing and the longer the treatment the more effect it has. It also serves to keep IDUs in contact with services; however, it seems less effective in reducing HCV spread. Needle and syringe programmes are available in most EU countries, but the scale and coverage seem to differ greatly and NSPs are still controversial, particularly in the US. In general, they have a preventive effect on IDU and risk behaviours and the spread of HIV, whereas the effect on HCV is less clear.

To be able to evaluate prevention measures and to improve the outcomes of modelling endeavours and cost-of-illness studies, high-quality and up-to-date epidemiological data are necessary. To meet this need, the EMCDDA has increased its efforts to collect prevalence and incidence data on HCV in IDUs in the EU. In Chapter 4, Wiessing et al. present the currently available prevalence data among IDUs in the EU. In all, 233 estimates were obtained from 63 sources in 111 study sites for the period 1996–2002. The unweighted median prevalence in the full samples is 65.8 %, with an inter-quartile range of 50.5 to 70.4 %, while among young injectors (aged less than 25 years) and new injectors (injecting for less than two years), medians of 30.8 and 47.6 % are found, respectively, suggesting high recent transmission. Of 52 time series, 21 show a significant decrease and 7 a significant increase, suggesting that decreases in prevalence among tested IDUs are more widespread than increases; however, this may depend on screening practices. The data suggest that geographic differences in prevalence and trends may exist; however, methods of data collection may confound these differences and the data are subject to a number of limitations. Estimates and trends in injecting drug use are also provided, suggesting that between two and five cases per 1 000 population aged 15 to 64 years are current or lifetime injectors among the active drug users in the EU, corresponding to some 500 000 to 1.25 million IDUs, and showing strongly diverging time trends and levels between countries in rates of injecting among opiate users in treatment. The HCV prevalence data collection may provide a simple and cost-effective indicator of HCV incidence and injecting risk behaviour, thereby extending in relevance to other diseases such as HIV and hepatitis B, and it may form a basis for targeted surveillance of blood-borne infections among IDUs.

Treatment options for IDUs with hepatitis C infection

Poynard (Chapter 2) gives a comprehensive overview of recent developments in diagnostics and treatment of HCV infection. He states that HCV infection is a major cause of chronic liver disease and should be detected and treated when necessary. Patients usually complain more about extrahepatic manifestations, especially rheumatic and cutaneous symptoms, which are frequent and impair quality of life. Treatment is now available that permits the eradication of the virus in 60 % of cases and reduces disease progression in others. Treatment response rates are 88 % for genotypes 2 and 3 and around 48 % for genotypes 1, 4, 5 and 6. Genotyping is important for the decision on the duration of combination therapy. Poynard suggests that liver biopsies are helpful for the decision about and the duration of therapy, but indications for biopsy should decrease because of the increasing validation of serum markers. There is increasing evidence that antibodies resolve in those who clear their infection and thus the rate of spontaneous clearance is underestimated. Patients with HIV coinfection have a worse natural history and are those most in need of treatment. If the patient is not at risk of cirrhosis, has no symptoms and is not at risk of transmitting the virus, there is no need to treat. However, patients without any fibrosis, and thus without risk of cirrhosis, represented only 7 % of 4 552 patients in a recent study (Metavir F0). Psychosis, severe depression, active injecting drug or alcohol use are contraindications for treatment; however, when drug use or alcohol use is reduced, treatment should be discussed on a case-by-case basis, including the benefit of preventing infecting others.

Foster (Chapter 3) provides an overview of methods and results of studies on quality of life among HCV-infected patients. Most HCV-infected patients are labelled asymptomatic; however, they often complain of a variety of extrahepatic symptoms, and reduced day-to-day functioning and quality of life. There are numerous quality of life measurement instruments, among which is the widely used SF36. All studies have shown a significant reduction in quality of life among HCV-infected persons, although there is wide variation. Among IDUs, quality of life may already be impaired, and HCV-infected drug users have usually lower scores than non-drug using patients. Treatment may temporarily reduce quality of life, due to side effects, and therefore some patients decline treatment, while others with less severe clinical symptoms may ask for treatment, evaluating the benefits and costs at the personal level. Attempts to increase the popularity of HCV treatment must involve an analysis of the patient's perception of benefits and costs. Knowledge of being infected can, by itself, reduce the quality of life, for example due to concerns of infecting others and of future consequences. Patients who know their infection have a much greater reduction in quality of life than those who are unaware of infection. HCV can infect the central nervous system, and infection of the brain is a possible explanation for some of the extrahepatic symptoms experienced by patients such as fatigue, malaise and non-specific pains and aches. Antiviral therapy can significantly improve the quality of life of HCV-infected patients, and the presence of significant symptoms associated with chronic hepatitis C should be regarded as an indication for combination therapy.

Analysing the dynamics of HCV and IDUs with mathematical models

Mathematical models are presented that provide insights into the dynamics of both HCV and IDU epidemics.

Kretzschmar and Wiessing (Chapter 5) present a compartmental model to describe the spread of HCV among IDUs. The model shows the existence of a threshold effect of needle sharing (10 times per year in the model; this could be different in reality), above which the prevalence of HCV carriers does not show important changes. This means that reduction of risk behaviour among IDUs should be very substantial before effects on prevalence or incidence will show. However, one feasible option for intervention seems to be massive treatment of infected IDUs. The model demonstrates that, at the threshold level of needle sharing, prevalence is highly sensitive to duration of infection, and higher rates of viral clearance will have a strong impact on total prevalence, both of carriers and of seropositives (see also Pollack and Heimer, Chapter 15). The effect of a core group of high-risk IDUs is investigated, showing that if these IDUs mainly share among themselves, the existence of such a core group will diminish the effects of prevention; however, if prevention can be specifically targeted to that group, a disproportionately large effect can be achieved. Introduction of 'time since injection' in the model shows that the high-risk individuals are infected soon after initiation of injecting and reach very high prevalence, as has often been observed in epidemiological studies. However, among the low-risk individuals, prevalence continues to rise over the course of many years, showing that: (a) prevention should aim at behaviour change before start of injecting; (b) behaviour change of high-risk IDUs might be too late to protect them from becoming infected, but it might reduce the risk for low-risk individuals; and (c) behaviour change of low-risk IDUs can protect them from infection, but can do little to reduce overall prevalence.

Rossi and Esposito (Chapter 6) present two nested compartmental models of both injecting drug use and HCV among IDUs. Qualitative results are presented based on Italian data, showing that: (a) drug use epidemics can spread fast and may reach endemic (steady) state after about seven years; (b) the impact of primary prevention is largest at the beginning and decreases afterwards; and (c) the impact of secondary prevention is highest at peak prevalence of drug use and decreases in the endemic phase. Regarding the HCV epidemic, the model shows that, for maximum impact, harm reduction measures should be implemented when an IDU epidemic is still in an early stage. The authors observe that the spread of infectious diseases in IDUs is primarily related to the hidden part of the drug user's career. This latency period of injecting drug use, that is the period between first drug use and first treatment, where IDUs have as yet no contact with healthcare services, is remarkably similar between different cities and is much longer in IDUs who start injecting at a younger age. This emphasises the need to implement specific interventions targeted at young drug users in order to both reduce their latency period and prevent the spread of infectious diseases.

In a mathematical model using optimal control theory and data on the US cocaine epidemic, it is shown that quick detection of a drugs epidemic is crucial to maximise the effect of prevention (Tragler, Chapter 7). Interventions considered are law enforcement (regarded as a prevention measure, through its price-increasing effect) and treatment. It is shown that in the early stages of a drug epidemic the most effective policy is massive prevention (in the model through law enforcement) and treatment, while in the case of an established epidemic, resources should progressively be shifted to treatment, although continued law enforcement can still moderate the size of the epidemic. Various extensions of the basic simple model are discussed, including the deterrent effect of 'heavy users' who, contrary to socially integrated 'light users', provide direct feedback to potential initiates regarding the negative consequences of problem drug use, and a 'memory effect' where prevalence of heavy use deters initiation with a time lag of many years, as well as age-structured models that can take into account age heterogeneity regarding initiation. The concepts of light and heavy users, with positive and negative feedback effects respectively on initiation, possibly with a long memory effect, are important to understand the long-term dynamics of (injecting) drug use, indicating that new generations of young persons, who have not experienced the devastating effects of an opiate or cocaine epidemic, may again become susceptible over the course of decades.

Estimating the economic costs of hepatitis C infection and injecting drug use

Economic evaluations are important for policy decisions as they may provide estimates of the economic impact of a disease or comparisons of resource consequences of alternative policy options. However, methods and approaches are still much in development, especially in estimating the wider costs of drug use to society, and in the monograph, several cost-evaluation methods are discussed. Estimates of the cost-effectiveness of treatment of IDUs with moderate or severe liver disease are presented first.

Wong et al. (Chapter 9) compare the risks and benefits of immediate antiretroviral treatment to natural history with no antiviral treatment, using a Markov model adapted to IDUs. IDUs are considered with moderate hepatitis or compensated cirrhosis. They note that, despite decreasing incidence of acute hepatitis C, the costs of HCV will continue to rise in the future. They also quote UK data indicating that, of 237 HCV-infected IDUs, therapy was indicated in 100, while only 50 actually initiated treatment (Jowett et al., 2001). The results of their model indicate that immediate antiviral treatment in this population would decrease the 20-year risk of compensated cirrhosis by 13 % and of liver-related mortality by 7 %. Long term, a 1.7-year gain in life expectancy, or 1.9 QALYs, is estimated compared with no therapy. More than two thirds of the USD 11 483 average treatment costs are offset by prevention of liver-disease-related complications. This is lower than results for non-IDUs, due to the assumed risk of relapse into IDU and reinfection with HCV. DQALYs and costs were USD 5 600 per DQALY gained compared with no antiviral therapy. They conclude that combination therapy is cost-effective, extends life and improves quality of life in this population. They note that, despite concerns regarding adherence, treatment tolerability and risk of reinfection, two European studies have demonstrated successful antiviral therapy in IDUs (Backmund et al., 2001; Jowett et al., 2001). They also mention a recent study that suggests the possible presence of protective HCV immunity (Mehta et al., 2002) and that could make reinfection 'less of a concern' among IDUs.

Estimating the direct healthcare costs of hepatitis C infection is a necessary step towards full economic evaluations such as cost-effectiveness analyses. Postma et al. (Chapter 8) estimate the direct healthcare costs of HCV infection in IDUs for the EU, using national-level estimates of HCV incidence, extrapolated from back-calculated IDU-related HIV incidence, in combination with a Markov disease progression model. They estimate that all incident HCV infections in IDUs in 1999 will cause EUR 1.43 billion of discounted future healthcare costs in the six high-impact countries alone (France, Germany, Italy, Portugal, Spain and the UK). This indicates almost a doubling of a previous estimate for 1995, where combination therapy was not considered. Extrapolated to the whole EU, the costs of HCV represent 0.23 % of the 2003 healthcare expenditures of the 15 EU countries.

Welte et al. (Chapter 10) discuss methods to estimate the indirect costs (lost productivity) of injecting drug use and they show estimates for paid and unpaid work loss in Germany and the Netherlands. The importance of the chosen perspective is elaborated in detail, showing how the relevance of certain costs may be different for the IDU, his or her family, the employer, social insurance or the society at large. They show how the indirect costs depend strongly on the chosen perspective and recommend that, in general, the societal perspective be chosen when possible as a reference perspective, while, depending on the focus of the study, additional perspectives should be applied. Calculating costs for different perspectives may help decide who should finance a measure. Different methods to estimate indirect costs (human capital approach, willingness-to-pay approach, friction cost method) give very different results, demonstrating the need for standardisation. For all perspectives, except those of the employer and social insurance, they recommend the human capital method as the most feasible approach.

Antoñanzas et al. (Chapter 11) present a review of studies on the social costs of injecting drug use. They discuss different methods used to measure costs and they propose a general model to calculate the social costs of drug use and related diseases. They note that, in most studies of social costs, potential benefits are disregarded, which is controversial both from the individual and from the societal perspective. The results show that there are major difficulties when comparing cost studies due to a lack of standard methods, a lack of understanding of causal relationships and determinants of drug use, and a lack of quality data. Most studies aggregate healthcare costs with no separation of diseases such as HIV or hepatitis B or C. The authors continue to give a preliminary prevalence-based estimate of the costs of HIV and HCV among IDUs in Spain of nearly EUR 240 million for HIV and EUR 135 million for HCV, the latter representing 5 % of total national expenditures on prescribed drugs and 1 % of the healthcare budget in Spain. They note that, when calculating costs due to mortality, the human capital approach underestimates the losses of the non-active population by focusing solely on lost productivity, while including lost productivity in social cost studies of a disease is controversial and discriminatory. They recommend the friction cost method as being more useful from a macroeconomic perspective. The studies ignore the external costs that IDUs cause to their relatives, which can involve significant healthcare costs (depression, stress) and lost productivity.

Jeanrenaud (Chapter 12) discusses a method to measure the costs of illicit drug use that covers not only direct (e.g. healthcare, police) and indirect (lost productivity) costs, but also intangible costs such as consequences on quality of life for the individual, pain and grief for his or her family, crime and loss of welfare of the community. He states that, until now, the social burden of illicit drugs has remained largely underestimated; for example, quality of life has a real economic value due to the fact that individuals are willing to sacrifice a substantial part of their income to raise it, while the costs of pain are clearly reflected in the huge world market for analgesics. He first presents an analytical framework with all the components of social costs, followed by a critical assessment of the two standard valuation methods, the human capital approach and the willingness-to-pay approach, after which he proposes a new method that combines both. Finally, he presents the costs of illicit drug consumption in Switzerland. He concludes that the adequate framework for measuring the costs of illicit drug use is that of a cost–benefit analysis rather than a cost-of-illness approach, while strongly questioning the rationale of studies that ignore the effects of drugs on quality of life, and he proposes revision of the international guidelines to include intangible costs.

Kopp and Blanchard (Chapter 13) present a prevalence-based study on the social costs of drug use in France in 1997. They limit the study to tangible costs that correspond to monetary losses and exclude intangible costs. They use the human capital approach to estimate production losses. They include a separate calculation of 'public expenditures', i.e. the budgetary costs borne by public organisations at State and regional levels plus social transfers such as the financial flows in the healthcare sector. They estimate a total cost of EUR 2 037 million excluding, and EUR 3 868 million to EUR 5 037 million including, the purchase costs of drugs, the first amounting to 0.16 % of GNP or an average per capita cost of EUR 35. In comparison, they mention estimates of the cost to society in France of alcohol and tobacco of nearly EUR 17 596 million and EUR 9 929 million, respectively.

Main outcomes and policy implications

- Methadone substitution treatment reduces injecting frequency and needle sharing and is cost-effective for HIV but not for HCV prevention. Although it does not prove cost-effective for HCV prevention if regarded in isolation or funded solely with that objective, the combined analysis of all MMT costs and outcomes would prove it a cost-effective public health intervention for IDUs.

- At high levels of coverage, different interventions will act in synergy and mutually reinforce one another's effects. Therefore, it remains critical to implement different prevention measures (including NSPs, HCV counselling and testing, and other drug treatment modalities) simultaneously and to attain high coverage with them all.

- Only one full economic evaluation was found regarding the cost-effectiveness of NSPs as a prevention measure for HCV and it concludes moderately positive, although other studies suggest NSPs are not cost-effective. However, given the large impact of NSPs on the transmission of HIV, it can be concluded that, even without inclusion of HCV prevention or referrals, NSPs represent a cost-effective public health intervention for IDUs.

- HCV therapy effectiveness has strongly improved and infection should be detected and treated when necessary. Screening of IDUs is indicated, possibly also extending to non-IDUs and partners of HCV-infected persons. Antiviral combination treatment should be offered to infected IDUs where indicated. In the considerations, the benefit of preventing infections to others should be included.

- Antiviral treatment is cost-effective for IDUs with moderate hepatitis or compensated cirrhosis. It extends life and improves the quality of life of HCV-infected patients. The presence of significant symptoms associated with chronic hepatitis C should be regarded as an indication for combination therapy. Studies have shown that IDUs can be treated successfully.

- Modelling studies show that reducing viral load in a population or shortening the average carrier duration by eliminating it in part of the population through substantial screening and treatment can have strong effects on HCV prevalence.

- Reduction of injecting risk behaviour has to be very substantial before an effect of HCV prevalence is to be expected. Targeting interventions at high-risk individuals can have a disproportionately large prevention effect. Interventions should aim to change behaviour before the start of injecting.

- With highly infectious diseases like hepatitis-C, specific prevention measures should be targeted at new and young injectors who may not yet be infected. Existing prevention programmes should be made accessible to them. Prevention before or at an early stage of exposure is more effective.

- Drug use epidemics can spread very fast and quick detection and early-stage prevention are crucial to maximise the impact of prevention. The impact of secondary prevention and treatment is highest at peak prevalence of drug use. Harm reduction should be implemented ideally before an IDU epidemic starts to increase.

- The future costs per year of new HCV infections are very substantial and may amount to 0.23 % of the EU healthcare budget. The current costs of illicit drug use amount to EUR 35 per capita in France, and are much lower than those of the use of alcohol or tobacco.

- In economic analyses, it is crucial to explicitly state what perspective is chosen; in general, the social perspective may be used as reference but additional perspectives should also be applied. Calculating costs for different perspectives can help decide who should finance a measure.

- Indirect cost analyses should include loss of unpaid work. Benefits should be included in economic evaluations; these should not be restricted to costs only.

- The intangible costs of drug use or related disease, including loss of quality of life, can be very substantial and economic evaluations should consider including these costs.

References

Backmund, M., Meyer, K., Von Zielonka, M., Eichenlaub, D. (2001), 'Treatment in hepatitis C infection in injection drug users', *Hepatology* 34: 188–93.

Commonwealth Department of Health and Ageing (2002), *Return on investment in needle and syringe programs in Australia — Report*, Commonwealth of Australia (available at: http://www.health.gov.au/pubhlth/publicat/document/roireport.pdf).

Hagan, H., McGough, J. P., Thiede, H., Weiss, N. S., Hopkins, S., Alexander, E. R. (1999), 'Syringe exchange and risk of infection with hepatitis B and C viruses', *American Journal of Epidemiology* 149: 203–13.

Jowett, S. L., Agarwal, K., Smith, B. C., Craig, W., Hewett, M., Bassendine, D. R., Gilvarry, E., Burt, A. D., Bassendine, M. F. (2001), 'Managing chronic hepatitis C acquired through intravenous drug use', *Quebec Journal of Medicine* 94: 153–8.

Mehta, S. H., Cox, A., Hoover, D. R., Wang, X. H., Mao, Q., Ray, S., Strathdee, S. A., Vlahov, D., Thomas, D. L. (2002), 'Protection against persistence of hepatitis C', *The Lancet* 359: 1478–83.

Pollack, H. A. (2001), 'Cost-effectiveness of harm reduction in preventing hepatitis C among injection drug users', *Medical Decision Making* 21: 357–67.

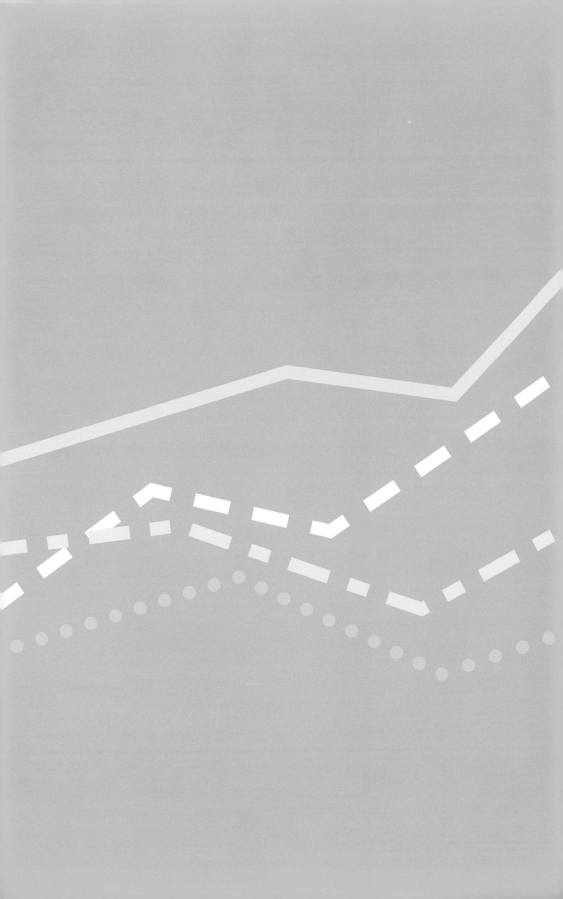

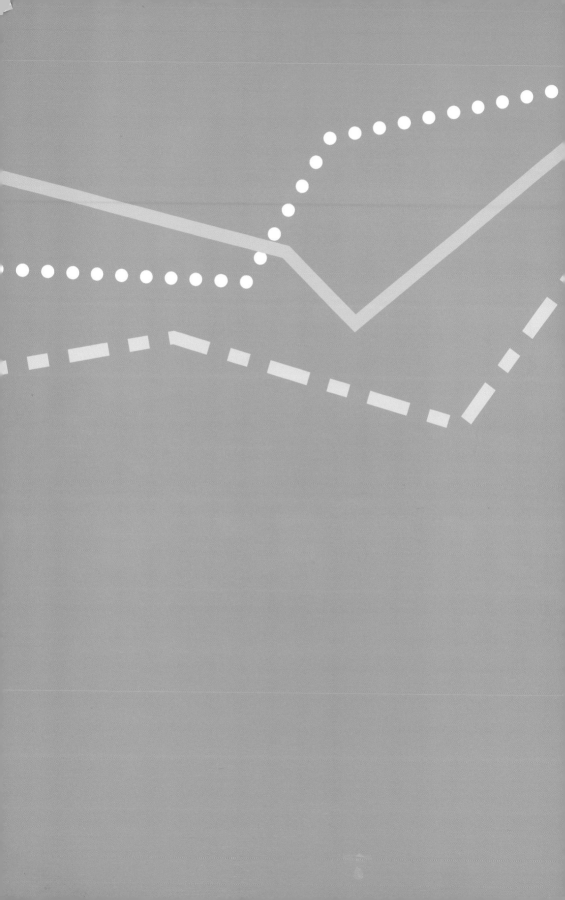

Contributors

Fernando Antoñanzas
Department of Economics
University of La Rioja
C/La Cigüeña, 60
E-26004 Logroño
Tel. (34) 941 29 93 87
Fax (34) 941 29 93 93
E-mail:
fernando.antonanzas@dee.unirioja.es

Nicolas Blanchard
Université Panthéon-Sorbonne (Paris 1)
106–112, boulevard de l'hopital
F-75013 Paris
E-mail: blanchard.nico@wanadoo.fr

Nicolino Esposito
Department of Mathematics
University of Rome Tor Vergata
Via della Ricerca Scientifica
I-133 Rome
Tel. (39) 672 59 46 11
Fax (39) 672 59 46 99
E-mail: nicola_esposito@yahoo.it

Graham Foster
DDRC
The Royal London Hospital
Turner Street
London E1 2AD
United Kingdom
Tel. (44-20) 78 82 72 42
E-mail: G.R.Foster@qmul.ac.uk

David Goldberg
Scottish Centre for Infection and
Environmental Health
Clifton House
Clifton Place
Glasgow G3 7LN
United Kingdom
Tel. (44-141) 300 11 04
Fax (44-141) 300 11 70
E-mail:
David.Goldberg@scieh.csa.scot.nhs.uk

Richard Hartnoll
Drug Research and Policy Analysis
Rua dos Ferreiros a Estrela, 73-3-E
P-1200-672 Lisboa
Tel. (351) 213 97 04 89
E-mail: richard.hartnoll@mail.telepac.pt

Gordon Hay
Centre for Drug Misuse Research
University of Glasgow
89 Dumbarton Road
Glasgow G11 6PW
United Kingdom
Tel. (44-141) 330 54 13
Fax (44-141) 330 28 20
E-mail: G.Hay@socsci.gla.ac.uk

Robert Heimer
Department of Epidemiology and Public
Health
Yale School of Medicine
60 College Street
New Haven, CT 06520-8034
United States of America
Tel. (1-203) 785 67 32
Fax (1-203) 785 75 52
E-mail: robert.heimer@yale.edu

Claude Jeanrenaud
Centre for Studies in Public Sector
Economics
Universities of Berne, Fribourg and
Neuchâtel and
Institute for Economic and Regional
Research
University of Neuchâtel
Pierre-à-Mazel 7
CH-2000 Neuchâtel
Tel. (41-32) 718 14 00
Fax (41-32) 718 14 01
E-mail: claude.jeanrenaud@unine.ch

Pierre Kopp
Université Panthéon-Sorbonne (Paris 1)
106–112, boulevard de l'hopital
F-75013 Paris
E-mail: pkopp@univ-paris.fr

Harold Pollack
Department of Health Management and
Policy
University of Michigan
School of Public Health
109 Observatory
Ann Arbor, MI 48109–2029
United States of America
Tel. (1-734) 936 12 98
Fax (1-734) 764 43 38
E-mail: haroldp@umich.edu

Thierry Poynard
Hôpital Pitié-Salpêtrière
Service d'hépato-gastro-entérologie
47–83, boulevard de l'hôpital
F-75651 Paris Cedex 23
Tel. (33) 142 16 10 02
Fax (33) 142 16 14 25
E-mail: tpoynard@teaser.fr

Roberto Rodríguez
Department of Economics
University of La Rioja
C/La Cigüeña, 60
E-26004 Logroño
Fax (34) 941 29 93 93
E-mail:
roberto.rodriguez@dee.unirioja.es

Carla Rossi
Department of Mathematics
University of Rome Tor Vergata
Via della Ricerca Scientifica
I-133 Rome
Tel. (39) 672 59 42 91/46 76
Fax (39) 672 59 46 99
E-mail: c.rossi@agora.it
rossi@axp.mat.unicoma2.it

Kirsty Roy
Blood Borne Viruses & STI Unit
Scottish Centre for Infection and
Environmental Health
Clifton House
Clifton Place
Glasgow G3 7LN
United Kingdom
Tel. (44-141) 300 11 73
Fax (44-141) 300 11 00
E-mail: Kirsty.Roy@scieh.csa.scot.nhs.uk

David Sapinho
82 rue Paul Vaillant Couturier
F-91270 Vigneux sur Seine
E-mail: dsapinho@hotmail.com

Uwe Siebert
Institute for Medical Informatics
Biometry and Epidemiology
University of Munich
Germany
and
Harvard Center for Risk Analysis
Harvard School of Public Health
Boston, MA
United States of America

Diana Sylvestre
Department of Medicine
University of California, San Francisco
San Francisco, CA
United States of America

Avril Taylor
School of Social Sciences
University of Paisley
University Campus Ayr
Beech Grove
Ayr KA8 0SR
United Kingdom
Tel. (44-1292) 88 62 05
E-mail: avril.taylor@paisley.ac.uk

Gernot Tragler
Institute for Econometrics, OR and
Systems Theory
University of Technology
Argentinierstraße 8/1192
A-1040 Vienna
Tel. (43-1) 58 80 11 19 20
Fax (43-1) 58 80 11 19 99
E-mail: tragler@eos.tuwien.ac.at

María Velasco
Soikos
C/Sardenya, 229–237, 6º, 4p
E-08013 Barcelona
Tel. (34) 932 31 40 66
Fax (34) 932 31 35 07
E-mail: maria@soikos.com

John Wong
Division of Clinical Decision Making
Department of Medicine
Tupper Research Institute
Tufts-New England Medical Center
Tufts University School of Medicine
750 Washington Street
Box 302
Boston, MA 02111
United States of America
Tel. (1-617) 636 56 95
Fax (1-617) 636 48 38
E-mail: jwong@tufts-nemc.org

**Department of Health Economics,
University of Ulm**

Hans-Helmut König
E-mail: Hans-
Helmut.Koenig@mathematik.uni-ulm.de

Reiner Leidl
E-mail:
Reiner.Leidl@mathematik.uni-ulm.de

Robert Welte
E-mail:
Robert.Welte@mathematik.uni-ulm.de

Department of Health Economics
University of Ulm
D-89069 Ulm
Tel. (49-731) 503 10 38
Fax (49-731) 503 10 32

EMCDDA

Lucas Wiessing
European Monitoring Centre for Drugs
and Drug Addiction
(EMCDDA)
Epidemiology Department
Rua da Cruz de Santa Apolónia, 23–25
P-1149-045 Lisbon
Tel. (351) 218 11 30 16
Fax (351) 218 13 79 43
E-mail: lucas.wiessing@emcdda.eu.int

GUIDE/GRIP

Jasper Bos
E-mail: j.bos@farm.rug.nl

Maarten Postma
E-mail: m.postma@farm.rug.nl

Department of Social Pharmacy,
Pharmaco-epidemiology and
Pharmacotherapy
Groningen University
Institute for Drug Exploration/
Groningen University Research Institute
of Pharmacy
(GUIDE/GRIP)
Antonius Deusinglaan 1
9713 AW Groningen
Netherlands
Tel. (31-50) 363 31 63
Fax (31-50) 363 26 12

RIVM

Ardine de Wit
E-mail: ardine.de.wit@rivm.nl

Johannes Jager
E-mail: hans.jager@rivm.nl

Mirjam Kretzschmar
E-mail: mirjam.kretzschmar@rivm.nl

Wien Limburg
E-mail: wien.limburg@rivm.nl

National Institute of Public Health
and the Environment (RIVM)
PO Box 1
3720 BA Bilthoven
Netherlands
Tel. (31-30) 274 91 11
Fax (31-30) 274 24 71

Abbreviations

EMCDDA	European Monitoring Centre for Drugs and Drug Addiction
EU	European Union
FTE	full-time equivalent
Ilid	legislation on illegal drugs
US	United States of America
WHO	World Health Organisation

Biomedical terms

ALT	alanine aminotransferase
DQALY	discounted quality-adjusted life year
ELISA	enzyme immunosorbant assay
HAV	hepatitis A virus
HBV	hepatitis B virus
HCC	hepatocellular carcinoma
HCV	hepatitis C virus
HIV	human immunodeficiency virus
HSV	herpes simplex virus
IDU	injecting drug user
MMT	methadone maintenance treatment
MU	million units
NSP	needle and syringe programme
PCR	polymerase chain reaction
PEG	pegylated
QALY	quality-adjusted life year
RIBA	recombinant immunoblot assay
RNA	ribonucleic acid
STD	sexually transmitted disease
tiw	three times a week

European Monitoring Centre for Drugs and Drug Addiction

EMCDDA Scientific Monograph Series No 7

Hepatitis C and injecting drug use: impact, costs and policy options

Luxembourg: Office for Official Publications of the European Communities

2004 — 389 pp. —16 x 24 cm

ISBN 92-9168-168-7

Price (excluding VAT) in Luxembourg: EUR 20